T0294740

2021

ADVANCES IN
SMALL ANIMAL CARE

EDITOR-IN-CHIEF

Philip H. Kass

SECTION EDITORS

David Levine

Denis J. Marcellin-Little

Elisa M. Mazzaferro

Laurel J. Gershwin

Larry D. Cowgill

ELSEVIER

Publishing Director, Medical Reference: Dolores Meloni
Editor: Stacy Eastman
Developmental Editor: Jessica Cañaberal

© 2021 Elsevier Inc. All rights reserved.

Photograph of Abyssinian kittens by Amy Buxton, copyright 2020; all other photos courtesy of Shutterstock, copyright 2020. This periodical and the individual contributions contained in it are protected under copyright by Elsevier and the following terms and conditions apply to their use:

Photocopying
Single photocopies of single articles may be made for personal use as allowed by national copyright laws. Permission of the Publisher and payment of a fee is required for all other photocopying, including multiple or systematic copying, copying for advertising or promotional purposes, resale, and all forms of document delivery. Special rates are available for educational institutions that wish to make photocopies for non-profit educational classroom use.
For information on how to seek permission visit www.elsevier.com/permissions or call: (+44) 1865 843830 (UK)/(+1) 215 239 3867 (USA).

Derivative Works
Subscribers may reproduce tables of contents or prepare lists of articles including abstracts for internal circulation within their institutions. Permission of the Publisher is required for resale or distribution outside the institution. Permission of the Publisher is required for all other derivative works, including compilations and translations (please consult www.elsevier.com/permissions).

Electronic Storage or Usage
Permission of the Publisher is required to store or use electronically any material contained in this periodical, including any article or part of an article (please consult www.elsevier.com/permissions). Except as outlined above, no part of this publication may be reproduced, stored in a retrieval system or transmitted in any form or by any means, electronic, mechanical, photocopying, recording or otherwise, without prior written permission of the Publisher.

Notice
No responsibility is assumed by the Publisher for any injury and/or damage to persons or property as a matter of products liability, negligence or otherwise, or from any use or operation of any methods, products, instructions or ideas contained in the material herein. Because of rapid advances in the medical sciences, in particular, independent verification of diagnoses and drug dosages should be made.

Although all advertising material is expected to conform to ethical (medical) standards, inclusion in this publication does not constitute a guarantee or endorsement of the quality or value of such product or of the claims made of it by its manufacturer.

Reprints: For copies of 100 or more of articles in this publication, please contact the Commercial Reprints Department, Elsevier Inc., 360 Park Avenue South, New York, NY 10010-1710. Tel: 212-633-3874; Fax: 212-633-3820; E-mail: reprints@elsevier.com.

Printed in the United States of America.

Editorial Office:
Elsevier, Inc.
1600 John F. Kennedy Blvd,
Suite 1800
Philadelphia, PA 19103-2899

International Standard Serial Number: 2666-4518
International Standard Book Number: 978-0-323-89704-4

ADVANCES IN SMALL ANIMAL CARE

EDITOR-IN-CHIEF

PHILIP H. KASS, BS, DVM, MPVM, MS, PhD
Diplomate, American College of Veterinary
Preventive Medicine
(Specialty in Epidemiology)
Vice Provost for Academic Affairs
Professor of Analytic Epidemiology
Department of Population Health and
Reproduction, School of Veterinary Medicine
Department of Public Health Sciences
School of Medicine, University of California, Davis
Davis, California, USA
phkass@ucdavis.edu

SECTION EDITORS

DAVID LEVINE PT, PhD, DPT, CCRP, FAPTA
Board-Certified Clinical Specialist in Orthopaedic
Physical Therapy
Professor and Walter M. Cline Chair of Excellence in
Physical Therapy
Department of Physical Therapy
The University of Tennessee at Chattanooga
Chattanooga, Tennessee, USA
david-levine@utc.edu

DENIS J. MARCELLIN-LITTLE, DEDV
Professor, Orthopedic Surgery
Department of Surgical and Radiological Sciences
School of Veterinary Medicine
University of California, Davis
Davis, California, USA
djmarcel@ucdavis.edu

ELISA M. MAZZAFERRO, MS, DVM, PhD,
DACVECC
Staff Criticalist
Cornell University Veterinary Specialists
Stamford, Connecticut, USA
emazzaferro@cuvs.org

LAUREL J. GERSHWIN, DVM, PhD, Dipl. ACVM
Distinguished Professor
Department of Pathology, Microbiology &
Immunology
School of Veterinary Medicine
University of California, Davis
Davis, California, USA
ljgershwin@ucdavis.edu

LARRY D. COWGILL, DVM, PhD, DACVIM (SAIM)
Professor, Department of Medicine & Epidemiology
School of Veterinary Medicine
Director, UC Veterinary Medical Center-San Diego
University of California-Davis
Davis, California, USA
ldcowgill@ucdavis.edu

ADVANCES IN SMALL ANIMAL CARE

CONTRIBUTORS

ANUSHA BALAKRISHNAN, BVSc, DACVECC
Triangle Veterinary Referral Hospital, Durham, North Carolina

JEFF BARNES
President, AimaLojic Animal Health, Rapid City, South Dakota

MICHELE BROADHURST, DC, CCSP, FIAMA, CCRP, CAC IVCA
Wellness 4 All Chiropractic Centre, Bloomfield, Colorado

MATTHEW BRUNKE, DVM, CCRP, CVPP, CVA, CCMT, DACVSMR
Veterinary Surgical Centers Rehabilitation, Vienna, Virginia

CHRISTOPHER G. BYERS, DVM, DACVECC, DACVIM (SAIM), CVJ
CriticalCareDVM.com

KATIE CAGEL-HOLTCAMP, PhD
Social Work Intern, Mississippi State University College of Veterinary Medicine, Starkville, Mississippi; Office of Academic Affairs, Mississippi State University, Mississippi State, Mississippi

DANA L. CLARKE VMD, DACVECC
Assistant Professor, Interventional Radiology & Critical Care, Department of Clinical Sciences and Advanced Medicine, University of Pennsylvania School of Veterinary Medicine, Philadelphia, Pennsylvania

LARRY D. COWGILL, DVM, PhD, DACVIM (SAIM)
Professor, Department of Medicine and Epidemiology, Associate Dean for Southern California Clinical Programs and Director, University of California Veterinary Medical Center-San Diego, School of Veterinary Medicine, University of California, Davis, Davis, California

JOSE DIAZ AUÑON, PhD
VP and Chief Scientist, ImmutriX Therapeutics, Inc, Rapid City, South Dakota

MARTI DRUM, DVM, PhD, DACVSMR
Department of Small Animal Clinical Sciences, University of Tennessee College of Veterinary Medicine, Knoxville, Tennessee

CEDRIC DUFAYET, DVM
Coordinator, Advanced Urinary Disease and Extracorporeal Therapies Service, University of California Veterinary Medical Center-San Diego, San Diego, California

TYLER J.M. JORDAN, DVM, DACVD
PhD Student, Department of Clinical Sciences, College of Veterinary Medicine, North Carolina State University, Postdoctoral Research Fellow, Department of Dermatology, School of Medicine, The University of North Carolina at Chapel Hill, Chapel Hill, North Carolina

PHILIP H. KASS, BS, DVM, MPVM, MS, PhD
Diplomate, American College of Veterinary Preventive Medicine (Specialty in Epidemiology); Vice Provost for Academic Affairs, Professor of Analytic Epidemiology, Department of Population Health and Reproduction, School of Veterinary Medicine, Department of Public Health Sciences, School of Medicine, University of California, Davis, Davis, California

DAVID LEVINE, PT, PhD, DPT, CCRP, FAPTA
Board-Certified Clinical Specialist in Orthopaedic Physical Therapy, Professor and Walter M. Cline Chair of Excellence in Physical Therapy, Department of

Physical Therapy, The University of Tennessee at Chattanooga, Chattanooga, Tennessee

DENIS J. MARCELLIN-LITTLE, DEDV
Veterinary Orthopedic Research Laboratory, School of Veterinary Medicine, University of California, Davis, Davis, California

DANI McVETY, DVM, CEO
Lap of Love Veterinary Hospice

EMILY McKAY, DPT, CCRP
Veterinary Orthopedic Research Laboratory, School of Veterinary Medicine, University of California, Davis, Davis, California

DARRYL L. MILLIS, MS, DVM
Department of Small Animal Clinical Sciences, University of Tennessee College of Veterinary Medicine, Knoxville, Tennessee

THANDEKA R. NGWENYAMA , DVM, DACVECC
Clinical Assistant Professor, Carlson College of Veterinary Medicine, Veterinary Clinical Sciences, Oregon State University, Corvallis, Oregon

KIRSTEN OLIVER, VN, DipAVN(surgical), RVT, CCRP, CVPP
VTS(physical rehabilitation), Veterinary Surgical Centers Rehabilitation, Vienna, Virginia

CATHERINE A. OUTERBRIDGE, DVM, MVSc, DACVIM (SAIM), DACVD
Professor of Clinical Dermatology, Department of Medicine and Epidemiology, School of Veterinary Medicine, University of California at Davis, Davis, California

PAULINE PRINCE, PhD, ABN
Coordinator of Clinical Services/Staff Psychologist, Office of Academic Affairs, Mississippi State University, Mississippi State, Mississippi

NOE REYES, DVM
ELIAS Animal Health, Olathe, Kansas

GARY W. WOOD, PhD
ELIAS Animal Health, Olathe, Kansas

ADVANCES IN SMALL ANIMAL CARE

CONTENTS

VOLUME 2 • 2021

Editorial Board, *iii*

Contributors, *v*

Preface: New Directions for the Journal's Second Year, *xi*
Philip H. Kass

Rehabilitation

Multifactorial Rehabilitation Planning in Companion Animals
Denis J. Marcellin-Little, David Levine, and Darryl L. Millis
- Introduction, *1*
- General features of rehabilitation programs, *1*
- Musculoskeletal tissue atrophy resulting from disuse, *3*
- Selecting management options during physical rehabilitation, *4*
- Proactive and retroactive forms of physical rehabilitation, *4*
  - *Logistics of Physical Rehabilitation, 5*
- Medical conditions, *5*
- Patient profile, *8*
- Ownership profile, *9*
- Care algorithms, *9*
- Clinics care points, *9*
- Disclosure, *10*

Cryotherapy in Small Animal Rehabilitation
David Levine and Denis J. Marcellin-Little
- Introduction, *11*
- Physiologic effects of cryotherapy, *11*
- Influences of cryotherapy on other rehabilitation treatments, *12*
- Application, risks, and precautions, *12*
- Types of cryotherapy devices, *12*
- Literature review, *13*
- Cryotherapy over coaptation devices, *15*
- Summary, *16*
- Clinics care points,*16*

Manual Therapy in Small Animal Rehabilitation
Matthew Brunke, Michele Broadhurst, Kirsten Oliver, and David Levine
- Introduction, *19*
  - *Soft-tissue mobilization, 19*
  - *Fascia, 20*
  - *Contraindications and precautions to soft-tissue mobilization, 21*
- Massage techniques, *21*
  - *Effleurage, 21*
  - *Petrissage, 21*
  - *Tapotement, 21*
  - *Cross-friction, 21*
  - *Myofascial release, 22*
  - *Ischemic compression, 22*
  - *Passive, active range of motion and stretching, 22*
- Additional manual techniques, *22*
  - *Dry needling, 23*
  - *Tui-na, 23*
- Review of joint mobilizations, *23*
  - *Recent research updates, 24*
- Summary, *26*
- Clinics care points, *26*
- Disclosure, *26*

The Role of Strengthening in the Management of Canine Osteoarthritis: A Review
Marti Drum, Emily McKay, David Levine, and Denis J. Marcellin-Little
- Introduction, *31*
- Strength training and aerobic activity in osteoarthritis, *33*
- Resistance training in osteoarthritis, *34*
- Aquatic therapy, *35*
  - *Principles of Aquatic Therapy, 36*

Swimming versus walking, 37
Summary, 37
Clinics care points, 37

Emergency and Critical Care

Crystalloids versus Colloids: Same Controversy, New Information
Christopher G. Byers
Introduction, 39
Significance, 39
Endothelial Glycocalyx, 40
Volume-Sparing Effects, 40
Normal Saline Versus Balanced Electrolyte Solutions, 41
Acute Kidney Injury and Colloids, 42
Coagulopathies and Colloids, 43
Albumin, 44
Present relevance and future avenues to consider or to investigate, 45
Summary, 45
Clinics care points, 45

Current and Future Practice in the Diagnosis and Management of Sepsis and Septic Shock in Small Animals
Thandeka R. Ngwenyama
Introduction, 49
Significance (in depth analysis), 51
Surviving Sepsis Campaign Guidelines for Management of Sepsis and Septic Shock, 51
Present relevance and future avenues to consider or to investigate, 53
Discussion, 54
Diagnosis, 54
Treatment, 56
Summary, 63
Clinics care points, 64

Current Standards and Practices in Small Animal Mechanical Ventilation
Anusha Balakrishnan
Initiating mechanical ventilation, 70
Modes of ventilation, 71
Application of positive end-expiratory pressure, 72
Suggested initial settings, 72
Monitoring the mechanically ventilated patient, 72
Equipment Care and Safety Checks, 73
Patient Care, 73
Complications of mechanical ventilation, 79
Weaning from mechanical ventilation, 79
Recovery from mechanical ventilation, 82
Clinics care points, 82

Medical and Surgical Management of Ureteral Obstructions
Dana L. Clarke
Introduction, 85
Etiology, 85
Diagnostic approach, 86
Medical management, 87
Surgical management, 88
Interventional management, 89
Postoperative management, 96
Ureteral intervention decision-making, 96
Clinics care points, 97
Disclosure, 97

Immunology

Current Knowledge on Canine Atopic Dermatitis: Pathogenesis and Treatment
Catherine A. Outerbridge and Tyler J.M. Jordan
Introduction, 101
Pathogenesis, 102
Genetics, 103
Environment, 103
Epidermal Barrier Dysfunction, 105
Immune Dysregulation, 105
Dysbiosis of the Cutaneous Microbiome, 106
Treatment, 106
The Role of Topical Therapies, 107
Systemic Anti-inflammatory and Antipruritic Therapies, 109
Allergen-Specific Immunotherapy, 111
Dietary Considerations, 111
Future avenues to consider, 111
Clinics care points, 111

Disclosure, *112*

Urology

Reevaluation of Prescription Strategies for Intermittent and Prolonged Renal Replacement Therapies

Cedric Dufayet and Larry D. Cowgill

Introduction, *117*
Current intermittent hemodialysis and intermittent hemodialysis hybrid prescription and delivery assessments, *119*
A reassessed paradigm for dialysis prescription and delivery, *120*
Therapeutic and prescription presumptions, *122*
Reprised urea reduction ratio approach and prolonged intermittent renal replacement therapy calculator to deliver renal replacement by fractional urea clearance, *125*
Prolonged Intermittent Renal Replacement Therapy with Hemofiltration, 127
Prolonged Intermittent Renal Replacement Therapy with Hemodialysis, 127
Prolonged Intermittent Renal Replacement Therapy with Hemodiafiltration, 127
Summary, *127*
Clinics care points, *127*

Activated Carbon Hemoperfusion and Plasma Adsorption: Rediscovery and Veterinary Applications of These Abandoned Therapies

Jeff Barnes, Larry D. Cowgill, and Jose Diaz Auñon

Introduction, *131*
Background, *131*
Hemoperfusion devices, *133*
Adsorption fundamentals, *133*
Legacy and modern sorbents, *135*
Use of hemoperfusion in drug overdose and poisoning, *136*
Volume of Distribution and Water Solubility, 136
Hemoperfusion in other disease conditions, *137*
Hemoperfusion; therapy delivery, *139*
Hemoperfusion; complications, *139*
Summary, *141*
Clinics care points, *141*
Funding, *142*
Disclosure, *142*

Vaccine-Enhanced Adoptive T-Cell Therapy to Treat Canine Cancers

Noe Reyes and Gary W. Wood

Introduction, *143*
General overview, background, and study rationale for vaccine-enhanced adoptive cell therapy, *144*
Vaccine-enhanced adoptive cell therapy in dogs: protocol and components, *147*
Individual Vaccine-Enhanced Adoptive Cell Therapy Components and Sequence, 147
Vaccine-Enhanced Adoptive Cell Therapy Use in Canine Osteosarcoma, 150
Significance and future directions, *152*
Clinics care points, *153*

Veterinarian Wellness

How to Toughen Them up Without Roughin' Them Up

Katie Cagel-Holtcamp and Pauline Prince

Introduction, *157*
Hazing in the workplace, *158*
Ways to teach the skill set without roughing up the students, *158*
Safety, *159*
Perspective, *159*
Open mindedness, *160*
Problem solving, *160*
Awareness of life experiences, *160*
Direct communication, *161*
Connective communication, *161*
Summary, *162*
Clinics care points, *162*
Disclosure, *162*

The Myth of Compassion Fatigue and the Reality of Emotional Fatigue

Dani McVety

Introduction, *163*
Compassion fatigue versus emotional fatigue, *164*
Emotional fatigue in veterinary medicine, *165*
Ethical Distress, 166
Client Frustrations, 166

Work-Life Imbalance, 167
High Debt-to-Income Ratio, 167
Euthanasia-Related Stress, 168
Separating emotional fatigue from compassion fatigue, *168*
Combating emotional fatigue, *169*
Remaining in Service to People and Pets, 169
Focusing on Priorities, 170
Reframing Conversations about Compassion Fatigue, 171
Summary, *171*
Clinics care points, *171*

Advances in Small Animal Care 2 (2021) xi–xii
ADVANCES IN SMALL ANIMAL CARE

Preface

New Directions for the Journal's Second Year

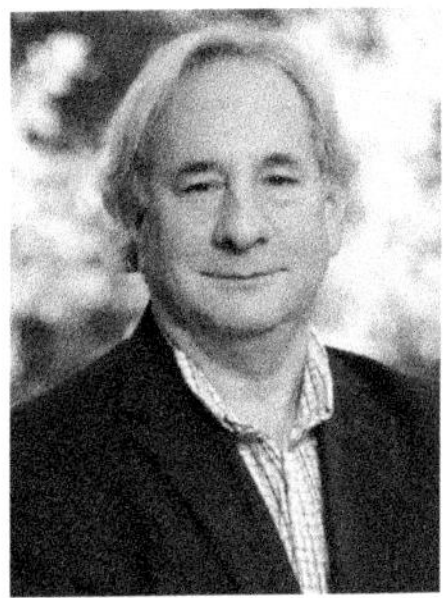

Philip H. Kass, BS, DVM, MPVM, MS, PhD
Editor

In this second issue of *Advances in Small Animal Care,* the scope of the articles has expanded beyond that of the first issue, which included behavior, imaging, gastroenterology, infectious disease, and nutrition, to now include entirely new subjects that are both topical and late-breaking: rehabilitation (including physical rehabilitation, cryotherapy, manual therapy, and strengthening exercising), emergency and critical care (crystalloid vs colloid therapy, sepsis and septic shock, mechanical ventilation, and ureteral obstruction), immunology (canine atopic dermatitis, vaccine cancer therapy), urology (renal replacement therapy, carbon hemoperfusion, and plasma adsorption), and veterinary wellness. Practitioners will find these first four sections particularly relevant, either for guidance on how scientific advances are moving into the mainstream of clinical veterinary medicine, or for what the future portends for entirely new avenues of medicine that, for now, may admittedly be technical and unfamiliar to most readers.

The last section on veterinary wellness is no less important, and one that it is hoped will be revisited in future issues. The American Veterinary Medical Association recently announced that one in six veterinarians have contemplated suicide, and that veterinarians are 2.7 times more likely to die from suicide than members of the general public. The causes are undoubtedly multifactorial, potentially starting with the myriad pressures of being a veterinary medical student, followed by the reality of an often crushing student debt to pay off, as well as the emotional stresses that are inherent in the work that veterinarians do as they interact with animals and their owners, and when self-affirming successes can often seem elusive. Two articles in this issue highlight some of these stresses at the educational and practitioner levels. Academicians and practitioners alike would do well to read these carefully, and I invite readers to submit their thoughts and proposals for additional topics in this area that is seemingly only now gaining the recognition it deserves.

I want to extend my gratitude to all the authors who provided these remarkable articles and offer a special thanks to the associate editors who oversaw and edited these submissions.

I also want to recognize with gratitude the invaluable contributions of this issue's current and past section editors, including Dr David Levine, Dr Denis J.

https://doi.org/10.1016/j.yasa.2021.08.001
2666-450X/21/ © 2021 Published by Elsevier Inc.

Marcellin-Little, Dr Elisa M. Mazzaferro, Dr Laurel J. Gershwin, Dr Larry D. Cowgill, and Dr Jennifer Brandt.

As this journal matures and its readership grows, it remains vitally important that we are providing the most up-to-date and topical resources for practitioners that bridge the gap between peer-reviewed scientific journals, publishing the discovery of new knowledge, and the textbooks that can be years in the making. I value your feedback about the contents of this issue and welcome suggestions for future issues if the topics can fortuitously fall into this exciting opportunistic publication niche.

Philip H. Kass, BS, DVM, MPVM, MS, PhD
Office of Academic Affairs
University of California, Davis
One Shields Avenue
Davis, CA 95616, USA

E-mail address: phkass@ucdavis.edu

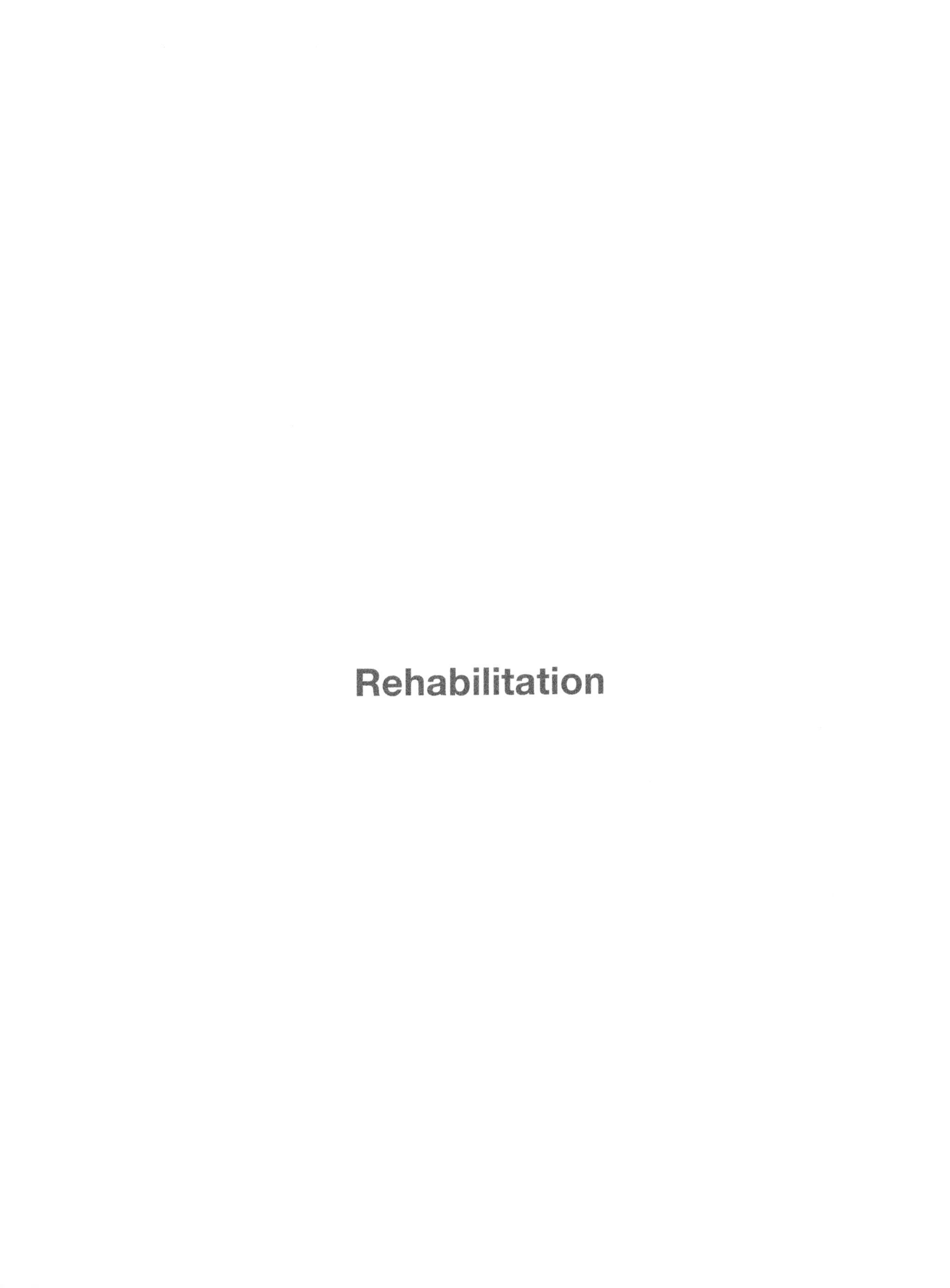

Rehabilitation

Advances in Small Animal Care 2 (2021) 1–10
ADVANCES IN SMALL ANIMAL CARE

Multifactorial Rehabilitation Planning in Companion Animals

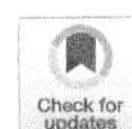

Denis J. Marcellin-Little, DEDV[a,*], David Levine, PT, PhD, DPT, CCRP, FAPTA[b], Darryl L. Millis, MS, DVM[c]

[a]Veterinary Orthopedic Research Laboratory, School of Veterinary Medicine, University of California, 1285 Veterinary Medicine DR, VM3A rm 4206, Davis, CA 95616, USA; [b]Department of Physical Therapy, 615 McCallie Avenue, University of Tennessee at Chattanooga, Chattanooga, TN 37403, USA; [c]Department of Small Animal Clinical Sciences, University of Tennessee College of Veterinary Medicine, C247 VTH, 2407 River Drive, Knoxville, TN 37996, USA

KEYWORDS

• Physical rehabilitation • Patient profile • Owner characteristics • Ergonomics • Electrophysical modalities • Manual therapy • Therapeutic exercise

KEY POINTS

- The design of a physical rehabilitation program is based on the medical condition and the anticipated progression of that condition, the profile of the patient, and the owner.
- The evaluation of the patient profile includes age, size, body condition, body conformation, demeanor, and anticipated role and activities.
- The evaluation of the owner profile includes their background knowledge, their ability and willingness to provide care, and their goals.
- The evaluation of the medical condition includes initial severity, impact on limb use and on locomotion, pain burden, chronicity, and anticipated progression.
- Physical rehabilitation programs rely on ergonomics, electrophysical modalities, manual therapy, and therapeutic exercise. Electrophysical modalities and manual therapy dominate therapy in the near term. Exercise dominates therapy in the midterm and long term.

INTRODUCTION

Physical rehabilitation focuses on the management of transient or permanent disability using ergonomics, electrophysical modalities, manual therapy, and therapeutic exercise. Rehabilitation programs may draw from some or all of these approaches. The selection of a rehabilitation program is a complex process that aims to maximize safety and efficacy, while streamlining the logistics and labor involved. Also, physical rehabilitation programs can be conducted as inpatient, outpatient, or at home. The purpose of this article is to describe the rehabilitation planning in companion animal rehabilitation, focusing on the relative importance of ergonomics, electrophysical modalities, manual therapy, and therapeutic exercise, and on the logistics of rehabilitation for situations that have resulted in disuse of musculoskeletal tissues and disability of the patient.

GENERAL FEATURES OF REHABILITATION PROGRAMS

Physical rehabilitation is planned based on the needs of the disabled patient. Rehabilitation patients may have sustained an injury, may have undergone surgery, or may have a chronic disease. Most patients have

*Corresponding author, *E-mail address:* djmarcel@ucdavis.edu

https://doi.org/10.1016/j.yasa.2021.06.001
2666-450X/21/ © 2021 Elsevier Inc. All rights reserved.

orthopedic or neurologic problems, some patients have systemic or chronic problems that interfere with their mobility or their ability to perform daily activities.

Rehabilitation can vary widely from inpatient care with multiple daily therapy sessions, outpatient care, home-based therapy, to intermittent oversight that relies on few interventions. The level of care in physical rehabilitation is generally based on patient or disease parameters: how severe the problem is, how rapidly it is progressing, and how debilitating it is (Table 1).

The severity of a problem influences rehabilitation planning; for example, a dog with patellar luxation may have unilateral or bilateral luxation that may be intermittent or constant. Unilateral, intermittent (grade 1 or 2) luxation can lead to skipping (intermittent and brief episodes of non–weight-bearing lameness). Surgery is likely to be relatively noninvasive. After surgery, the patient is likely to be weight-bearing and only have modest rehabilitation needs. By comparison, a dog with bilateral and permanent (grade 4) luxation may have such internal rotation of the tibia relative to the femur that the quadriceps femoris no longer extends the stifle joint and may act as a flexor of the stifle. Over time, the dog may lose stifle extension and quadriceps length, and may alter its posture by shifting weight forward. Surgery is likely to be invasive and may be staged or done bilaterally, and stifle joint extension is likely to remain limited immediately after surgery. The patient is likely to need extensive rehabilitation to regain stifle joint extension and recover proper limb use and posture.

The rate of progression of a problem influences rehabilitation planning. A femoral fracture in a skeletally immature dog or cat carries a risk of quadriceps contracture that has been reported to be as high as 16% in 1 study of 28 cats with a femoral fracture [1]. Quadriceps contractures are challenging to manage when discovered promptly and are irreversible if left untreated for a few weeks. The potential rapid progression of a distal femoral fracture toward quadriceps contracture warrants frequent examination (daily, in the immediate postoperative period), combined with rehabilitation (protection from postoperative trauma, promotion of limb use, and stretching). Although most orthopedic problems do not progress as rapidly as a contracture of the quadriceps femoris muscle (approximately 2–3 weeks from onset to irreversible contracture), most orthopedic problems increase in impact and complexity when left untreated.

The most common complication in orthopedic patients is the onset of limb disuse resulting from sustained chronic pain most often caused by a partial failure of fixation, low-grade infection, or joint subluxation or instability. In most instances, limb disuse progresses over a period of 2 months to severe muscle atrophy, potential loss of joint motion, and local hyperesthesia. The physical rehabilitation examination should evaluate early limb disuse of musculoskeletal tissues and pain. This evaluation may be performed as early as the day after injury or surgery in some situations (such as a distal femoral physeal fracture in a puppy), or 10 to 14 days after injury or surgery in less critical

TABLE 1
Risks and Impact of Common Problems Managed Using Physical Rehabilitation

Problem	Risks	Impact
Fracture		
Long bone fracture	Potential high-energy injury	Tissue trauma, muscle damage
Articular fracture	Joint surface and capsule damage	Loss of joint motion, osteoarthritis
Cranial cruciate ligament injury	Chronicity, bilateral injury	Limb disuse, osteoarthritis
Patellar luxation	Loss of quadriceps extensor function	Loss of stifle joint motion, disuse
Femoral head ostectomy	Chronic joint instability	Loss of hip extension, limb disuse
Osteoarthritis	Inflammation, capsular fibrosis	Loss of joint motion, limb disuse
Disc herniation	Loss of motor function, deep pain	Loss of muscle mass (lower motor neuron), loss of mobility
Degenerative myelopathy	Progressive loss of motor function	Progressive loss of mobility
Fibrocartilaginous embolism	Loss of motor function, deep pain	Loss of muscle mass (lower motor neuron), loss of mobility

situations (such as after a tibial plateau leveling osteotomy in a patient with a chronic cruciate ligament rupture). Although patients with acute or rapidly developing conditions may be re-evaluated daily in some situations, patients with slowly progressive chronic problems are reevaluated less frequently.

The physical rehabilitation examination of neurologic conditions follows a pattern similar to orthopedic physical rehabilitation: patients with acute neurologic problems and rapidly evolving problems are evaluated immediately and often daily, and patients with slowly progressive problems are evaluated less often. Acute and rapidly evolving problems include the early postoperative period after intervertebral disc herniation, fibrocartilaginous embolic myelopathy, and spinal cord myelomyelacia. Slowly progressive problems include disc protrusion, the long-term recovery after intervertebral disc herniation, and degenerative myelopathy.

The level of disability resulting from injury or disease impacts rehabilitation needs. There is no standard or global measure of impairment or disability in companion animals for many conditions. Impairment includes being nonambulatory or being unable to perform daily activities (also described as activities of daily living). Large nonambulatory dogs are a major management burden for most owners, warranting a more comprehensive rehabilitation plan, and potentially requiring inpatient care. Severe impairment includes the loss of limb use (often described as limb disuse). Orthopedic problems that result in an initial loss of ambulation include pelvic and long bone fractures affecting multiple limbs. In the presence of cofactors or comorbidities, some dogs with joint pain or joint instability in multiple limbs may become nonambulatory. Some examples include large or overweight dogs with bilateral cranial cruciate ligament rupture or severe patellar luxation, or elbow joint osteoarthritis and pain secondary to elbow dysplasia. Severe impairment can include a partial loss of mobility that interferes with daily activities. For example, a dog may need to climb a set of stairs to go indoors and may be unable to do so as a consequence of chronic pain or loss of strength. Severe impairment may also include a loss of ability to posture to urinate or defecate, or a loss of ability to eat and drink. As described elsewhere in this article, limb disuse most often results from sustained chronic pain resulting from a biological problem (infection, loss of joint motion) or a mechanical problem (failure of fixation, joint instability). For working dogs and some sporting dogs, being unable to work or engage in sporting activity creates a major hardship for handlers or owners and might be construed as major disability. Fortunately, the majority of orthopedic and neurologic problems warranting physical rehabilitation are not associated with major impairment.

MUSCULOSKELETAL TISSUE ATROPHY RESULTING FROM DISUSE

The consequences of the severity of the problem, the progression of the problem, and how debilitating the problem is all affect the magnitude and severity of atrophy of musculoskeletal tissues. Muscle, cartilage, ligaments, tendons, and bone all undergo atrophy as a result of disuse or disability. In addition, fibrosis of tissues, especially joint capsule and muscle, must be considered when planning a rehabilitation program to improve the function of patients. Depending on the length of time atrophy is allowed to occur, or the severity of tissue atrophy, changes may be reversible or permanent. These factors have been reviewed previously [2,3]. Although the primary focus of rehabilitation is directed to the main tissues that are affected, such as a fractured bone or tendon repair, knowledge of the timing and magnitude of atrophy or the other tissues is key to preventing or reversing deleterious changes. As a general rule, muscles are among the first tissues to undergo atrophy, usually within 7 to 10 days of injury or after surgery, and are often the most noticed. For example, after acute rupture of a cranial cruciate ligament, muscle mass may decrease by one-third in the affected limb within 4 to 6 weeks if no rehabilitation is performed [4]. Recovery of muscle mass is more gradual over the course of several months, and attention should be paid to aerobic and strengthening exercises to restore more normal function. Neurogenic muscle atrophy as a result of lower motor neuron conditions is more severe and rapid and is generally permanent if neurologic function is not restored [5]. Cartilage atrophy also occurs with limb disuse, including decreased cartilage matrix and cartilage thickness and stiffness [6,7]. The restoration of cartilage function is possible, but the therapists should use caution when implementing a rehabilitation program to avoid continued deleterious changes that may occur from loading the joints too rapidly or with too much intensity early in the rehabilitation period [8]. Tendons lose strength and stiffness over several weeks and return to strength and stiffness generally occurs over several months with appropriate, gradually increased loading stresses [9]. The bulk of ligaments respond similarly to tendons regarding disuse and rehabilitation. However, the insertion site of ligaments on bones responds much more slowly, primarily because of bone loss and because recovery of bone mineral content and density at the insertion sites is slow. In some instances, the ligament–bone junction may take a year or more to recover [10]. Bone is usually the slowest tissue to respond to decreased loading stresses and recovery. Bone atrophy generally takes 2 weeks to begin after injury or disuse, atrophy may continue for several weeks after loading of the bone occurs, and it may take months to regain lost bone mineral content [4]. If bone atrophy lasts for months, such as in a patient with deep pain negative intervertebral disc herniation patient, loss of bone mineral may be permanent, even if function is restored [11].

SELECTING MANAGEMENT OPTIONS DURING PHYSICAL REHABILITATION

Physical rehabilitation relies on 5 categories of actions and interventions: the rehabilitation assessment, electrophysical modalities, manual therapy, ergonomics, and therapeutic exercise. The rehabilitation assessment is done in all patients and is the basis for the selection of the 4 types of interventions (Fig. 1).

Electrophysical modalities include cold and heat, sensory and motor electrical stimulation, and energy such as ultrasound, electromagnetic field, acoustic shockwaves, and photons delivered to tissues. Manual therapy includes passive range of motion, massage, stretching, and joint mobilization. Ergonomics includes the use of specific resting and ambulation surfaces, external coaptation, and ambulation assistance. Therapeutic exercises are all forms of activity used to achieve specific therapeutic purposes such as strengthening, stretching, enhancing balance, and proprioception. Many rehabilitation plans draw from these 4 categories of therapy; however, because time and resources are most often limited, programs emphasize aspects of therapy over others based on therapeutic needs (Table 2). Also, clinicians have a responsibility to streamline and simplify therapy as much as possible to minimize the burden of care on the patient and owners, to maximize compliance, and to minimize cost. Electrophysical modalities are most often selected in the short term after injury or surgery to manage pain and inflammation. Manual therapy is used to stretch (improve range of motion) and is also used to decrease edema and provide pain relief via massage. Ergonomics is used to protect patients and to assist with the delivery of electrophysical modalities and therapeutic exercises. Exercise is key to preserving or recovering strength and mobility. The emphasis shifts over time, generally from electrophysical modalities in the short term, to manual therapy in the midterm, and to therapeutic exercise in the long term. The therapy plan informs who should be delivering therapy, where it should occur and how often it should take place.

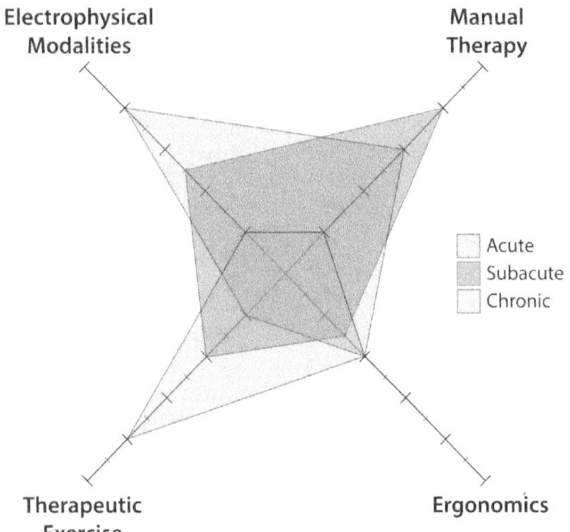

FIG. 1 The use of electrophysical modalities, manual therapy, ergonomics, and therapeutic exercise during physical rehabilitation varies over time. As an example, when considering physical rehabilitation at 3 stages of recovery after stabilization of a cranial cruciate injury, a shift in emphasis over time is visible from electrophysical modalities in the acute phase (*green*), to manual therapy in the midterm (*red*), and to therapeutic exercise in the long term (*blue*).

PROACTIVE AND RETROACTIVE FORMS OF PHYSICAL REHABILITATION

Physical rehabilitation can occur in preparation for an activity, including work or sport (conditioning), can occur proactively after an injury or surgery, or can occur retroactively when recovery after an injury or surgery is suboptimal.

Conditioning is the most proactive form of therapy. It relies on the principles of specificity and overload [12]. According to the specificity principle, activities during conditioning should match the type of activities a dog is being conditioned to do. According to the overload principle, activities should fatigue muscles to trigger metabolic changes that will enhance future performance. Conditioning takes place in the absence of injury and at a rate that ensures an increase in performance without the onset of injury. The conditioning rate varies based on the type of activity and the trainer or owner objectives and priorities.

TABLE 2
Use of Various Aspects of Physical Rehabilitation to Achieve Specific Medical Goals

Therapeutic Purpose	Electrophysical Modalities	Manual therapy	Ergonomics	Exercise
Prevent or eliminate edema	+++	+++	++	+
Prevent or alleviate pain	+++	++	+	+
Preserve or recover joint motion	-	++	-	++
Preserve or recover muscle strength	-	-	+	+++
Preserve or recover mobility	-	-	++	+++

Key: +++, primary and predictably efficacious therapeutic option; ++, efficacious therapeutic option; +, secondary and possibly efficacious option; -, minor or indirect benefits.

Proactive physical rehabilitation follows an injury or surgery and includes therapeutic steps that are implemented during recovery and in the absence of complications. Proactive physical rehabilitation usually is divided into 3 phases, starting with the acute phase, which focuses on minimizing pain, decreasing inflammation, and promoting the onset of limb use, therefore decreasing the likelihood of the onset of limb disuse. The acute phase usually lasts 7 to 14 days.

The subacute phase of proactive physical rehabilitation focuses on increasing limb use and joint motion. It lasts 2 to 4 weeks. The chronic phase focuses on completing healing and recovering muscle mass. It may last 1 to 3 months. Proactive physical rehabilitation is based on regular visits that ensure the appropriate transition from one phase to the next. It provides the opportunity to educate owners regarding recovery and enhances the safety of that recovery.

Retroactive physical rehabilitation is used to address the failure to recover from an injury or surgery. It is generally implemented to manage limb disuse, that is, to recover limb use, recover the loss of muscle mass, or recover joint motion. Retroactive rehabilitation requires a more complex assessment of the cause of limb disuse. Mechanical factors and pain may contribute to the need for retroactive rehabilitation. The pain patterns, which are more complex in patients with limb disuse owing to local amplification of pain perception, regional and central sensitization, hyperalgesia, and allodynia are analyzed. The impairment in strength (loss of muscle mass) and joint motion are evaluated. Pain is treated first. A specific set of activities is developed that ensures appropriate limb use when standing, walking, and trotting. Parameters explored include the type of constraint (harness type, leash length, the position of the handler relative to the dog during exercise), the type of activity (intensity, duration, frequency), and the exercise environment (location, ground surface). Retroactive physical rehabilitation is more complex and less predictably successful than proactive physical rehabilitation.

Logistics of Physical Rehabilitation

For acute care, physical rehabilitation is often done daily as an inpatient or an outpatient. In subacute care, physical rehabilitation is often offered as outpatient care, 1 to 3 times per week. For chronic care, physical rehabilitation visits often occur weekly or every other week. The frequency of physical rehabilitation visits is increased when patients have severe problems, including the loss of locomotion, limb disuse, and severe sustained pain. Frequency is also increased when managing rapidly evolving problems, such as a loss of joint motion in a skeletally immature patient. The frequency of physical rehabilitation is also increased when a dog is not meeting progress milestones at anticipated time points and when owners are unable or unwilling to participate in rehabilitation care, but are seeking rehabilitation. It may be most effective to hospitalize a patient who needs daily rehabilitation care or whose transportation to and from home is challenging.

MEDICAL CONDITIONS

Several aspects of medical problems greatly impact rehabilitation planning, including the anticipated duration, the anticipated pain, and the anticipated impact.

The duration of medical conditions warranting rehabilitation varies widely from brief and transient to permanent. Problems with brief duration include acute orthopedic injury such as low-energy fractures, acute joint luxations, or acute tendon ruptures. Relatively young patients undergoing uncomplicated tibial plateau leveling (to manage a cranial cruciate ligament injury) or undergoing a total hip replacement also fit in this category [13]. Neurologic patients with acute disc herniation who have motor function after surgery also fit in this category. For those patients, pain and inflammation can be managed with relatively few interventions, for example, with cold therapy and passive range of motion but without the need for more labor-intensive electrophysical modalities such as therapeutic ultrasound or transcutaneous electrical stimulation. Pain and inflammation are expected to subside substantially within 1 week, and limb use and mobility are expected to return within a few days. In the subacute rehabilitation period, joint motion is unlikely to be impacted significantly, and therefore a focus on stretching is unnecessary. In the chronic rehabilitation period, the dog may look and feel normal; however, their musculoskeletal tissues are relatively weak and are still undergoing remodeling. The exercise program restricts high-impact activity to avoid excessive stress on healing tissues while promoting low-impact activities that prevent muscle atrophy and promote normal limb use, a normal posture, and a normal gait. Because many owners and dogs are unfamiliar with control, educating owners to balance dog control and activity restriction on the one hand, and the promotion of low-impact activity on the other hand, is often challenging. Overall, physical rehabilitation for focal and transient problems is predictably successful and should be affordable to most owners, owing to its relative simplicity. Alternatively, chronic problems warranting physical rehabilitation can affect patients in the long term or may result in permanent deficits in function. These chronic problems may include slowly progressive conditions resulting in pain and inflammation, or neurologic compromise. Problems such as severe osteoarthritis affecting multiple limbs, long-term joint subluxation or luxation, musculoskeletal tissue fibrosis with loss of joint motion, permanent or progressive neurologic compromise, fracture nonunions, chronic low-grade musculoskeletal tissue infection, loose total joint components, and some forms of neoplasia fit in this category. Because the objective of rehabilitation shifts from curing to managing the patient (optimizing quality of life, preserving mobility), the presence of long-term or permanent disability greatly influences the physical rehabilitation plan.

The pain burden on rehabilitation patients varies widely and has a profound impact on rehabilitation planning. It is, therefore, critically important to evaluate pain in rehabilitation patients. A mild pain experience treated without delay can often be managed with a nonsteroidal anti-inflammatory drug combined with rest, without extensive use of electrophysical modalities and manual therapy. In contrast, the treatment of severe acute or postoperative pain and the treatment of sustained chronic pain must be more comprehensive, multifocal, and integrated with the pharmacologic pain management. Whenever possible, the cause of sustained chronic pain should be identified and eliminated. Subjectively, sustained chronic pain is particularly likely in a patient with neoplasia and failure of fixation after the stabilization of a fracture. Sustained chronic pain happens in a subset of patients with joint disease such as cruciate ligament injury, patellar luxation, or elbow and hip dysplasia. Sustained chronic pain also occurs after surgery for these and other conditions, and seems to be more likely when surgery addresses the problem only partially. As an example, a femoral head ostectomy can lead to severe limb disuse possibly because of the addition of acute pain (from surgery) on chronic pain (from hip dysplasia), and possibly because the pseudoarthrosis resulting from the removal of the femoral head has physical limitations, such as lack of stability under load, restriction of motion, or chronic inflammation.

The anticipated impact of a medical problem on limb use and mobility has a major impact on physical rehabilitation planning. Limb use is likely to be compromised in patients with problems affecting joint motion, including loss of joint motion or an excess of joint motion. Subjectively, the loss of joint motion is more detrimental to limb use than excess joint motion. Loss of joint motion can be primary developmental or secondary. Primary loss of motion can be neurologic or orthopedic (Fig. 2) [14]. A mild loss of motion generally has no negative impact on limb use. For example, with hip dysplasia, a modest loss of hip extension is likely. That loss has no clear detrimental impact on limb use [15]. Loss of joint motion has a profound impact when the loss is severe. For example, a loss of carpal extension of 50° precludes the use of a forelimb [14,16]. Loss of joint motion also has a profound impact when severe pain is perceived at the end of joint motion, such as in some dogs with severe patellar luxation or partial tear of the cranial cruciate ligament.

Evaluation of full joint motion and the response to full joint motion are therefore key aspects of the rehabilitation assessment [17]. Joint motion may be evaluated subjectively during palpation. When abnormal motion is detected, it can be measured objectively using goniometry or photography [18]. Excess motion is most often the consequence of joint laxity or luxation. The most common developmental joint luxation is hip

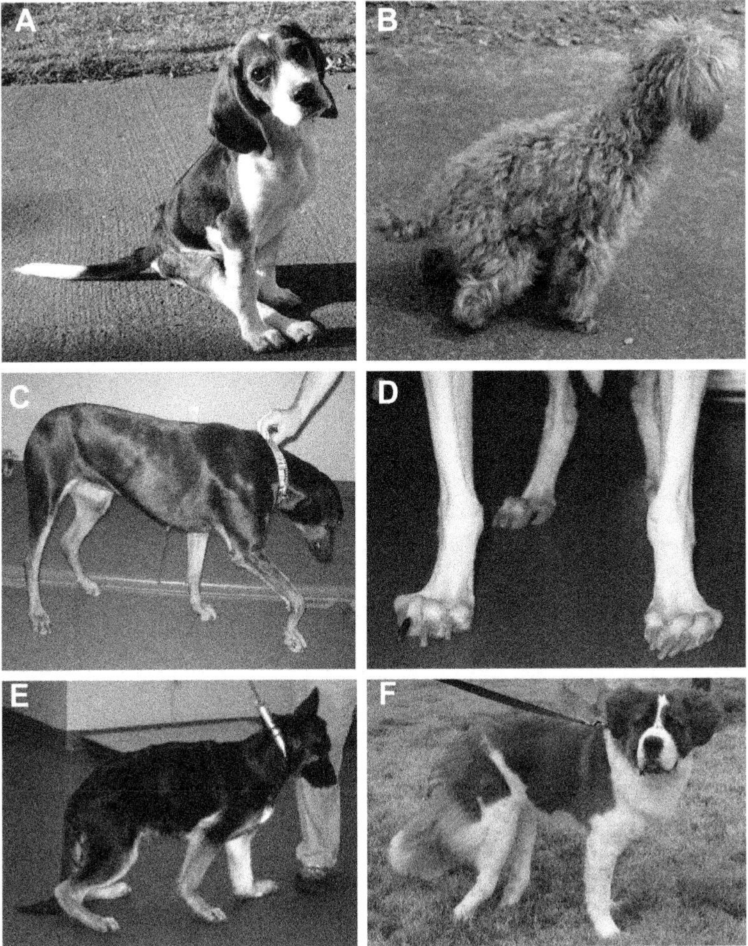

FIG. 2 Loss of joint motion can affect all joints and has a profound impact on physical rehabilitation of dogs. Subjectively, the stifle joint is most vulnerable, as seen in a young Beagle after a bite to the thigh region (loss of flexion, **A**) or a Miniature Poodle with bilateral grade 4 patellar luxation (loss of extension, **B**). Loss of motion can also occur in the carpus, as seen a young Doberman with a developmental loss of extension associated with a lack of length in the flexor carpi ulnaris muscle (**C**) or in a Whippet with a lack of digit extension, resulting from a lack of length in the digital flexor muscles (**D**). Excess motion also impacts physical rehabilitation. Subjectively, the carpus and tarsus are most vulnerable to excess joint motion compared with other major joints. A young German Shepherd has lax carpi (**E**) and a young Saint Bernard has hyperextended tarsi as a consequence of hip dysplasia (**F**).

luxation secondary to excessive hip laxity. Other developmental joint luxations include shoulder luxation, most often medially, in small dogs. Elbow luxation or, more specifically, lateral or caudolateral luxation of the radial head relative to the humerus may be seen in young dogs. Often, these dogs have a large, heavy body and are chondrodystrophic (Bulldogs). In the tarsus, hyperextension can result from a cranial weight shift present in large dogs with severe hip pain. The tarsus become more and more extended over time and that excessive extension interferes with limb use. Large dogs with angular deformities of the distal portion of the femur can have intertarsal rotational subluxation, where the pes rotates externally in relation to the tarsus. Mobility also has a major impact on rehabilitation. Baseline mobility may be compromised owing to chronic joint disease (osteoarthritis) affecting multiple limbs, excess weight, a large size, or systemic or neurologic problems. Postinjury mobility may be compromised by a loss of limb use, particularly when multiple limbs are affected. Common causes of loss of mobility include intervertebral disc herniation, pelvic

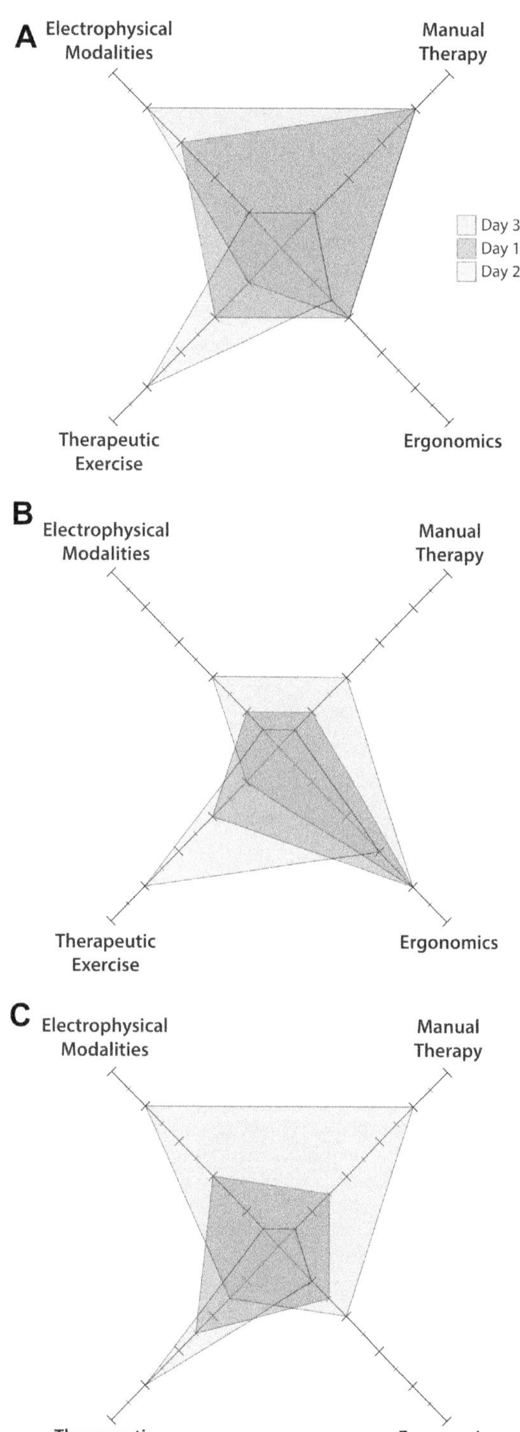

FIG. 3 Care algorithms representing the reliance on the 4 key aspects of rehabilitation: electrophysical modalities, manual therapy, therapeutic exercise, and ergonomics over time for various patients commonly receiving physical rehabilitation. For a patient undergoing surgery to stabilize a cranial cruciate ligament-deficient stifle joint (**A**), the initial emphasis of care (at day 3, acute phase, green shaded area) would be placed on electrophysical modalities (cold, therapeutic ultrasound, TENS, photobiomodulation) and manual therapy (passive range of motion, massage). At day 14 (subacute phase, red shaded area), the emphasis would shift to manual therapy (stretching) and therapeutic exercise. At day 28 (chronic phase, blue shaded area) the emphasis would shift further to therapeutic exercise. For a dog recovering from surgery to manage herniation on an intervertebral disc (**B**), the emphasis of care would initially be placed on ergonomics (eg, nursing care, ambulation assistance) with some care involving electrophysical modalities and manual therapy. At day 14, the emphasis on ergonomics would remain, with an increase of emphasis toward therapeutic exercise. At day 28, the emphasis would shift to therapeutic exercise while continuing the focus on ergonomics (ambulation assistance). For a dog recovering from surgery to manage a fracture (**C**), the initial emphasis of care would be on electrophysical modalities (cold, TENS, therapeutic ultrasound) and manual therapy (passive range of motion and massage). That emphasis would shift progressively to exercise at days 14 and 28.

fractures or bilateral long bone fractures, and bilateral cranial cruciate ligament injury, the latter in dogs with a baseline compromise in mobility. The loss of muscle mass, in the absence of chronic pain, may not lead to limb disuse or to the loss of mobility.

PATIENT PROFILE

Physical rehabilitation planning is influenced by the patient's profile, including age, size, conformation, and anticipated functions and activities. Skeletally immature dogs are high-risk patients because young dogs undergo rapid growth and rapid tissue turnover. Although healing in growing dogs is rapid, limb disuse, loss of joint motion, and tissue loss also have a rapid onset. Bone loss can develop rapidly as a consequence of limb disuse or joint immobilization. Mechanically, bone and fracture repairs are fragile relative to bone and fracture repairs in adult dogs, potentially incentivizing clinicians to protect repairs with a bandage or splint. However, bandages and splints carry a high risk of complications in growing dogs. Growing dogs have an exaggerated connective tissue response to injury, relative to adult dogs. That response may lead to fibrosis of the joint capsule, adhesions between tissue planes, and to the invasion of limb compartments, including muscles, with rapidly maturing fibrous tissue. Muscle and joint laxity (carpal hypertension, flaccid digits) can occur after a brief period of limb disuse. Growing dogs tend to have excitable personalities, making the control of their activity and the delivery of nursing and rehabilitation care more challenging. Owners and therapists may have difficulties with manual therapy and therapeutic exercises because of growing dogs' brief attention span and low obedience level. In addition, growing dogs can possibly be at indirect risk because owners may subconsciously think that youth positively impacts the likelihood of rapid and complete healing, when experience suggests that growing dogs have a higher complication rate than adult dogs after injury or surgery [19]. It is also possible that the bond between owners and growing dogs may not be as strong as the bond with adult dogs who may be more likely to be considered long-term family members; this factor may result in less attention to rehabilitation of younger dogs performed by the owner. Geriatric patients are also at risk because of the greater likelihood of orthopedic comorbidities and possibly a lack of drive during recovery.

Patient size influences the physical rehabilitation plan. Small patients are at an increased risk of fracture, such as of the radius, and other injuries. Subjectively, small patients are also at risk of limb disuse, possibly because they can ambulate effectively on 3 legs. The demeanor of small patients can complicate the planning of a therapeutic program. Very large dogs also present challenges in physical rehabilitation. They are at risk of becoming nonambulatory and they are difficult to manage, often requiring the efforts of several people. Their large size also complicates the planning of a therapeutic exercise program. Overweight dogs also have complicated physical rehabilitation plans because overweight and obese dogs are at risk of becoming nonambulatory and require therapeutic exercise tailored to their mobility and fitness. Dogs with chondrodystrophic conformation also need oversight during rehabilitation because of potential comorbidities (upper airway syndrome, limb deformity, elbow joint subluxation, patellar luxation). The patient's demeanor influences physical rehabilitation. Poorly socialized or aggressive dogs may be best suited for hands-off rehabilitation based mostly on therapeutic exercise provided by the owner, whereas shy dogs may be best suited for hand-on rehabilitation with manual therapy.

OWNERSHIP PROFILE

The ownership profile impacts physical rehabilitation. Owners have variable background knowledge in medical problems, physical restrictions and risks, commitment to recovery, and ability to engage in hands-on (massage, passive range of motion, cold therapy, stretching) and hands-off (therapeutic exercise) activities. Also, an owner's intent for their dog to engage in work or sporting activities varies widely. Finally, an owner's ability and willingness to incur the costs of care vary widely. The rehabilitation clinician adapts care, including the type of care (inpatient, outpatient, or home-based therapy) and visit frequency and duration to the level of owner involvement, abilities and expectations.

CARE ALGORITHMS

The development of a rehabilitation program is based on the intent of the clinician to incorporate various aspects of physical rehabilitation: electrophysical modalities, manual therapy, therapeutic exercise, and ergonomics (Fig. 3). Reliance on electrophysical modalities and manual therapy is initially high. Reliance on therapeutic exercise is initially modest and increases overtime to become the dominant form of therapy. Reliance on ergonomics is often biphasic: initially high in trauma and in neurologic patients and high over the long term in patients with chronic and progressive diseases.

CLINICS CARE POINTS

- Physical rehabilitation programs are particularly critical when managing patients with severe conditions that interfere with limb use and mobility, that carry a heavy pain burden, and that have a rapid progression.
- Physical rehabilitation programs are particularly important in patients with profiles that are associated with an increased complication rate, such as very small and very large dogs, skeletally immature and geriatric dogs, dogs with a heavy body condition, and chondrodystrophic dogs.
- Physical rehabilitation is simpler and more predictably efficacious when implemented proactively, when chronicity is minimal, and before the onset of complications.

ACKNOWLEDGMENTS

The authors thank Chrisoula Toupadakis Skouritakis, PhD, for assistance with illustrations.

DISCLOSURE

The authors report no conflict of interest.

REFERENCES

[1] Fries CL, Binnington AG, Cockshutt JR. Quadriceps contracture in four cats: a complication of internal fixation of femoral fractures. Vet Comp Orthop Traumatol 1988;1:38–43.

[2] Kirkby Shaw K, Alvarez L, Foster SA, et al. Fundamental principles of rehabilitation and musculoskeletal tissue healing. Vet Surg 2020;49:22–32.

[3] Millis DL. Responses of musculoskeletal tissues to disuse and remobilization. In: Millis DL, Levine D, editors. Canine rehabilitation and physical therapy. Philadelphia, PA: Saunders; 2014. p. 92–153.

[4] Francis DA, Millis DL, Head LL. Bone and lean tissue changes following cranial cruciate ligament transection and stifle stabilization. J Am Anim Hosp Assoc 2006;42:127–35.

[5] Gordon T, Mao J. Muscle atrophy and procedures for training after spinal cord injury. Phys Ther 1994;74:50–60.

[6] Palmoski M, Perricone E, Brandt KD. Development and reversal of a proteoglycan aggregation defect in normal canine knee cartilage after immobilization. Arthritis Rheum 1979;22:508–17.

[7] McDonough AL. Effects of immobilization and exercise on articular cartilage-a review of literature. J Orthop Sports Phys Ther 1981;3:2–5.

[8] Palmoski MJ, Brandt KD. Running inhibits the reversal of atrophic changes in canine knee cartilage after removal of a leg cast. Arthritis Rheum 1981;24:1329–37.

[9] Yasuda K, Hayashi K. Changes in biomechanical properties of tendons and ligaments from joint disuse. Osteoarthr Cartil 1999;7:122–9.

[10] Noyes FR. Functional properties of knee ligaments and alterations induced by immobilization: a correlative biomechanical and histological study in primates. Clin Orthop Relat Res 1977;210–42.

[11] Jortikka MO, Inkinen RI, Tammi MI, et al. Immobilisation causes longlasting matrix changes both in the immobilised and contralateral joint cartilage. Ann Rheum Dis 1997;56:255–61.

[12] Marcellin-Little DJ, Levine D, Taylor R. Rehabilitation and conditioning of sporting dogs. Vet Clin North Am Small Anim Pract 2005;35:1427–39.

[13] Marcellin-Little DJ, Doyle ND, Pyke JF. Physical rehabilitation after total joint arthroplasty in companion animals. Vet Clin North Am Small Anim Pract 2015;45:145–65.

[14] Marcellin-Little DJ, Levine D. Principles and application of range of motion and stretching in companion animals. Vet Clin North Am Small Anim Pract 2015;45:57–72.

[15] Greene LM, Marcellin-Little DJ, Lascelles BD. Associations among exercise duration, lameness severity, and hip joint range of motion in Labrador Retrievers with hip dysplasia. J Am Vet Med Assoc 2013;242:1528–33.

[16] Kwan TW, Marcellin-Little DJ, Harrysson OL. Correction of biapical radial deformities by use of bi-level hinged circular external fixation and distraction osteogenesis in 13 dogs. Vet Surg 2014;43:316–29.

[17] Levine D, Millis DL, Marcellin-Little DJ. Introduction to veterinary physical rehabilitation. Vet Clin North Am Small Anim Pract 2005;35:1247–54, vii.

[18] Jaegger G, Marcellin-Little DJ, Levine D. Reliability of goniometry in Labrador Retrievers. Am J Vet Res 2002;63:979–86.

[19] Bardet JF. Quadriceps contracture and fracture disease. Vet Clin North Am Small Anim Pract 1987;17:957–73.

Advances in Small Animal Care 2 (2021) 11–18

ADVANCES IN SMALL ANIMAL CARE

Cryotherapy in Small Animal Rehabilitation

David Levine, PT, PhD, DPT, CCRP, FAPTA[a,*], Denis J. Marcellin-Little, DEDV[b]

[a]Department of Physical Therapy, 615 McCallie Avenue, The University of Tennessee at Chattanooga, Chattanooga, TN 37403, USA; [b]Veterinary Orthopedic Research Laboratory, School of Veterinary Medicine, University of California, 1285 Veterinary Medicine DR, VM3A rm 4206, Davis, CA 95616, USA

KEYWORDS

• Cryotherapy • Cold compression device • Ice pack • Vasoconstriction

KEY POINTS

- Cryotherapy causes a decrease in blood flow to the area, which may decrease the amount of hemorrhage and edema, and a decrease local tissue metabolism and enzyme-mediated tissue damage
- Cryotherapy can decrease pain and improve function in the postoperative patient
- Careful consideration should be taken to choose the proper application and timing of cryotherapy to achieve an optimal effect and to understand how it may facilitate or hinder a positive outcome

INTRODUCTION

Cryotherapy, taken from the Greek "kryo" meaning cold and "therapeía" for therapy or cure, is the use of cold for therapeutic purposes. Used by the Egyptians as early as 2500 BC to treat inflammation, by Hippocrates to treat pain and inflammation, and by Napoleon's surgeon to facilitate amputations in the battlefield, cryotherapy has been continually used throughout history for a variety of medical conditions [1,2]. The principle of PRICE (protection, rest, ice, compression, elevation) has been the mainstay of medical treatment of acute inflammation in sports medicine and orthopedics since these fields were founded [3]. The origins of cryotherapy in small animal practice evolved from the human practice, and it has now become commonplace. Cryotherapy can be applied in several ways, the most common being cold packs, ice packs, and cold compression devices. Although cryotherapy is a standard practice of care, the evidence describing its clinical effects is limited. Cryotherapy is used not only during the acute and subacute phases of tissue injury and healing to mitigate the effects and sequelae of tissue injury or surgery but also after exercise during rehabilitation to minimize adverse secondary inflammatory responses [4–9]. Cryotherapy is frequently used to treat overuse injuries such as tendonitis [10,11].

This article discusses the current literature regarding cryotherapy as a treatment of acute soft tissue injuries in small animal practice. The physiologic responses caused by cryotherapy; the benefits, potential risks, and adverse effects; common methods of application of cryotherapy; and are reviewed and recommendations for clinical practice are discussed.

PHYSIOLOGIC EFFECTS OF CRYOTHERAPY

In response to cooling, acutely inflamed tissues exhibit a slowed metabolic rate, inhibition of inflammatory enzymatic reactions, and reduced release of histamine. These

The authors have no conflict to disclose.

*Corresponding author, *E-mail address:* David-Levine@utc.edu

https://doi.org/10.1016/j.yasa.2021.07.002
2666-450X/21/ Published by Elsevier Inc.

physiologic responses serve to limit tissue damage [12]. The vasoconstriction associated with cold application limits edema formation and hemorrhage [13–15]. Pain may be lessened due to reduced pressure on nociceptive receptors through edema reduction as well as through reduced nerve conduction velocity [16]. As these effects are most relevant to acute inflammation, cold is most effective when applied during the acute phase of trauma, typically in the first 72 hours after injury or surgery. Cryotherapy may also be useful in chronic pain situations such as experienced with osteoarthritic joints to reduce pain, edema, collagenolysis, synovial inflammation, and joint destruction [10,17–20]; this is possibly because inflammation is a common feature of osteoarthritis, particularly for periodic symptom flares [21]. As a result of its analgesic effect, cryotherapy may permit decreased use of pain medications [22,23]. Cryotherapy is used in postoperative treatment of swelling and pain, in musculoskeletal injury, muscle spasm, and after exercise to prevent edema or pain [4,24–30].

The primary basis for cryotherapy in the management of acute injuries is grounded on several principles: the decrease in tissue metabolism that occurs when the temperature is lowered; the decrease in blood flow to the area (vasoconstriction), which may decrease the bleeding and hemorrhage into the area; and relieving pain [10,25,31–33]. The decrease in blood flow slows edema formation after injury or surgery [31]. The cooling of the tissue reduces the metabolic rate of the treated tissue, decreases the rate of reactions related to the acute inflammatory process, causes the inhibition of enzymatic effects related to inflammation, and minimizes the release of histamine, which reduces tissue damage [15,34]. At a temperature of 30°C or lower, cartilage-degrading enzymes (protease, hyaluronidase, collagenase) are inhibited. The vasoconstriction of blood vessels also may help to decrease pain by decreasing pressure on nociceptors, which may be stimulated as a result of increased tissue swelling and edema, as well as by other physiologic means such as decreased nerve conduction velocity [35]. For optimal benefits, cryotherapy should be applied within the first few hours that follow tissue injury [36] (Box 1).

Cryotherapy can reduce inflammatory pain through several mechanisms. Cold decreases skin and the underlying tissue temperature and reduces blood flow to the cooled tissues via a sympathetic vasoconstrictive reflex [37]. Reduction in blood flow reduces edema and slows the delivery of inflammatory mediators [37]. Cryotherapy also produces a local anesthetic effect by decreasing the threshold of tissue nociceptors and the conduction velocity of sensory nerves [38].

INFLUENCES OF CRYOTHERAPY ON OTHER REHABILITATION TREATMENTS

Cryotherapy may also have a positive influence on the effectiveness of therapeutic laser treatments, given its effects on blood flow and the saturation of blood chromophores in the tissue. Where tissue perfusion is reduced with cryotherapy, the absorption of laser energy may be improved, so that deeper structures may receive greater laser energy [39]. Some have raised concerns about a potential negative impact of cryotherapy on the efficacy of platelet-rich plasma injections because of the decrease in local metabolic activity; however, this has not been studied in a clinical setting.

APPLICATION, RISKS, AND PRECAUTIONS

Before the application of cryotherapy, tissues should be checked for the level of sensation, and if decreased or absent, care must be used to prevent injury. The skin should also be checked for redness, burns, scabs, or wounds because these may alter the thermal transmission or affect the method of treatment. The area to be treated may need to be cleaned to remove dirt or any other substance on the skin that could decrease conductance or alter uniformity of conduction. If the application of cold is over a postsurgical site, a clean towel or other barrier should be placed between the cryotherapy device and the skin to minimize the risk of infection. Cryotherapy devices such as cold packs or cold compression sleeves should be disinfected between patients to minimize the risk of nosocomial bacterial infection.

TYPES OF CRYOTHERAPY DEVICES

Cryotherapy is most commonly applied using cold packs, ice packs, and cold compression devices. Other forms of cryotherapy can include ice massage and vapocoolant sprays that cause immediate evaporation of the liquid upon hitting the skin, effectively cooling tissues via evaporation, similarly to sweating. Commercial cold packs are available in many sizes and are kept in a freezer until ready for use (Fig. 1). A variety of available cryotherapy devices are pictured in Fig. 2. Most of these devices are applied for 10 to 20 minutes to achieve adequate tissue cooling. Cold compression devices combine the effects of cryotherapy with compression around an injured tissue to help further reduce edema (Figs. 3 and 4). The cold and compression is applied intermittently and repeatedly in the early postoperative period [7].

BOX 1
Physiologic Effects of Cryotherapy

- Decreased blood flow to the area (vasoconstriction)
- Decreased hemorrhage and edema
- Decreased local tissue metabolism and enzyme-mediated tissue damage
- Decreased pain via decreased pressure on pain receptors, decreased concentration of proteolytic enzymes, and decreased nerve conduction velocity

LITERATURE REVIEW

Most protocols for cryotherapy in veterinary patients have been adapted from human studies and have historically been used after surgery and to manage acute musculoskeletal injuries. Little is known about the optimal technique, magnitude and depth of cooling, duration of application for specific injuries or locations on the body, and duration of tissue cooling in dogs. In a study evaluating cryotherapy on the epaxial region of dogs, muscle temperature was measured at depths of 0.5, 1.0, and 1.5 cm during application of frozen gel packs applied for 5, 10, or 20 minutes. Five minutes after application, only the 0.5 cm depth had significantly cooled compared with the controls. Temperatures at all depths were significantly cooler at 10 minutes compared with the controls, and tissue temperatures continued to decrease at 20 minutes, when maximal cooling occurred. Maximal temperature decreases at 0.5 cm, 1.0 cm, and 1.5 cm depth were 8.2°C, 6.5°C, and 4.7°C, respectively. Superficial tissues had the greatest cooling, and the effect decreased with greater tissue depth. The investigators suggested that although the deeper tissues were not in direct contact with the cooling apparatus, the tissue temperature decreased by transfer of heat from the deep to the superficial layers, ultimately requiring longer contact time for sufficient cooling [28]. Clinically, this study supplies evidence that a treatment time of 10 to 20 minutes seems optimal for tissue cooling.

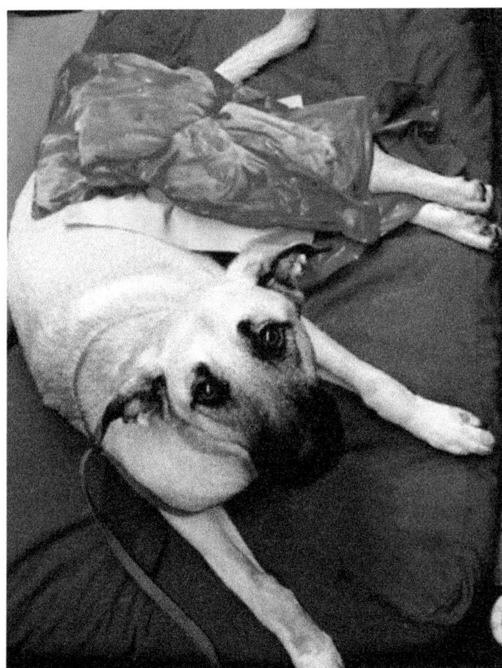

FIG. 1 Commercial cold packs applied to the medial and lateral aspects of the stifle joint after surgery.

A study evaluating the effects of cold compression therapy (CCT) applied immediately postoperatively after stifle joint surgery (vs a soft padded bandage [SPB]) examined functional outcome measures including limb use, range of motion, and nociceptive thresholds, in addition to the time to return to normothermia after surgery [7]. The cold compression unit was used for 30 minutes every 2 hours after surgery until the next morning, and the control group received an SPB after surgery. When comparing the CCT to the SPB at 24 hours postoperatively, dogs undergoing CCT had more stifle joint flexion ($P<.01$) and weight bearing ($P<.001$) after surgery than dogs with SPB. Return to normothermia was slightly delayed in the CCT group, with temperatures ~0.5°C lower 120 minutes after surgery ($P = .013$). The investigators concluded that CCT had a positive short-term impact on stifle flexion and early weight bearing after stifle surgery, relative to bandaging.

Appendicular injuries are common in canine patients and are frequently treated with cryotherapy in the acute stage. Many of the affected target tissues, including muscles and joints, are located under several centimeters of soft tissue. One previous study evaluated temperature change in canine superficial tissues of the skin and subcutaneous tissue (0.3 cm), intramuscular

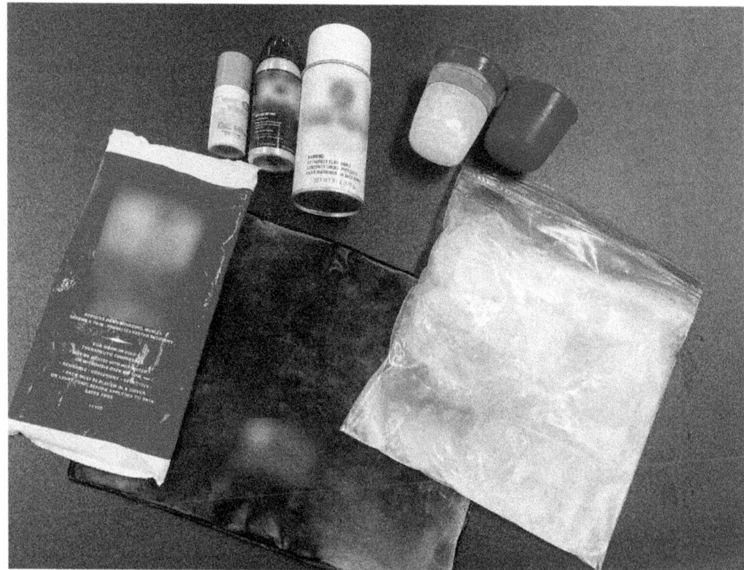

FIG. 2 Cryotherapy options (clockwise starting top right): ice massage cups, alcohol-water slush plastic bags, commercial cold wraps, and fluoromethane cold spray.

tissues (2.5 cm), and periosteal tissue layers (4.0 cm) by applying a cold gel pack to the lateral aspect of the femur for 30 minutes. The temperature at the skin, subcutaneous tissues, intramuscular tissues, and periosteal tissues decreased 16.2C, 11.2C, 5.0C, and 4.0C, respectively. The period of rewarming was also noted to be slower in deeper tissues compared with superficial tissues [40]. This study concluded that the superficial tissues experienced a more significant cooling effect, with maximum temperature decrease occurring at 30 minutes. Merrick and colleagues [41,42] found that thermal treatment modalities that go through a change of state (eg, change from ice to water) absorb significantly more heat from superficial tissues than those that do not (eg, gel pack), resulting in greater transfer of thermal energy and possibly a greater change in tissue temperature.

Less is known about the effect of the hair coat on tissue temperature changes during cryotherapy. Most patients receiving cryotherapy during the acute postoperative period have their hair clipped; however, dogs that sustained nonsurgical injuries may have cryotherapy included in their treatment protocol. One study compared the depth of effective cooling using cold packs on the caudal thigh muscles of dogs at 1.0 and 3.0 cm depth and the influence of hair on tissue cooling

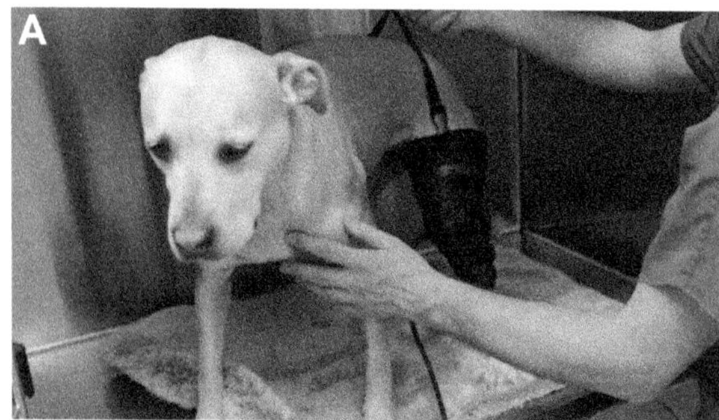

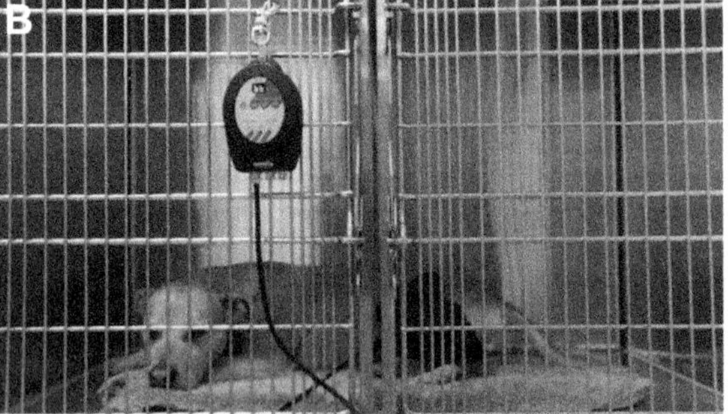

FIG. 3 (*A*) A cold compression unit is delivering cold to a dog stifle joint after surgery. Cold is delivered via a refrigerated gel pack. (*B*) The unit has a battery operated pump providing air pressure for compression.

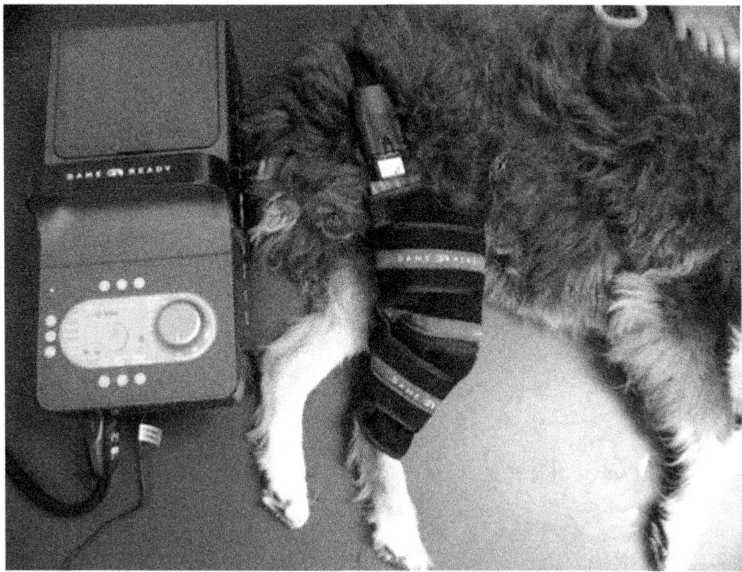

FIG. 4 A cold compression unit; ice water is stored in the unit and circulated through the compression sleeve.

[4]. Similar to previous studies, tissue temperature reduction was larger at 1.0 cm depth than at 3.0 cm depth [28,40]. All depths had a significant decrease in temperature; however, the surface and superficial muscle tissue reached significantly cooler temperatures than deeper muscle tissue. The cooling effect between the haired and clipped limbs was not statistically significant; however, short-haired dogs (mixed-breed hounds) were used in this study. This finding lends support to achieving significant cooling over nonclipped limbs in short-haired dogs. Another interesting finding in this study was that the surface temperature of the haired limbs was significantly cooler 20 minutes after the ice pack was removed than that of the clipped limbs. The investigators hypothesized that this may have resulted in an insulating effect with measurement of hair/trapped air temperature rather than a measurement of true skin temperature [4].

Studies in humans evaluating cryotherapy after musculoskeletal surgery have revealed conflicting evidence regarding the effectiveness of treatment. One study in postoperative shoulders found that the application of cryotherapy resulted in significantly less swelling and pain in patients who received treatment immediately after surgery [43]. However, another study evaluating patients after anterior cruciate ligament reconstruction did not find any significant difference in range of motion, use of pain medication, or length of hospital stay between patients receiving cryotherapy and those who did not [44]. Cryotherapy has also been evaluated in human knees with osteoarthritis and has been found to reduce interleukin-1β, interleukin-6, and vascular endothelial growth factor in the synovial fluid [18].

CRYOTHERAPY OVER COAPTATION DEVICES

Coaptation devices such as SPBs are sometimes placed on the limbs following injury or surgery. As cryotherapy is useful during the acute inflammatory phase, it would be beneficial to apply cryotherapy over coaptation devices without the need to remove and reapply these devices. Several studies in people have addressed the use of cryotherapy over casts or bandages, and although specific studies are not available in animals, these findings may serve as guidelines for use in animals.

One study of humans evaluated the magnitude of temperature changes at the skin over the ankle after the application of ice bags to the surface of various casts and bandages over the ankle [45]. This study compared the effectiveness of ice packs on decreasing skin temperature under a plaster cast, a fiberglass cast, an ACE wrap (elastic bandage), and a Robert Jones dressing over a 90-minute time frame. Decreases in skin temperature respectively were 14.6°C, 13.3°C, 11.3°C, and 4.6°C.

BOX 2
General Recommendations for Cryotherapy

- Apply as soon as possible after injury or surgery
- Use a cloth between the cold and the skin and mold the cold pack to the tissue surface by pressing gently
- Apply for at least 10 minutes (10–20 minute is optimal for cold packs)
- Apply every 2 to 4 hours if possible for the first 24 hours. As signs of inflammation subside, reduce the frequency to 2 to 3 times each day

Although skin temperature under dressings and casts decreased significantly relative to the baseline temperatures in all groups, the smallest decreases happened with the Robert Jones bandage and the greatest temperature decrease occurred with the plaster cast [45]. A similar study concluded that synthetic or plaster casts do not eliminate tissue cooling when crushed ice packs are applied to the surface of the casts, but the time required for maximum cooling was approximately 1 hour, and bulky dressings inhibit adequate cooling [46]. These studies only evaluated skin temperature, so effects of cooling on deeper tissues are unknown.

SUMMARY

Cryotherapy can be a powerful adjunct in the rehabilitation of musculoskeletal injuries in dogs. Successful management depends on an accurate assessment of the dog's presenting problems at the beginning of each treatment session. Careful consideration should be taken to choose the proper therapeutic modality to achieve an appropriate effect and understand how the modality chosen may facilitate or hinder a positive outcome (Box 2). Cryotherapy is most useful during the acute inflammatory stages of tissue healing. Two recent papers on cranial cruciate surgery in dogs have demonstrated the effectiveness of postoperative cryotherapy to minimize inflammation [9,27].

CLINICS CARE POINTS

- Cryotherapy is most beneficial during the acute inflammatory stages of tissue healing.
- Understanding of the mode of application and the timing of application is important in the application of cryotherapy.
- Cryotherapy should be applied in most cases for 10 to 20 minutes for adequate cooling.

REFERENCES

[1] Freiman A, Bouganim N. History of cryotherapy. Dermatol Online J 2005;11(2):9.
[2] Adams F. The genuine works of hippocrates. New York: William Wood and Company; 1929. p. 741–2.
[3] Landry GL, Gomez JE. Management of soft tissue injuries. Adolesc Med 1991;2(1):125–40.
[4] Janas K, Millis D, Levine D, et al. Effects of cryotherapy on temperature change in caudal thigh muscles of dogs. Vet Comp Orthop Traumatol 2021. https://doi.org/10.1055/s-0041-1723786.
[5] Dambros C, Martimbianco AL, Polachini LO, et al. Effectiveness of cryotherapy after anterior cruciate ligament reconstruction. Acta Ortop Bras 2012;20(5):285–90.
[6] Martimbianco AL, Gomes da Silva BN, de Carvalho AP, et al. Effectiveness and safety of cryotherapy after arthroscopic anterior cruciate ligament reconstruction. A systematic review of the literature. Phys Ther Sport 2014;15(4):261–8.
[7] Szabo SD, Levine D, Marcellin-Little DJ, et al. Cryotherapy improves limb use but delays normothermia early after stifle joint surgery in dogs. Front Vet Sci 2020;7:381.
[8] von Freeden N, Duerr F, Fehr M, et al. Comparison of two cold compression therapy protocols after tibial plateau leveling osteotomy in dogs. Tierarztl Prax Ausg K Kleintiere Heimtiere 2017;45(4):226–33.
[9] Drygas KA, McClure SR, Goring RL, et al. Effect of cold compression therapy on postoperative pain, swelling, range of motion, and lameness after tibial plateau leveling osteotomy in dogs. J Am Vet Med Assoc 2011;238(10):1284–91.

[10] Zhang J, Pan T, Wang JH. Cryotherapy suppresses tendon inflammation in an animal model. J Orthop Translat 2014;2(2):75–81.
[11] Knobloch K, Grasemann R, Spies M, et al. Intermittent KoldBlue cryotherapy of 3x10 min changes mid-portion Achilles tendon microcirculation. Br J Sports Med 2007;41(6):e4.
[12] McMaster WC. A literary review on ice therapy in injuries. Am J Sports Med 1977;5(3):124–6.
[13] Knight KL. A re-examination of Lewis' cold-induced vasodiltation in the finger and ankle. J Athl Train 1980;15: 238–50.
[14] Knight KL. Cryotherapy in sport injury management. Champaign, Illinois: Human Kinetics; 1995.
[15] Ravindhran B, Rajan S, Balachandran G, et al. Do ice packs reduce postoperative midline incision pain, NSAID or narcotic use? World J Surg 2019;43(11):2651–7.
[16] Algafly AA, George KP. The effect of cryotherapy on nerve conduction velocity, pain threshold and pain tolerance. Br J Sports Med 2007;41(6):365–9.
[17] Barbosa GM, Cunha JE, Cunha TM, et al. Clinical-like cryotherapy improves footprint patterns and reduces synovial inflammation in a rat model of post-traumatic knee osteoarthritis. Sci Rep 2019;9(1):14518.
[18] Guillot X, Tordi N, Mourot L, et al. Cryotherapy in inflammatory rheumatic diseases: a systematic review. Expert Rev Clin Immunol 2014;10(2):281–94.
[19] Ihsan M, Watson G, Abbiss CR. What are the physiological mechanisms for post-exercise cold water immersion in the recovery from prolonged endurance and intermittent exercise? Sports Med 2016;46(8):1095–109.
[20] Peres D, Sagawa Y Jr, Dugué B, et al. The practice of physical activity and cryotherapy in rheumatoid arthritis: systematic review. Eur J Phys Rehabil Med 2017;53(5): 775–87.
[21] Greene MA, Loeser RF. Aging-related inflammation in osteoarthritis. Osteoarthritis Cartilage 2015;23(11): 1966–71.
[22] Quinlan P, Davis J, Fields K, et al. Effects of localized cold therapy on pain in postoperative spinal fusion patients: a randomized control trial. Orthop Nurs 2017; 36(5):344–9.
[23] Yu SY, Chen S, Yan HD, et al. Effect of cryotherapy after elbow arthrolysis: a prospective, single-blinded, randomized controlled study. Arch Phys Med Rehabil 2015; 96(1):1–6.
[24] Piana LE, Garvey KD, Burns H, et al. The cold, hard facts of cryotherapy in orthopedics. Am J Orthop (Belle Mead NJ) 2018;47(9):1–13.
[25] Kirkby Shaw K, Alvarez L, Foster SA, et al. Fundamental principles of rehabilitation and musculoskeletal tissue healing. Vet Surg 2020;49(1):22–32.
[26] Wang H, Olivero W, Wang D, et al. Cold as a therapeutic agent. Acta Neurochir (Wien) 2006;148(5):565–70 [discussion 569–70].
[27] Rexing J, Dunning D, Siegel AM, et al. Effects of cold compression, bandaging, and microcurrent electrical therapy after cranial cruciate ligament repair in dogs. Vet Surg 2010;39(1):54–8.
[28] Millard RP, Towle-Millard HA, Rankin DC, et al. Effect of cold compress application on tissue temperature in healthy dogs. Am J Vet Res 2013;74(3):443–7.
[29] Kieves NR, Bergh MS, Zellner E, et al. Pilot study measuring the effects of bandaging and cold compression therapy following tibial plateau levelling osteotomy. J Small Anim Pract 2016;57(10):543–7.
[30] Davis MS, Marcellin-Little DJ, O'Connor E. Comparison of postexercise cooling methods in working dogs. J Spec Oper Med 2019;19(1):56–60.
[31] Deal DN, Tipton J, Rosencrance E, et al. Ice reduces edema. A study of microvascular permeability in rats. J Bone Joint Surg Am 2002;84(9):1573–8.
[32] Bocobo C, Fast A, Kingery W, et al. The effect of ice on intra-articular temperature in the knee of the dog. Am J Phys Med Rehabil 1991;70(4):181–5.
[33] Sasaki R, Sakamoto J, Kondo Y, et al. Effects of cryotherapy applied at different temperatures on inflammatory pain during the acute phase of arthritis in rats. Phys Ther 2020. https://doi.org/10.1093/ptj/pzaa211.
[34] Ho SS, Coel MN, Kagawa R, et al. The effects of ice on blood flow and bone metabolism in knees. Am J Sports Med 1994;22(4):537–40.
[35] Halar EM, DeLisa JA, Brozovich FV. Nerve conduction velocity: relationship of skin, subcutaneous and intramuscular temperatures. Arch Phys Med Rehabil 1980;61(5): 199–203.
[36] Kwiecien SY, McHugh MP. The cold truth: the role of cryotherapy in the treatment of injury and recovery from exercise. Eur J Appl Physiol 2021. https://doi.org/10.1007/s00421-021-04683-8.
[37] Malanga GA, Yan N, Stark J. Mechanisms and efficacy of heat and cold therapies for musculoskeletal injury. Postgrad Med 2015;127(1):57–65.
[38] Nadler SF, Weingand K, Kruse RJ. The physiologic basis and clinical applications of cryotherapy and thermotherapy for the pain practitioner. Pain Physician 2004;7(3): 395–9.
[39] Haslerud S, Naterstad IF, Bjordal JM, et al. Achilles tendon penetration for continuous 810 nm and super-pulsed 904 nm lasers before and after ice application: an in situ study on healthy young adults. Photomed Laser Surg 2017;35(10):567–75.
[40] Akgun K, Korpinar MA, Kalkan MT, et al. Temperature changes in superficial and deep tissue layers with respect to time of cold gel pack application in dogs. Yonsei Med J 2004;45(4):711–8.
[41] Merrick MA, Knight KL, Ingersoll CD, et al. The effects of ice and compression wraps on intramuscular temperatures at various depths. *J Athl Trainl* 1993;28(3):236–45.
[42] Merrick MA, Jutte LS, Smith ME. Cold modalities with different thermodynamic properties produce different surface and intramuscular temperatures. J Athl Train 2003;38(1):28–33.

[43] Speer KP, Warren RF, Horowitz L. The efficacy of cryotherapy in the postoperative shoulder. J Shoulder Elbow Surg 1996;5(1):62–8.
[44] Konrath GA, Lock T, Goitz HT, et al. The use of cold therapy after anterior cruciate ligament reconstruction. A prospective, randomized study and literature review. Am J Sports Med 1996;24(5):629–33.
[45] Weresh MJ, Bennett GL, Njus G. Analysis of cryotherapy penetration: a comparison of the plaster cast, synthetic cast, Ace wrap dressing, and Robert-Jones dressing. Foot Ankle Int 1996;17(1):37–40.
[46] Metzman L, Gamble JG, Rinsky LA. Effectiveness of ice packs in reducing skin temperature under casts. Clin Orthop Relat Res 1996;330:217–21.

Advances in Small Animal Care 2 (2021) 19–30
ADVANCES IN SMALL ANIMAL CARE

Manual Therapy in Small Animal Rehabilitation

Matthew Brunke, DVM, CCRP, CVPP, CVA, CCMT, DACVSMR[a,*],
Michele Broadhurst, DC, CCSP, FIAMA, CCRP, CAC IVCA[b],
Kirsten Oliver, VN, DipAVN(surgical), RVT, CCRP, CVPP, VTS(physical rehabilitation)[a],
David Levine, PT, PhD, DPT, CCRP, FAPTA[c]
[a]Veterinary Surgical Centers Rehabilitation, Vienna, VA, USA; [b]Wellness 4 All Chiropractic Centre, Bloomfield, CO, USA; [c]Department of Physical Therapy, The University of Tennessee at Chattanooga, Chattanooga, TN, USA

KEYWORDS

• Manual therapy • Dog • Joint mobilization • Massage • Soft tissue mobilization • Veterinary rehabilitation • Dry needling • Maitland

KEY POINTS

- Soft-tissue mobilization focuses on massage and myofascial trigger point therapy to provide pain mitigation and improve comfortable range of motion.
- Joint mobilization focuses on the interaction of the physiologic and accessory movements in a joint, providing pain relief and improving range of motion.
- Once either treatment is used, it is critical to then initiate a therapeutic exercise program to improve coordination and strength.

INTRODUCTION

Manual therapy is used in the rehabilitation process for patient assessment and treatment. Manual therapy techniques include soft-tissue mobilization (STM), focusing on soft tissues such as muscle and fascia, and joint mobilization. The goals of manual techniques are commonly to reduce pain, increase joint motion, improve lymphatic return, and improve function. While the use of manual techniques is common, evidence to support its use is lacking in veterinary medicine. This article reviews soft-tissue and joint mobilization, with a focus on its applications in small animal practice.

Soft-tissue mobilization

STM is a form of manual therapy in which techniques are applied by the hands to tissues such as muscles, fascia, ligaments, tendons, joint capsules, and bursas [1–5]. STM can also be performed with instruments, which is termed instrument-assisted soft-tissue mobilization (IASTM) [6,7]. STM and IASTM can be used to increase range of motion (ROM) in joints [8,9], increase blood supply [10,11], increase lymphatic flow [12,13], and reduce pain [14–16].

STM is used to manage skeletal muscle abnormalities including tightness, adaptive shortening, adhesions, edema, pain, and trigger points [17–22]. Normal muscle tissue is soft, pliable, and flexible; it has an elastic quality. Underlying structures should easily be palpable through the muscles with no pain or tenderness on palpation. Taut muscle bands may feel ropey or cord-like that can vary in size from thin strings to thick bands. These tight, contracted muscles often feel painful or tender on palpation, the muscle itself is less elastic and supple, and, in

*Corresponding author, *E-mail address:* drmattbrunke@gmail.com

https://doi.org/10.1016/j.yasa.2021.07.008
2666-450X/21/ © 2021 Elsevier Inc. All rights reserved.

severe cases, one may be unable to palpate underlying structures [23–27].

Trigger points found in muscle can be defined as a hyperirritable locus within a taut band of skeletal muscle, located in the muscular tissue and/or its associated fascia [28]. Myofascial trigger points (MFTPs) can be located both in muscle and in fascia. Trigger points can form in any muscle of the body; however, certain muscles are more prone to MFTPs because of mechanical strain and overuse. Commonly seen locations for MFTPs in humans include the upper trapezius and levator scapulae [29,30]. A study of MFTPs in 48 dogs reported their most common occurrence in the triceps brachii, infraspinatus, peroneus longus, gluteus medius, iliocostalis lumborum, adductor-pectineus, and quadriceps femoris muscles. Thoracic limb trigger points were often unilateral, while trigger points of the pelvic limb were commonly bilateral [31]. Myofascial dysfunction may be due to an acute or gradual onset, from muscle strain or from long-standing muscle overuse or overload. MFTPs may result in an increase, as a result of nerve sensitization, of the accumulation of cellular metabolites, a decrease in blood flow, and impaired lymphatic drainage [24,27,29,30,32–36]. Referral from MFTPs tends to be away from the affected muscle in specific and predictable pain patterns. In humans, relationships between active MFTPs and their referred pain patterns are well established [17].

Often, the pain associated with MFTPs can result in a referred pain pattern and other signs and symptoms such as visual disturbances, nausea, dizziness, tearing of the eyes, skin temperature changes, tinnitus, and others [29,30,35,37–39]. MFTPs can be active or latent, both leading to tightness through the muscle, pain and tenderness on palpation, and a resultant muscle weakness. Active MFTPs are spontaneously painful and can refer pain at any time, while latent MFTPs are only painful and refer pain when stimulated, for example, with digital pressure [17,29,35,37,38].

MFTPs can be visualized by magnetic resonance imaging and sonographic elastography [23,32,40–42], which has shown that active MFTPs are commonly larger than latent MFTPs and feature a reduction in blood flow [32]. MFTPs are physiologic contractures, characterized by local ischemia and hypoxia [32,43], a significantly lower pH (active MFTPs only), a chemically altered milieu (active MFTPs only) [25,36,44], local and referred pain [35,37,38], and altered muscle activation patterns [45,46]. Although latent MFTPs are not spontaneously painful, recent research has shown that they do contribute to nociception; therefore, they are included in patients' treatment plan.

MFTPs are associated with dysfunctional motor endplates [26,47], endplate noise [22], and an increased release of acetylcholine [24,27,48–50]. MFTPs activate muscle nociceptors and are peripheral sources of persistent nociceptive input, thus contributing to the development of peripheral and central sensitization [33,34,51,52]. Stimulation of MFTPs activates the periaqueductal gray matter and anterior singular cortex in the brain [39,53,54] and enkephalinergic, serotonergic, and noradrenergic inhibitory systems associated with A-δ (A delta) fibers through segmental inhibition [55,56].

Fascia

A fundamental understanding of fascia and its role in tissue injury and return to proper function is needed to understand STM. Fascia is part of the connective tissue system that permeates the body, forming a whole-body continuous three-dimensional matrix of structural support [57]. Every muscle fiber and every muscle belly is surrounded by facia, and it penetrates and surrounds all organs, muscles, bones, and nerve fibers and transmits almost 40% of the force of a muscle contraction [58]. Fascial planes are sensory organs that communicates with the CNS [58,59]. Muscle spindle cells that help regulate muscle function are found in fascia [60]. If a fascia is too dense and unable to slide over or within muscle, spindle cells cannot provide normal feedback to the CNS [58]. This can lead to abnormalities in muscle function and eventually to pain and dysfunction [58,59,61]. Fascia evolves into tough, flexible supporting structures such as ligaments and tendons and forms the bursae that reduces friction and allows free movement over joints [59]. Fascia also produces scar tissue after an injury and that helps to stabilize the injured area throughout healing [59,61,62].

Fascia also separates muscles from each other so that they can slide past each other as they contract in different directions. Muscles are covered by specific types of deep fascia, called epimysial or aponeurotic fascia [59,62,63]. In the limbs, a thin layer of epimysial fascia called the epimysium covers the surface of each muscle [64]. It surrounds the entire surface of the muscle belly and separates it from adjoining muscles [64]. It gives form to all the muscles of the limbs [64]. Aponeurotic fascia aids in transmitting the force of the muscles it covers and is innervated predominantly in the superficial layer [58,59,64]. Fascia helps with delivery of fluids, nutrients, and oxygen as well as removal of toxins and waste [60,61]. Electrical impulses flow through it, and it is postulated that the energy or life force known as "chi" in Chinese medicine flows through it as well [65].

Maintenance and repair of fascia is adversely affected by poor or unbalanced nutrition [58]. Chronic pain or stress impacts the fascia by causing constant tension in the muscles, resulting in a reduction in blood flow, causing the fascia to become stiff and dry [57,63,64,66,67]. When fascia is inflamed, an inflammatory response changes it from a soft, pliable gel to a stiff solid material, changing its electrical conductivity. Changes in fascial pliability impact the animal's ability to ambulate and result in compensations and biomechanical changes [59]. Stiffened fascia leads to poor posture and abnormal or dysfunctional biomechanics as well as lowered strength and endurance [59]. With an inefficient or painful nervous system, this leads to reactive or unusual behavior [64]. As a natural part of healing, scar tissue forms at the site of damage and then remodels and subsides during the repair process [58,60]. Poor circulation, lack of movement, inadequate nutrition, and other factors do not allow the healing process to be completed [58], leaving behind adhesions (ie, tissue planes that are stuck together) and stiffness. Those adhesions are fascial trigger points and have referral pain patterns [64]. Chronic overwork or reinjuring an area can also affect the fascia [66]. If an animal is trained into an aberrant way of standing or moving, worked beyond his/her ability to recover completely, or kept in a constant state of tension, the fascia can be stressed along with overused muscles, tendons, and ligaments [68].

Contraindications and precautions to soft-tissue mobilization

Contraindications and precautions to manual and massage therapy include the presence of an open wound, infection, acute soft-tissue trauma, over or around an area of malignancy, acute gastrointestinal disorders, skin disease, thermoregulatory conditions, and acute nerve or neuralgia [4,5,69].

It is important to also point out that apart from thermal, chemical, and mechanical nociceptors in the skin, there are also four specialized receptors that are triggered during massage (18).

1. Pacini's receptors: found in the dermis and are stimulated with low-frequency vibration and pressure [70].
2. Ruffini's receptors: found in the dermis and are stimulated with skin stretch [70].
3. Merkel's receptors: found in the epidermis and are stimulated with pressure [70].
4. Meissner's receptors: found in the dermis and are stimulated with stroking, light, tactile touch [70].

MASSAGE TECHNIQUES

Effleurage

The term is derived from the French word "effleurer" meaning to touch lightly (Fig. 1). This massage technique is typically used to open and close a massage session. The therapist uses long, unbroken strokes using the thenar eminence of hand which conforms to the surface of the underlying tissue being treated. Application of this technique follows the direction of tissue fibers. This technique is a gentle, easy introduction for the patient to get used to touch and can aide in relaxation. Effleurage improves blood flow and decreases venous stasis [23,42].

Petrissage

The term is derived from the French word "petrir" meaning to knead (Fig. 2). This technique involves lifting the tissue away from the underlying structures with the intention of improving tissue elasticity and stimulating local lymph and blood circulation. Techniques include kneading, skin rolling, and gentle wringing of the tissue. Petrissage can stimulate deeper tissue fibers and decrease the tone in superficial tissues [23,41,71].

Tapotement

The term is derived from the French word "tapoter" meaning to tap (Fig. 3). This technique uses the rhythmic percussion of tissue using a cupped hand, fingertips, or the hypothenar eminence (lateral aspect) of the hand. It is used to stimulate sensory endings, stimulating muscle tone, and aide in the removal of waste products and congestion (eg, coupage) [23,71].

Cross-friction

Cross-friction or deep tissue massage has been used in human soft-tissue injuries extensively and was developed in an empirical way by James Cyriax, a British physician [72] (Fig. 4). The purpose of cross-friction

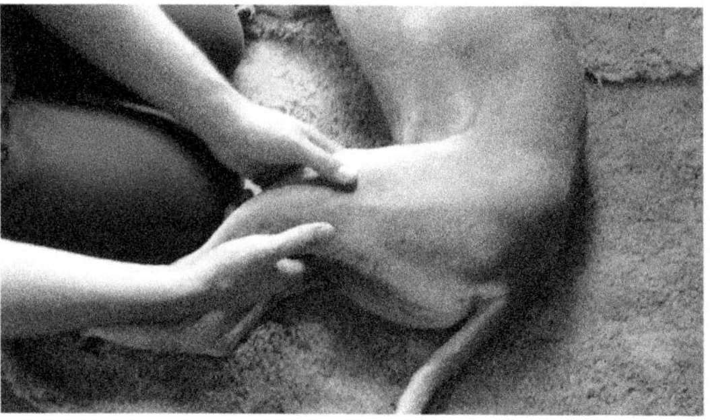

FIG. 1 Effleurage massage technique.

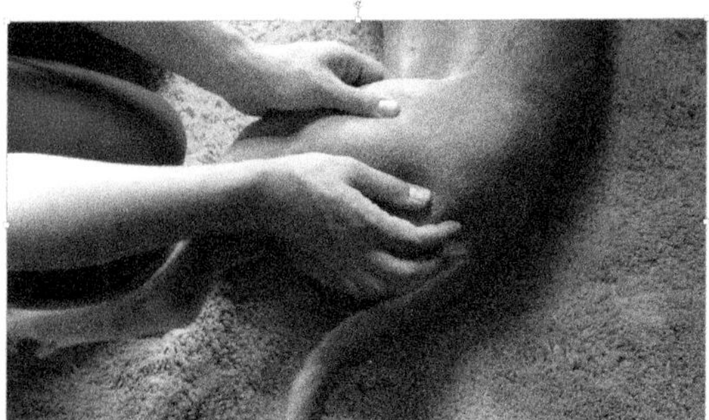

FIG. 2 Petrissage massage technique.

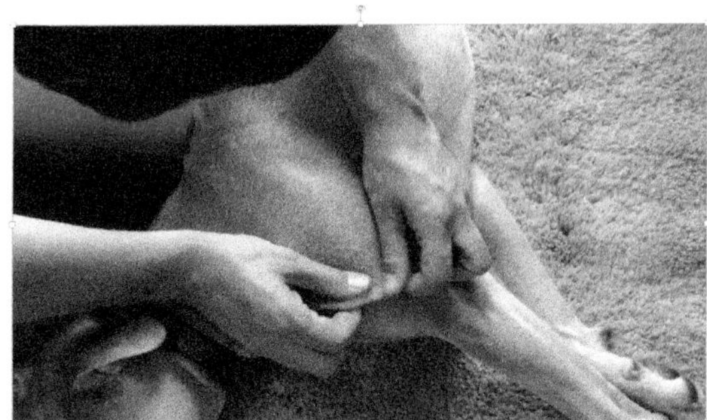

FIG. 4 Vibration/friction massage technique.

massage is to maintain the mobility of the involved soft-tissue structure and prevent adhesions from forming [72]. The principle is fairly simple — when there is inflammation in the soft tissues, there is a disruption of the direction of the fibers. Normally, all muscle and tendon fibers are parallel to each other. With inflammation, the fibers lie in disarray, and proper functioning of the soft tissue is impossible unless they are realigned. The application of a sweeping manual force perpendicular to the fibers will assist in the realignment of the fibers [72]. This motion is applied to the tendon or muscle, and the soft-tissue slack of the skin must be overcome. The sweeping motion is applied for a total of 5 minutes in acute phases [72]. The goals of this treatment are to provide movement to tissue itself and to improve blood supply to the area [72].

Myofascial release

This manual technique is used for treating primary muscle immobility and discomfort by the relaxation of tight muscles [17,27,47,73], thereby improving blood, oxygen, and lymphatic circulation and stimulating the stretch reflex within the muscle [73]. Techniques used involve the application of a sustained gentle pressure on the tissue to improve range of motion and reduce pain [17,27,73]. A sustained low load or gentle pressure will allow the fascia to slowly elongate and effectively "unwind" [19,74].

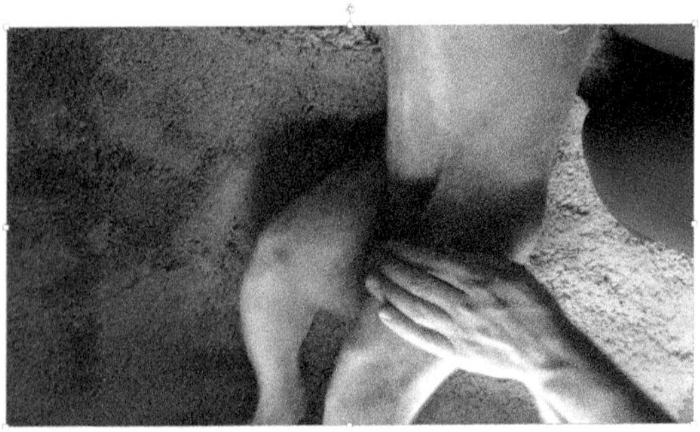

FIG. 3 Tapotement massage technique.

Ischemic compression

This technique requires the use of the fingers or the flat of the hand or palm placed over a larger area of hyperactivity using a moderate to deep amount of pressure sustained over 60–90 seconds [75]. This technique may restore blood flow, decrease muscle tension and pain, and promote healing [75].

Passive, active range of motion and stretching

Range of motion is often performed in the acute phase of healing after soft-tissue injury [76,77]. Range of motion should be applied slowly and deliberately to the affected joint and the joint above and below the affected joint if possible. For example, if a dog is suffering from bicipital tendonitis, range of motion should be performed to the shoulder, elbow, and carpus in a flexion and extension movement.

ADDITIONAL MANUAL TECHNIQUES

IASTM uses specifically designed instruments, with edges and angles, to effectively detect and treat myofascial restrictions [78,79]. Scar tissue and adhesions can limit range of motion leading to a negative input on sensory motor firing rate [78]. This perpetuates the dysfunctional cycle of the CNS, pain, and decreased movement [78]. IASTM effectively aides in the reduction of these cycles and thus improves tissue healing, improving tissue pliability and elasticity [78,79]. Care, caution, and training should be employed when using IASTM because "over energetic" use may cause pain, bruising, and tissue trauma [78,79]. An excellent understanding of muscle anatomy and biomechanics is required to prevent patient injury. The target tissue for this treatment is the fibroblasts which synthesize, organize, and remodel collagen. Appropriate tools may alleviate the repetitive stress and strain on the therapist [79]. The angles and surfaces of the different tools provide a variety of treatment options, thus allowing the therapist to easily move from parallel to perpendicular planes of treatment [78,79]. Duration of treatment must be guided by the patient's comfort and tolerance, but typically an area may be treated for 90 seconds to 4 minutes [78,79].

Dry needling

Dry needling can be defined as a skilled intervention that uses a thin, solid filament needle to penetrate the skin and stimulate underlying MFTPs for the treatment of myofascial pain and muscle dysfunction [17,33]. The American Physical Therapy Association defines dry needling as an invasive technique used by physical therapists (and other practitioners, where allowed by state or country laws) to treat myofascial pain that uses a dry needle, without medication or injection, which is inserted into areas of the muscle known as trigger points [80].

There is some evidence that excessive muscle tension, as seen, for example, in spasticity, can be alleviated with dry needling [74,81]. Scar tissue has been linked to myofascial pain [82] and fibroblasts [83,84]. Fibroblasts are specialized contractile cells within the fascia that are of particular interest, as they synthesize, organize, and remodel collagen, dependent on the tension between the extracellular matrix and the cell [66,85]. Dry needling, especially when used in combination with stimulation of the needle, can place fibroblasts in a high-tension matrix, at which point the fibroblast changes shape and assumes a lamellar shape and increases its collagen synthesis and cell proliferation [86,87]. Dry needling has been shown to directly activate fibroblasts through mechanical manipulation of the needle [56,88,89], which in turn activates the release of cytokines and other proinflammatory mediators [54,90–93]. Dry needling can play a substantial role in the process of mechanotransduction, which is described as the process by which the body converts mechanical loading into cellular responses [20,39,49,94–97]. Fibroblast activation with a solid filament has been shown to result in pain neuromodulation [55,90].

Some similarities exist between dry needling and the Traditional Chinese Medicine (TCM) style of acupuncture. Acupuncture is based on meridians, the movement of qi optimally in the body and the Jing-Luo system. It consists of many complex channels and focuses on transporting qi, nourishing the body, coordinating the Zang-Fu organs [66], and connecting the whole body, as well as preventing the invasion of pathogens and resisting illness and disease [65].

Tui-na

Tui-na, from the Chinese "tui" meaning to push and "na" meaning to lift or squeeze. This technique is based on TCM principles to bring balance to the body by improving the body's defensive life force, or Wei-Qi. Tui-na uses specific manipulation systems such as "Bai-dong-fa" (swinging), "Mo-ca-fa" (friction), "Ji-ya-fa" (squeezing), "Zhen-dong-fa" (trembling), and "Kou-ji-fa" (percussion), performed on or around acupuncture points, along the body meridians, or in qi pathways [98].

Joint mobilization

Manual therapy techniques are skilled hand movements intended to improve tissue extensibility; increase ROM; induce relaxation; mobilize or manipulate soft tissue and joints; modulate pain; and reduce soft-tissue swelling, inflammation, or restriction [2]. Mobilizations are passive movements that are oscillatory or sustained stretch performed in such a manner that the patient can prevent the motion if so desired. These motions are performed anywhere within the available range of motion. Maitland techniques have been described in both the human and veterinary literature [2,99,100]. Those techniques will be discussed here, but for in depth details, other sources are recommended. The goal of this article is to briefly review those techniques and provide recent evidence-based medicine to advocate for their use within the scope of veterinary physical rehabilitation.

Mobilizations can be applied in dogs to vertebral and appendicular joints [2,69]. Studies in human literature often looked at them as an addition to traditional therapies (exercise, rest, placebo, or pharmaceutical intervention) [99,101,102]. In those studies, manual therapy has often been found to be superior to traditional techniques. Research parameters have included subjective and objective outcomes measures (pain scores, goniometric measurements, functional scales, and so forth). Joint mobilizations have been used in equine patients for a variety of conditions, including coffin joint disorders and spinal pain [103].

REVIEW OF JOINT MOBILIZATIONS

Joint mobilizations are performed in a loose-packed position, always on an awake patient. The loose-packed position is defined as the position of a joint in which the joint surfaces are not congruent and the joint capsule is lax [104]. For orientation, the practitioner's hands are placed on either side of the joint. The hand on the proximal side of the joint does *not* move (stabilizing hand), and the hand on the distal side of the joint performs the motion (mobilizing hand). They are typically done for 15 to 30 seconds and then followed either with stretching or some form (passive or active, open chain or closed chain) exercise [2].

These techniques include both physiologic and accessory motions. Physiologic motions are the normal, active motion that is available at a joint. Examples of physiologic motion include internal rotation, abduction, flexion, and extension. Accessory motions are those movements that cannot be performed actively. These include rotations, spins, glides, and rolls.

Mobilizations are dependent on the joint anatomy. There are two orientations described: concave-on-convex and convex-on-concave. With concave-on-convex movement, the articular surfaces move in the *same* direction of the shaft of the bone [69]. An example of this is when the distal radius is moved on the stationary carpal bones, the concave surface of the radius rolls and slides on the convex proximal row of carpal bones. Conversely, the convex-on-concave motions are those in which the articular surface moves in the *opposite* direction of the shaft of the bone. When the shoulder joint is flexed in a dog by moving the humerus, the convex surface of the humerus is slides and spins on the concave glenoid of the scapula.

Joint End Feels

Table 1 describes common end feels in joint mobilization. The end feel is evaluated during passive range of motion and is the feeling perceived by the practitioner at the very end of the available ROM. What is felt at the end of range of motion is the "end feel." The end feel can provide valuable information about joint pathologies [69].

Maitland mobilizations are graded on a scale of I-IV and are determined by their movement in the joint with regard to resistance. Refer to Fig. 5 for a visualization of these parameters. In these cases, R1 represents the initial point at which resistance is noted in the joint, and R2 the resistance at the end of available range of motion. Grade I mobilizations are small-amplitude movements performed in pain-free range of motion. These are done at a rate of 3 to 4 oscillations per second while working in the *opposite* direction of painful movement. They are typically performed for 15 to 30 seconds. For example, for pain with extension, perform grade I into flexion. Grade II mobilizations are large-amplitude movements performed in a pain-free range approaching R1 but should not cause pain. They are also done at a rate of 3 to 4 oscillations per second, working in a direction *opposite* to painful movement. For example, for pain with flexion, perform grade II into extension. Grade III mobilizations are large-amplitude movements that occur at 50% of the distance between R1 and R2 near the end of range of restricted motion (bumping R2). While they are done at 3 to 4 oscillations per second, the practitioner should be aware that they may cause slight discomfort for patient. Finally, grade IV mobilizations are small-amplitude movements that occur at 50% of the distance between R1 and R2, near the end of range of motion, at 3 to 4 oscillations per second. As a general rule, if pain is being treated and physiologic mobilization grades I and II cause pain, then accessory grades I and II should be performed. Additionally, if 50% of physiologic active ROM is not available secondary to pain, then the use of accessory grades I and II to treat pain (50/50 rule) is recommended [69].

Contraindications to joint mobilizations include, but are not limited to, spinal instability, bacterial infection, malignancy, systemic localized infections, sutures, recent fracture, cellulitis, fever, hematoma, open wound at treatment site, osteomyelitis, inappropriate end feel, constant severe pain, pain unrelieved by rest, and severe irritability [104].

Recent research updates

The relief of pain is an important component in manual therapy. Recent research by Salgado and colleagues showed that 40 oscillations per minute alleviated knee pain in an experimental model of murine complex regional pain syndrome type I. This is a chronic painful condition that frequently develops after a deep tissue injury, such as a fracture or sprain, without nerve injury. Treated animals received a total of 9 minutes of MT divided into 3 series of 3 minutes each with a 30-second interval between series. A limitation to this study is that the mice had to be sedated for the treatment, which is not recommended in human or veterinary clinical practice [105].

Clayton and colleagues showed in horses that the use of dynamic cervical flexion exercises increased the range of motion of the neck when compared to those same angulations in a neutral standing position. These exercises can be taught to the horse via a rehabilitation program and can be actively done to improve range of motion in the animal [106].

A systematic review on carpal tunnel syndrome showed that in each study where joint mobilization was used, positive effects in pain, function, or additional

TABLE 1
Joint end feels

Name	Description	Example
Bony or hard	Bone approximates bone, resulting in an abrupt, hard stop.	Loss of elbow flexion with end-stage elbow arthritis
Soft-tissue approximation	Motion is stopped by compression of soft tissues. Abnormal if occurs too early in the range due to edema.	Normal stifle flexion
Capsular or firm	A firm but slightly yielding stop occurs due to tension in joint capsule or ligaments. Abnormal if occurs too early in the ROM.	Normal carpal extension
Springy block	A rebound is felt at the limit of motion – motion stops and then rebounds. Abnormal may indicate joint effusion or a joint mouse	Entrapped, torn medial meniscus
Empty	No end point is felt because the patient stops the motion due to pain; no resistance felt. Abnormal indicates presence of sharp pain	Always abnormal, sciatic nerve entrapment as a result of a migrating pin

From Saunders DG, Walker JR, and Levine D. Chapter 26: Joint Mobilization. In: Millis D, Levine D, eds. Canine Rehabilitation and Physical Therapy. 2nd ed. Elsevier; 2014: 447-463.

outcomes were noted. In most cases, the intervention group integrating joint mobilization performed better than the comparison group not receiving joint techniques. It is important to note that this review did not identify any studies where joint mobilizations were used as the sole therapy [102].

Romanowski and colleagues [107] looked at mobilizations for knees in human patients with rheumatoid arthritis, compared to exercise. After intervention, the manual therapy group showed a significantly greater reduction in the visual analog scale than the control group. However, there were no significant differences in the Knee Society Score and Oxford Knee Score between the groups.

Two recent studies both looked at the ankle joint using the Mulligan technique (mobilization with movement, MWM). Meyer and colleagues showed that, in patients with a history of ankle sprain and decreased dorsiflexion of the ankle, MWM significantly improved the dorsiflexion range of motion (DFROM) in the ankle and indicated that after 2 sets of MWMs, no further improvements were identified [108].

Another ankle study compared Maitland techniques by a practitioner to self-mobilization with Mulligan concept [99]. Study subjects received either Maitland grade III anterior-to-posterior talocrural joint mobilizations or weight-bearing lunge Self-Mob. Each intervention consisted of four 2-minute sets, with a 1-minute rest between sets. Dynamic balance, isometric strength, and perceived function significantly improved in both groups after the intervention. The DFROM significantly improved in the Self-Mob group. While self-mobilization is not possible in veterinary rehabilitation, similar techniques could be achieved through an owner-guided home exercise program.

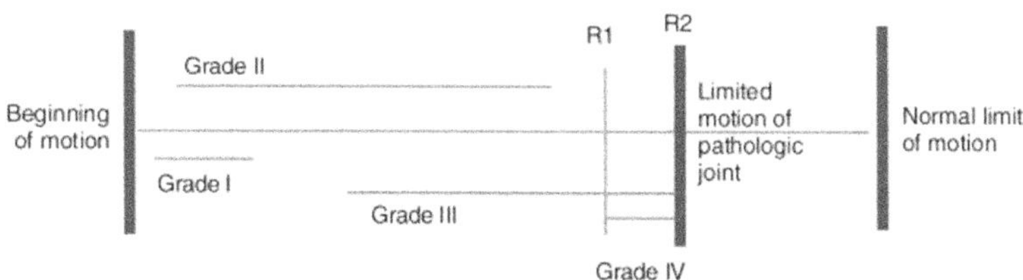

FIG. 5 Maitland mobilizations. (*From* Saunders DG, Walker JR, and Levine D. Chapter 26: Joint Mobilization. In: Millis D, Levine D, eds. Canine Rehabilitation and Physical Therapy. 2nd ed. Elsevier; 2014: 447-463.)

Joint mobilizations have been studied extensively in the literature for the glenohumeral joint and talocrural joint (ankle). Consequently, joint mobilizations have been established as an effective means of improving ROM within these joints. However, there is a lack of extant research to suggest these effects may apply within another critical joint in the body, the hip. When using a mobilization belt and observing functional outcomes, a prospective study found improvement in multiple planes of motion for the hip joint [101]. In another recent study looking at the hip, range of motion was shown to increase in cadavers after joint mobilizations. The improvements in hip ROM appear to be related to the changes in the strain on capsular-ligament tissue after high-force long-axis distraction mobilization [109].

SUMMARY

Manual therapy is one component in the recovery process but provides a variety of methods to assist the patient. Through the reduction of pain and improvement in joint motion, progression to weight-bearing and strengthening can then commence. While further research is always needed, the fundamental principles of manual therapy do provide a benefit in the animal rehabilitation process.

CLINICS CARE POINTS

1. Soft-tissue mobilization
   a. The indication for massage is muscle tension secondary to spinal and joint disease.
   b. By increasing blood flow in the treated area, massage not only increases the elasticity of tendons and ligaments but also improves joint and muscle function.
   c. Early massage therapy after trauma and/or surgery helps prevent or improve congestion in the affected area and prevents adhesions.
   d. In neurologic patients with paresis and paralysis, massage is used to improve muscle tone and sensory awareness.
   e. Mainly in sports medicine but also in therapeutic indications, massage is used to prepare the muscles and connective tissues for training; in the cool-down phase after training, massage accelerates muscle recovery.
2. Joint mobilization – Relationship between pain and stiffness
   a. Grades I-II: for joints with pain dominance
   b. Grades III-IV: for joints with dominant hypomobility and limited pain
   c. If pain is being treated and physiologic mobilization grades I and II cause pain
      i. Accessory grades I and II should be performed
   d. If 50% of physiologic active ROM is not available secondary to pain
      i. Use accessory grades I and II to treat pain (50/50 rule)
   e. When treating stiffness, a grade III or IV accessory motion is commonly followed by either a grade III or IV physiologic mobilization, or sometimes by sustained stretching.
   f. Sixty seconds of an accessory motion, for example, would be followed by 60 seconds of physiologic mobilization (or by a 20- to 30-second stretch 2–3 times).
   g. Sustained stretch versus grade III-IV oscillations. Either of these may be used to help increase range of motion. Some animals will prefer one over another, and this gives the clinician some options.

DISCLOSURE

The authors state that they have nothing to disclose.

REFERENCES

[1] Hughes GA, Ramer LM. duration of myofascial rolling for optimal recovery, range of motion, and performance: a systematic review of the literature. Int J Sports Phys Ther 2019;14:845–59.

[2] Saunders DG, Walker JR, Levine D. Joint mobilization. Vet Clin North Am Small Anim Pract 2005;35: 1287–316, vii–viii.

[3] Kalichman L, Ben David C. Effect of self-myofascial release on myofascial pain, muscle flexibility, and strength: a narrative review. J Bodyw Mov Ther 2017; 21:446–51.

[4] Formenton MR, Pereira MAA, Fantoni DT. Small animal massage therapy: a brief review and relevant observations. Top Companion Anim Med 2017;32:139–45.

[5] Corti L. Massage therapy for dogs and cats. Top Companion Anim Med 2014;29:54–7.

[6] Nazari G, Bobos P, MacDermid JC, et al. The effectiveness of instrument-assisted soft tissue mobilization in athletes, participants without extremity or spinal conditions, and individuals with upper extremity, lower extremity, and spinal conditions: a systematic review. Arch Phys Med Rehabil 2019;100:1726–51.

[7] Seffrin CB, Cattano NM, Reed MA, et al. Instrument-assisted soft tissue mobilization: a systematic review and effect-size analysis. J Athl Train 2019;54:808–21.

[8] Sharman MJ, Cresswell AG, Riek S. Proprioceptive neuromuscular facilitation stretching : mechanisms and clinical implications. Sports Med 2006;36:929–39.

[9] Young C, Argáez C. CADTH rapid response reports. *Manual Therapy for chronic non-cancer Back and neck pain: a Review of clinical effectiveness*. Ottawa, ON: Canadian Agency for Drugs and Technologies in Health; 2020.

[10] Chatchawan U, Jarasrungsichol K, Yamauchi J. Immediate effects of self-thai foot massage on skin blood flow, skin temperature, and range of motion of the foot and ankle in type 2 diabetic patients. J Altern Complement Med 2020;26:491–500.

[11] Weerapong P, Hume PA, Kolt GS. The mechanisms of massage and effects on performance, muscle recovery and injury prevention. Sports Med 2005;35:235–56.

[12] Guerero RM, das Neves LMS, Guirro RRJ, et al. Manual lymphatic drainage in blood circulation of upper limb with lymphedema after breast cancer surgery. J Manipulative Physiol Ther 2017;40:246–9.

[13] Zebrowska A, Trybulski R, Roczniok R, et al. Effect of physical methods of lymphatic drainage on postexercise recovery of mixed martial arts athletes. Clin J Sport Med 2019;29:49–56.

[14] Bervoets DC, Luijsterburg PA, Alessie JJ, et al. Massage therapy has short-term benefits for people with common musculoskeletal disorders compared to no treatment: a systematic review. J Physiother 2015;61:106–16.

[15] Furlan AD, Giraldo M, Baskwill A, et al. Massage for low-back pain. Cochrane Database Syst Rev 2015;(9) Cd001929.

[16] Yeun YR. Effectiveness of massage therapy for shoulder pain: a systematic review and meta-analysis. J Phys Ther Sci 2017;29:936–40.

[17] Travell JG, Simons DG. Myofascial pain and dysfunction: the trigger point manual. Baltimore, Maryland: Williams and Wilkins; 1983.

[18] Ajimsha MS, Al-Mudahka NR, Al-Madzhar JA. Effectiveness of myofascial release: systematic review of randomized controlled trials. J Bodyw Mov Ther 2015;19:102–12.

[19] Anandkumar S, Manivasagam M. Effect of fascia dry needling on non-specific thoracic pain - A proposed dry needling grading system. Physiother Theor Pract 2017;33:420–8.

[20] Dommerholt J, Huijbregts P. Myofascial trigger points – pathophysiology and evidence-informed diagnosis and management. Sudbury, Massachusetts: Jones and Bartlett Publishers; 2011.

[21] Kraus-Hansen AE. Trigger points in 48 dogs with myofascial pain syndromes. Vet Surg 1992;21:87.

[22] Kuan TS, Hsieh YL, Chen SM, et al. The myofascial trigger point region: correlation between the degree of irritability and the prevalence of endplate noise. Am J Phys Med Rehabil 2007;86:183–9.

[23] Chen Q, Bensamoun S, Basford JR, et al. Identification and quantification of myofascial taut bands with magnetic resonance elastography. Arch Phys Med Rehabil 2007;88:1658–61.

[24] Hong CZ, Simons DG. Pathophysiologic and electrophysiologic mechanisms of myofascial trigger points. Arch Phys Med Rehabil 1998;79:863–72.

[25] Shah JP, Gilliams EA. Uncovering the biochemical milieu of myofascial trigger points using in vivo microdialysis: an application of muscle pain concepts to myofascial pain syndrome. J Bodyw Mov Ther 2008;12:371–84.

[26] Simons DG, Hong CZ, Simons LS. Endplate potentials are common to midfiber myofacial trigger points. Am J Phys Med Rehabil 2002;81:212–22.

[27] Simons DG. New views of myofascial trigger points: etiology and diagnosis. Arch Phys Med Rehabil 2008;89:157–9.

[28] Travell JG, Simons DG. Myofascial pain and dysfunction: the trigger point manual. Baltimore, Maryland: Williams and Wilkins; 1983.

[29] Alvarez DJ, Rockwell PG. Trigger points: diagnosis and management. Am Fam Physician 2002;65:653–60.

[30] Barbero M, Cescon C, Tettamanti A, et al. Myofascial trigger points and innervation zone locations in upper trapezius muscles. BMC Musculoskelet Disord 2013;14:179.

[31] Janssens LA. Trigger points in 48 dogs with myofascial pain syndromes. Vet Surg 1991;20:274–8.

[32] Ballyns JJ, Shah JP, Hammond J, et al. Objective sonographic measures for characterizing myofascial trigger points associated with cervical pain. J Ultrasound Med 2011;30:1331–40.

[33] Dommerholt J. Dry needling - peripheral and central considerations. J Man Manip Ther 2011;19:223–7.

[34] Fernández-de-las-Peñas C, Cuadrado ML, Arendt-Nielsen L, et al. Myofascial trigger points and sensitization: an updated pain model for tension-type headache. Cephalalgia 2007;27:383–93.

[35] Fernández-de-Las-Peñas C, Ge HY, Alonso-Blanco C, et al. Referred pain areas of active myofascial trigger points in head, neck, and shoulder muscles, in chronic tension type headache. J Bodyw Mov Ther 2010;14:391–6.

[36] Shah JP, Danoff JV, Desai MJ, et al. Biochemicals associated with pain and inflammation are elevated in sites near to and remote from active myofascial trigger points. Arch Phys Med Rehabil 2008;89:16–23.

[37] Fernández-Carnero J, Fernández-de-Las-Peñas C, de la Llave-Rincón AI, et al. Prevalence of and referred pain from myofascial trigger points in the forearm muscles in patients with lateral epicondylalgia. Clin J Pain 2007;23:353–60.

[38] Fernández-de-Las-Peñas C, Ge HY, Arendt-Nielsen L, et al. The local and referred pain from myofascial trigger points in the temporalis muscle contributes to pain

profile in chronic tension-type headache. Clin J Pain 2007;23:786–92.
[39] Niddam DM, Chan RC, Lee SH, et al. Central modulation of pain evoked from myofascial trigger point. Clin J Pain 2007;23:440–8.
[40] Ballyns JJ, Turo D, Otto P, et al. Office-based elastographic technique for quantifying mechanical properties of skeletal muscle. J Ultrasound Med 2012;31:1209–19.
[41] Chen Q, Basford J, An KN. Ability of magnetic resonance elastography to assess taut bands. Clin Biomech (Bristol, Avon) 2008;23:623–9.
[42] Sikdar S, Shah JP, Gebreab T, et al. Novel applications of ultrasound technology to visualize and characterize myofascial trigger points and surrounding soft tissue. Arch Phys Med Rehabil 2009;90:1829–38.
[43] Brückle W, Suckfüll M, Fleckenstein W, et al. [Tissue pO2 measurement in taut back musculature (m. erector spinae)]. Z Rheumatol 1990;49:208–16.
[44] Shah JP, Phillips T, Danoff JV, et al. A novel microanalytical technique for assaying soft tissue demonstrates significant quantitative biomechanical differences in 3 clinically distinct groups: normal, latent and active. Arch Phys Med Rehabil 2003;84:E4.
[45] Lucas KR, Rich PA, Polus BI. Muscle activation patterns in the scapular positioning muscles during loaded scapular plane elevation: the effects of Latent Myofascial Trigger Points. Clin Biomech (Bristol, Avon) 2010;25:765–70.
[46] KR L, BI P, PS R. Latent myofascial trigger points: their effects on muscle activation and movement efficiency. J Bodyw Mov Ther 2004;8:160–6.
[47] Simons DG. Review of enigmatic MTrPs as a common cause of enigmatic musculoskeletal pain and dysfunction. J Electromyogr Kinesiol 2004;14:95–107.
[48] Gerwin RD, Dommerholt J, Shah JP. An expansion of Simons' integrated hypothesis of trigger point formation. Curr Pain Headache Rep 2004;8:468–75.
[49] McPartland JM, Simons DG. Myofascial trigger points: translating molecular theory into manual therapy. J Man Manip Ther 2006;14:232–9.
[50] Bukharaeva EA, Salakhutdinov RI, Vyskocil F, et al. Spontaneous quantal and non-quantal release of acetylcholine at mouse endplate during onset of hypoxia. Physiol Res 2005;54:251–5.
[51] Mense S. How do muscle lesions such as latent and active trigger points influence central nociceptive neurons? J Musculokelet Pain 2010;18:348–53.
[52] Xu YM, Ge HY, Arendt-Nielsen L. Sustained nociceptive mechanical stimulation of latent myofascial trigger point induces central sensitization in healthy subjects. J Pain 2010;11:1348–55.
[53] Niddam DM, Chan RC, Lee SH, et al. Central representation of hyperalgesia from myofascial trigger point. Neuroimage 2008;39:1299–306.
[54] Svensson P, Minoshima S, Beydoun A, et al. Cerebral processing of acute skin and muscle pain in humans. J Neurophysiol 1997;78:450–60.
[55] Langevin HM, Bouffard NA, Badger GJ, et al. Dynamic fibroblast cytoskeletal response to subcutaneous tissue stretch ex vivo and in vivo. Am J Physiol Cell Physiol 2005;288:C747–56.
[56] Langevin HM, Bouffard NA, Badger GJ, et al. Subcutaneous tissue fibroblast cytoskeletal remodeling induced by acupuncture: evidence for a mechanotransduction-based mechanism. J Cell Physiol 2006;207:767–74.
[57] Wilke J, Schleip R, Yucesoy CA, et al. Not merely a protective packing organ? A review of fascia and its force transmission capacity. J Appl Physiol (1985) 2018;124:234–44.
[58] Pavan PG, Stecco A, Stern R, et al. Painful connections: densification versus fibrosis of fascia. Curr Pain Headache Rep 2014;18:441.
[59] Schleip R, Klingler W. Active contractile properties of fascia. Clin Anat 2019;32:891–5.
[60] Stecco C, Macchi V, Porzionato A, et al. The fascia: the forgotten structure. Ital J Anat Embryol 2011;116:127–38.
[61] Willard FH, Vleeming A, Schuenke MD, et al. The thoracolumbar fascia: anatomy, function and clinical considerations. J Anat 2012;221:507–36.
[62] Barrett JG, Hao Z, Graf BK, et al. Inflammatory changes in ruptured canine cranial and human anterior cruciate ligaments. Am J Vet Res 2005;66:2073–80.
[63] Benjamin M. The fascia of the limbs and back–a review. J Anat 2009;214:1–18.
[64] Garfin SR, Tipton CM, Mubarak SJ, et al. Role of fascia in maintenance of muscle tension and pressure. J Appl Physiol Respir Environ Exerc Physiol 1981;51:317–20.
[65] Mayor DFaM. M. S. Energy medicine east and west: a natural history of qi'. Churchill Livingstone Elsevier; 2011.
[66] Findley TW. Fascia research from a clinician/scientist's perspective. Int J Ther Massage Bodywork 2011;4:1–6.
[67] Wilke J, Macchi V, De Caro R, et al. Fascia thickness, aging and flexibility: is there an association? J Anat 2019;234:43–9.
[68] Wright B. Management of chronic soft tissue pain. Top Companion Anim Med 2010;25:26–31.
[69] Levine D, Torraca D, Brunke M. Joint mobilization in canines. In: B B, editor. Essential Facts of physical rehabilitation and sports medicine in companion animals. 1st edition. Babenhausen, Germany: VBS GmbH; 2019. p. 191–202.
[70] Iheanacho F, Vellipuram AR. Physiology, Mechanoreceptors. In: StatPearls. Treasure Island (FL): StatPearls Publishing LLC.; 2020.
[71] Poppendieck W, Wegmann M, Ferrauti A, et al. Massage and performance recovery: a meta-analytical review. Sports Med 2016;46:183–204.
[72] Loew LM, Brosseau L, Tugwell P, et al. Deep transverse friction massage for treating lateral elbow or lateral knee tendinitis. Cochrane Database Syst Rev 2014;11:CD003528.
[73] McKenney K, Elder AS, Elder C, et al. Myofascial release as a treatment for orthopaedic conditions: a systematic review. J Athl Train 2013;48:522–7.

[74] Whisler SL, Lang DM, Armstrong M, et al. Effects of myofascial release and other advanced myofascial therapies on children with cerebral palsy: six case reports. Explore (NY) 2012;8:199–205.

[75] Cagnie B, Castelein B, Pollie F, et al. Evidence for the use of ischemic compression and dry needling in the management of trigger points of the upper trapezius in patients with neck pain: a systematic review. Am J Phys Med Rehabil 2015;94:573–83.

[76] Kirkby Shaw K, Alvarez L, Foster SA, et al. Fundamental principles of rehabilitation and musculoskeletal tissue healing. Vet Surg 2020;49:22–32.

[77] Baltzer WI. Rehabilitation of companion animals following orthopaedic surgery. N Z Vet J 2020;68: 157–67.

[78] Gamboa AJ, Craft DR, Matos JA, et al. functional movement analysis before and after instrument-assisted soft tissue mobilization. Int J Exerc Sci 2019;12:46–56.

[79] Ikeda N, Otsuka S, Kawanishi Y, et al. Effects of instrument-assisted soft tissue mobilization on musculoskeletal properties. Med Sci Sports Exerc 2019;51: 2166–72.

[80] Broadhurst M. A clinicians guide to myofascial pain in the canine patient 2020.

[81] DiLorenzo L, Traballesi M, Morelli D. Hemiparetic shoulder pain syndrome treated with deep dry needling during early rehabilitation: a prospective, open-label, randomized investigation. J Musculoskelet Pain 2004; 12:25–34.

[82] Lewit K, Olsanska S. Clinical importance of active scars: abnormal scars as a cause of myofascial pain. J Manipulative Physiol Ther 2004;27:399–402.

[83] Iqbal SA, Sidgwick GP, Bayat A. Identification of fibrocytes from mesenchymal stem cells in keloid tissue: a potential source of abnormal fibroblasts in keloid scarring. Arch Dermatol Res 2012;304:665–71.

[84] Eto H, Suga H, Aoi N, et al. Therapeutic potential of fibroblast growth factor-2 for hypertrophic scars: upregulation of MMP-1 and HGF expression. Lab Invest 2012;92:214–23.

[85] Grinnell F. Fibroblast biology in three-dimensional collagen matrices. Trends Cell Biol 2003;13:264–9.

[86] Hicks MR, Cao TV, Campbell DH, et al. Mechanical strain applied to human fibroblasts differentially regulates skeletal myoblast differentiation. J Appl Physiol (1985) 2012;113:465–72.

[87] Langevin HM, Bouffard NA, Fox JR, et al. Fibroblast cytoskeletal remodeling contributes to connective tissue tension. J Cell Physiol 2011;226:1166–75.

[88] Fu ZH, Wang JH, Sun JH, et al. Fu's subcutaneous needling: possible clinical evidence of the subcutaneous connective tissue in acupuncture. J Altern Complement Med 2007;13:47–51.

[89] Fu ZH, Chen XY, Lu LJ, et al. Immediate effect of Fu's subcutaneous needling for low back pain. Chin Med J (Engl) 2006;119:953–6.

[90] Chiquet M, Renedo AS, Huber F, et al. How do fibroblasts translate mechanical signals into changes in extracellular matrix production? Matrix Biol 2003;22: 73–80.

[91] Langevin HM, Storch KN, Snapp RR, et al. Tissue stretch induces nuclear remodeling in connective tissue fibroblasts. Histochem Cell Biol 2010;133:405–15.

[92] Evans HE, De Lahunta A. Miller's anatomy of the dog. 4th edition. St. Louis, Missouri: Elsevier; 2013.

[93] J D, JP S. Myofascial pain syndrome. In: Fishman SM, Ballantyne JC, Rathmell JP, editors. Bonica's pain management. 4th edition. Baltimore, Maryland: Lippincott, Williams & Wilkins; 2010. p. 450–71.

[94] Hägglund M, Waldén M, Bahr R, et al. Methods for epidemiological study of injuries to professional football players: developing the UEFA model. Br J Sports Med 2005;39:340–6.

[95] Mueller-Wohlfahrt HW, Haensel L, Mithoefer K, et al. Terminology and classification of muscle injuries in sport: the Munich consensus statement. Br J Sports Med 2013;47:342–50.

[96] Evans J, Levesque D, Shelton GD. Canine inflammatory myopathies: a clinicopathologic review of 200 cases. J Vet Intern Med 2004;18:679–91.

[97] Shelton GD. Routine and specialized laboratory testing for the diagnosis of neuromuscular diseases in dogs and cats. Vet Clin Pathol 2010;39:278–95.

[98] Wei X, Wang S, Li L, et al. Clinical Evidence of Chinese Massage Therapy (Tui Na) for cervical radiculopathy: a systematic review and meta-analysis. Evid Based Complement Alternat Med 2017;2017:9519285.

[99] Burton CA, Arthur RJ, Rivera MJ, et al. the examination of repeated self-mobilizations with movement and joint mobilizations on individuals with chronic ankle instability. J Sport Rehabil 2020;1–9.

[100] Pennetti A. A multimodal physical therapy approach utilizing the Maitland concept in the management of a patient with cervical and lumbar radiculitis and Ehlers–Danlos syndrome-hypermobility type: a case report. Physiother Theor Pract 2018;34:559–68.

[101] Brun A, Sandrey MA. The effect of hip joint mobilizations using a mobilization belt on hip range of motion and functional outcomes. J Sport Rehabil 2020; 1–9.

[102] Sault JD, Jayaseelan DJ, Mischke JJ, et al. The utilization of joint mobilization as part of a comprehensive program to manage carpal tunnel syndrome: a systematic review. J Manipulative Physiol Ther 2020;43: 356–70.

[103] Haussler KK. Joint mobilization and manipulation for the equine athlete. Vet Clin North Am Equine Pract 2016;32:87–101.

[104] Bogaerts E, Van der Vekens E, Verhoeven G, et al. Intraobserver and interobserver agreement on the radiographical diagnosis of canine cranial cruciate ligament rupture. Vet Rec 2018;182:484.

[105] Salgado ASI, Stramosk J, Ludtke DD, et al. Manual therapy reduces pain behavior and oxidative stress in a murine model of complex regional pain syndrome type I. Brain Sci 2019;9:197.

[106] Clayton HM, Kaiser LJ, Lavagnino M, et al. Dynamic mobilisations in cervical flexion: Effects on intervertebral angulations. Equine Vet J Suppl 2010; 688–94.

[107] Romanowski MW, Špiritović M, Romanowski W, et al. Manual therapy (Postisometric Relaxation and Joint Mobilization) in knee pain and function experienced by patients with rheumatoid arthritis: a randomized clinical pilot study. Evid Based Complement Alternat Med 2020;2020:1452579.

[108] Meyer JE, Rivera MJ, Powden CJ. the evaluation of joint mobilization dosage on ankle range of motion in individuals with decreased dorsiflexion and a history of ankle sprain. J Sport Rehabil 2020;1-6.

[109] Estébanez-de-Miguel E, González-Rueda V, Bueno-Gracia E, et al. The immediate effects of 5-minute high-force long axis distraction mobilization on the strain on the inferior ilio-femoral ligament and hip range of motion: a cadaveric study. Musculoskelet Sci Pract 2020;50:102262.

Advances in Small Animal Care 2 (2021) 31–38
ADVANCES IN SMALL ANIMAL CARE

The Role of Strengthening in the Management of Canine Osteoarthritis

A Review

Marti Drum, DVM, PhD, DACVSMR[a,*], Emily McKay, DPT, CCRP[b], David Levine, PT, PhD, DPT, CCRP, FAPTA[c], Denis J. Marcellin-Little, DEDV[b]

[a]Department of Small Animal Clinical Sciences, University of Tennessee College of Veterinary Medicine, Knoxville, TN, USA; [b]Veterinary Orthopedic Research Laboratory, School of Veterinary Medicine, University of California, Davis, Davis, CA, USA; [c]Department of Physical Therapy, University of Tennessee at Chattanooga, Chattanooga, TN, USA

KEYWORDS

• Exercise • Osteoarthritis • Physical training • Treatment

KEY POINTS

- Prevalence of osteoarthritis is significant and anticipated to continue to increase.
- Osteoarthritis is considered a serious disease because of its significant impact on quality of life.
- Osteoarthritic pain can limit the activity level, causing further loss of strength.
- Exercise plays a key role in the management of osteoarthritis.
- A moderate to large treatment effect is seen with strengthening exercises for osteoarthritis.
- Benefits from strengthening exercise can be seen in the short (3 months) and long (12 months) term after completion of an exercise program, but several weeks to months of exercise are needed for the benefits to become apparent.
- Osteoarthritis may make exercise difficult due to increased sensitivity to pain.
- Patients improve to a greater degree with more supervised exercise sessions (>12) compared with self-directed home therapy programs or intermittent supervised sessions.

INTRODUCTION

Prevalence of canine osteoarthritis (OA) ranges from 20% in dogs older than 1 year up to 80% in dogs older than 8 years [1], whereas the Centers for Disease Control and Prevention estimates 25% of Americans have OA and 80% of people older than 55 years have symptomatic OA [2]. Another parallel between humans and dogs is the high rate of hip and stifle joint OA [3]. Core treatments defined by the Osteoarthritis Research Society International (OARSI) for knee OA include land-based exercise, strength training, weight management, water-based exercise, self-management, and education [4]. Strength training is defined as physical training designed to improve strength and endurance. Strengthening exercises in humans generally include push-pull training, power lifting, explosive dynamic training, and muscular isolation exercises. It can be difficult to impossible to accomplish technically equivalent strengthening exercises in canine patients. However, with some creativity, specialized equipment, and a willing canine patient, strengthening exercises can be successfully performed (Figs. 1 and 2). Although a small

The authors have no conflict to disclose.

*Corresponding author, *E-mail address:* mdrum@utk.edu

https://doi.org/10.1016/j.yasa.2021.07.003
2666-450X/21/ © 2021 Elsevier Inc. All rights reserved.

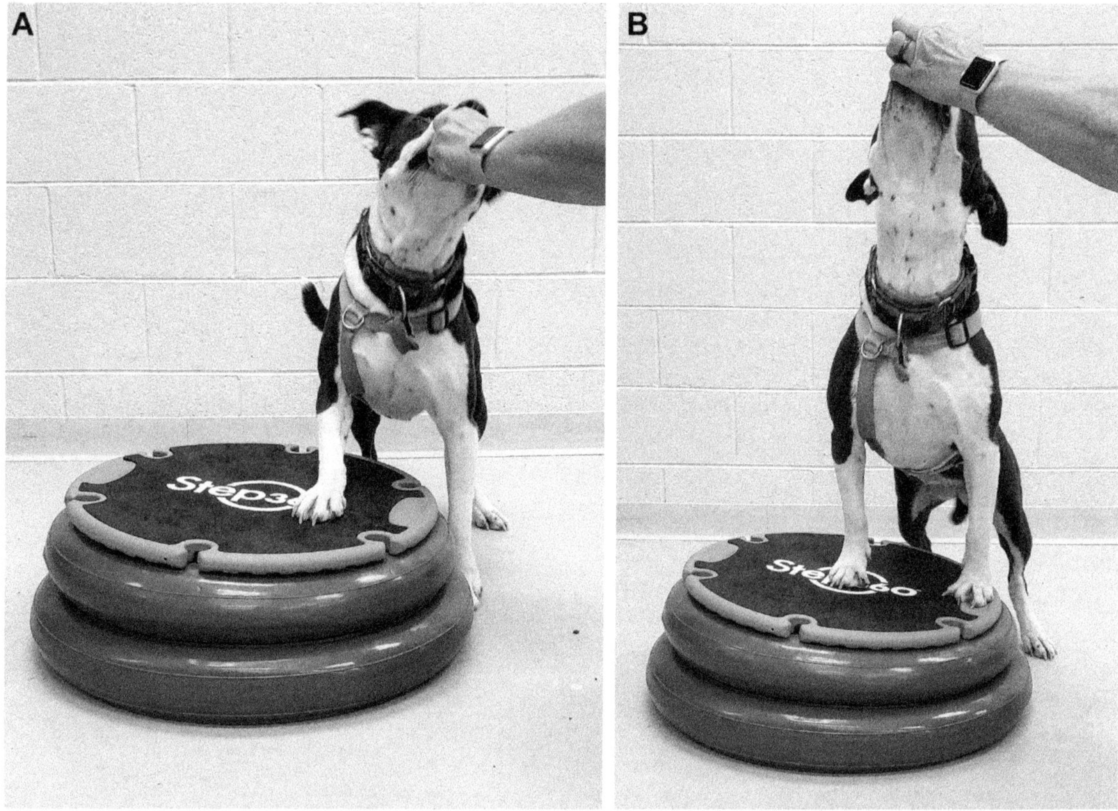

FIG. 1 Exercise equipment is used to strengthen lateral forelimb and shoulder extensor muscles (**A, B**).

number of studies have begun to evaluate muscle activity during selected exercises used for canine strengthening [5–7], no studies have evaluated the effect of strengthening exercises for treatment of canine OA. Spontaneous OA in dogs can be a preclinical model for human OA. Similarly, clinical trials of strength training in humans can be translated to exercise-based treatment of canine OA.

The OARSI considers strength training for treatment of knee OA an appropriate therapy based on a "good-quality" 2011 meta-analysis of lower limb and quadriceps resistance-based exercises [8]. A moderate treatment effect was found on pain control (standardized mean difference [SMD] = 0.38) and functional mobility (SMD = 0.41) in comparison to untreated arthritis controls. It is worthwhile to note that strength programs included both weight-bearing and non-weight-bearing strength exercises performed in a group setting or on an individual basis. Land-based exercises in human knee OA provide short-term pain relief for 2 to 6 months in humans, and the magnitude of treatment effect is similar to nonsteroidal antiinflammatory drugs [9]. Interestingly, within the review greater improvements were noted in studies with a higher number (greater than 12 sessions) of supervised, face-to-face interactions with patients, compared with self-directed home programs or infrequent provider visits.

A Cochrane Review [10] of general exercise to manage OA, including strength exercises, demonstrated a 6% improvement in the Western Ontario and McMaster Universities Osteoarthritis Index (WOMAC) scores for pain and function in the exercise group. Interestingly, before instituting a prescribed exercise program, study subjects believed movement was beneficial for joints but also experienced pain with movement and were concerned the movement may be causing harm. The barrier to exercise can also be greater in these patients with OA due to pain sensitization [11], especially severe knee OA. Thus, patients avoid activity, resulting in further pain and stiffness. Likewise, osteoarthritis in dogs most commonly presents with a chief complaint

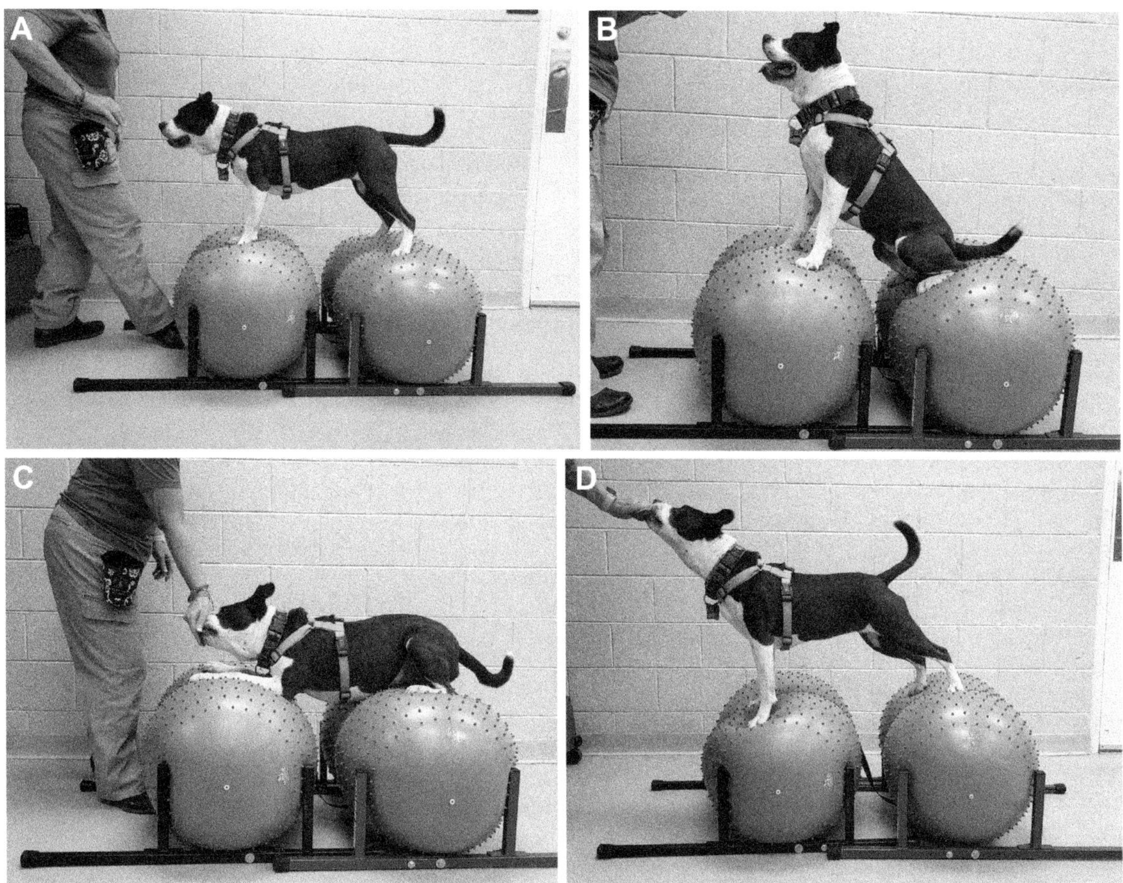

FIG. 2 Canine fitness equipment is used to strengthen hind limb and forelimb muscles using an ordered sequence of exercises (**A–D**).

of lameness, decreased mobility and reluctance to walk [12]. Pet owners frequently eliminate exercise due to lack of knowledge whether exercise is beneficial or detrimental to their dog's lameness. Educating clients regarding modifying exercise, either in duration or type of activity, is a key component of the physical management of canine OA, similar to the reassurance and enjoyable exercise programs used in the management of human OA. Of note from the Cochrane Review is the lengthy duration (35–45 weeks) of the exercise programs before maximum results were observed. There have not been any studies regarding length of exercise program (in weeks) for managing canine OA, but a study evaluating duration of daily exercise and lameness in Labradors with hip dysplasia [13] found that daily exercise for more than 60 minutes was superior to daily exercise for less than 20 minutes, regardless of exercise type. Although it seems logical that chronic diseases require consistent treatment over the long term to yield significant effects, it is imperative that the veterinary team effectively communicate that recommended regular exercises be maintained for several months, or even indefinitely, to maximize improvements in mobility and pain outcomes.

STRENGTH TRAINING AND AEROBIC ACTIVITY IN OSTEOARTHRITIS

Exercise and weight loss are essential pieces in the OA management puzzle. The magnitude of effect exercise contributes to OA management is equivalent to that seen with nonsteroidal anti-inflammatory drug treatment, with fewer adverse events [14]. However, adherence to exercise programs, particularly weight-bearing exercises, is more challenging than dosing of medications for arthritis. A study of OA in Spain [15] evaluated overweight patients participating in an isometric strength training program of the quadriceps and lower limb muscles in combination with non–weight-bearing aerobic (experimental) or loaded aerobic exercise (control). Interestingly, adherence to the load-bearing aerobic control program was much lower (41%) than the non–weight-bearing experimental program (59%), which complicated the interpretation of the significance of the self-reported quality of life improvements noted in the experimental group difficult. It is also worth noting that no differences were noted in the pain, stiffness, and function (WOMAC) score in either group over 6 months. A separate meta-analysis of 3-times-weekly strength training with or without aerobic activity concluded muscle strengthening exercises, with or without aerobic training, were effective for short-term pain control of knee OA [16]. The meta-analysis included 8 studies. A large treatment effect (SMD = −0.94) of exercise on pain scores in knee OA was found. All 8 studies found a significant benefit of exercise versus controls (*P*<.001). Furthermore, non–weight-bearing strength exercise had the largest treatment effect (SMD = −1.42) followed by weight-bearing strength exercise (SMD = −0.71) and aerobic exercise (SMD = −0.45).

RESISTANCE TRAINING IN OSTEOARTHRITIS

Meta-analysis of 8 randomized controlled trials in older adults (mean group age >65 years) found a moderate treatment effect on patients performing lower limb progressive resistance training (PRT) programs [17]. The moderate treatment effect was found for both lower limb strength and pain (SMD = 0.33 and −0.35, respectively). Further, the treatment effect of exercise on strength in older adults without OA was much larger, indicating that weakness is interrelated to OA either by cause, effect, or both. Importantly, treatment effect on function following PRT was greater in the OA group compared with non-OA patients. Examining high-intensity versus low-intensity exercise has demonstrated that both approaches improve pain and function over control groups, and no differences were found between exercise groups [18]. This is an important finding, because it is already challenging to engage dogs in a resistance-based training program, let alone starting geriatric arthritic dogs in a high-resistance training program. Lastly, comparing dynamic versus isometric strength programs using resistance bands also proved to be beneficial for function and pain, relative to control groups [14]. Resistance band strengthening would likely be the most challenging type of exercise to simulate in dogs, except at light resistance band training, as some dogs will refuse to walk or move even with light resistance bands, and most dogs refuse to move when moderate to heavy resistance bands are used. The take-home message of these meta-analyses is that, at least in the short term, there is no single type of strength training program superior to others, as long as the program provides progressive overload. The program intensity should be customized to patient tolerance.

Meta-analysis [19] of studies evaluating resistance training to evaluate intensity of exercises for specific arthritic joint movements have not clearly identified whether low- or high-intensity exercises are superior to specific types of exercises. Within low-intensity exercises, a small treatment effect for knee extension and a moderate treatment effect for knee flexion compared with controls was found in high-quality studies with short-term follow-up. Medium-term studies were of low quality for the same exercises and found no difference between controls. Only a single study of long-term follow-up of low-intensity knee flexion exercises was available. It was considered to be of high-quality data and showed a strong treatment effect. Insufficient studies for meta-analysis of low-intensity strengthening of the hip were available, but a single study [20] of hip abduction and flexion low-intensity exercises did show a short-term benefit in knee load. High-intensity exercise for knee extension strength in OA was favorable in the short term with a moderate effect, whereas knee flexion exercises had a large treatment effect. Intermediate-term data from these studies were of low quality but did report a medium to large effect. Long-term data were not reported.

Although no studies evaluating exercises by category (exercise intensity, aerobic vs resistive, closed vs open chain) have been performed in dogs, a few studies of therapeutic exercises commonly prescribed in dogs have been evaluated [7,21–24]. These selected therapeutic exercises improve hip or knee strength using flexion and/or extension-based activities. However, none of these studies evaluated whether the exercises were effective in diseased states. Sit-to-stand exercises are commonly recommended for hip strengthening due to activation quadriceps and gluteal musculature. Kinematic evaluation of sit-to-stand exercises was used to demonstrate decreased hip extension in dogs during this exercise [6]; This is of particular note since hip movement in canine hip OA has demonstrated decreased hip extension, and sit to stand exercises may inherently reduce stress during hip extension [25,26]. Unfortunately, there have not been any studies that demonstrate improvement in hip extension using

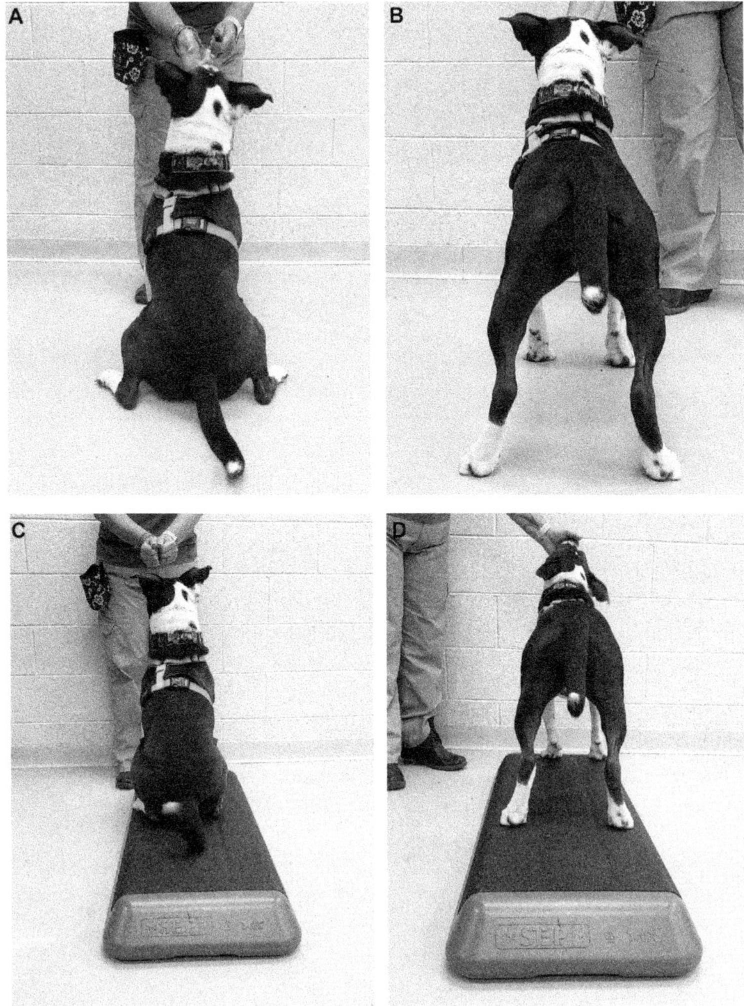

FIG. 3 A dog has poor posture when sitting (**A**) and standing on regular ground (**B**). Posture is improved when an aerobic step is used to encourage proper "tuck sit" posture (**C**) followed by standing (**D**). The standing posture is also improved.

sit-to-stand exercises in dogs with OA. It should be noted that correct form is important during this exercise for proper strengthening of target muscles (Fig. 3).

AQUATIC THERAPY

Research has shown that exercise alone has proved to be effective in preserving independence while slowing the progression of musculoskeletal degeneration [27]. In particular, aquatic physiotherapy has been considered a safe and effective method for treating OA of the knee in humans [27]. In a randomized control trial, 38 participants were assigned to 2 separate groups, aquatic exercise and nonexercise control [28]. The exercise group participated in a 12-week aquatic exercise program with data collected at baseline, 6 weeks, and 12 weeks. Aquatic exercise demonstrated a statistical significance in improving knee and hip flexibility, strength, and aerobic fitness.

Aquatic therapy can include a variety of therapies that occur in water but this article focuses on therapeutic exercise in water. In humans, aquatic exercise is commonly recommended for later stages of OA, as land-based exercise becomes more challenging [29]. In later stages of OA, pain and inefficient muscle control around the joint are encountered, along with joint instability, which can lead to decreased functional ability [29]. There is no single treatment that can improve strength and function while reducing pain, but aquatic exercise has proved to be one of a variety of forms of treatment in helping patients with OA [29]. By incorporating the hydrodynamic principles and prescribing the appropriate amount of loading, aquatic exercise can be a successful treatment option in small animals with OA as well.

Principles of Aquatic Therapy

Buoyancy

Movement in water has been reported to be easier and less painful than on land [28]. The buoyancy of the water allows for increased support of joints and muscles, allowing for people with arthritis to exercise with less effort and increased range of motion. The buoyancy of the water also supports the painful limb to aid in weight-bearing during exercise allowing for increased movement with reduced pain [29]. Loading the leg is different when performing the same functional exercise in water versus on land; load and resistance depend on the depth of the water.

Depth

Load and limb resistance depend on the depth of the water (Fig. 4). Aquatic exercise can be used for muscle strengthening by using the turbulence and depth of the water to your advantage. For instance, exercising in water at the same speed as land will be more difficult because of the amount of resistance the patient has to fight when propelling through the water [29]. Aquatic exercise must be designed with the appropriate training load for the patient in order to achieve desired strength gains [29,30]. Strengthening the muscles surrounding the arthritic joint aids in the reduction of pain. Focusing solely on the reduction of pain without muscle strengthening would do a disservice to the patient. Overall, muscle strengthening leads to increased joint stability, which results in decreased pain.

Hydrostatic pressure

Hydrostatic pressure is the pressure from the water, surrounding the immersed limb. Water pressure around the limb is higher than diastolic pressure, which aids in venous return. This encouragement of venous return helps in reducing swelling/edema, which results in improved range of motion and decreased pain. Furthermore, hydrostatic pressure can provide increased nonnoxious sensory input, resulting in decreased pain sensation [28].

Water temperature

The temperature of the water can decrease pain sensation in addition to promoting relaxation and therefore, decreasing muscle spasms and tightness. Warm water transfers heat to the immersed body part, whereas colder temperatures aid in reducing delayed onset muscle soreness postexercise, speeding up recovery following more strenuous exercise. Aquatic exercise normally occurs in thermoneutral water, allowing for the combination of keeping the limb warm while benefiting from the hydrostatic pressure.

By implementing the hydrodynamic principles used in aquatic exercise for humans, discussed earlier, we can achieve the same benefits in the canine patient.

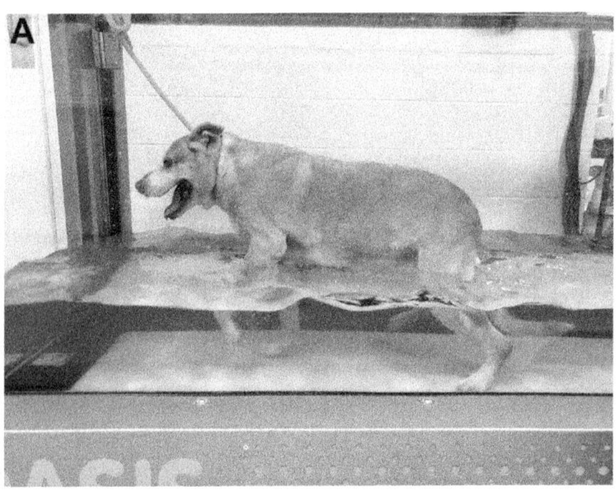

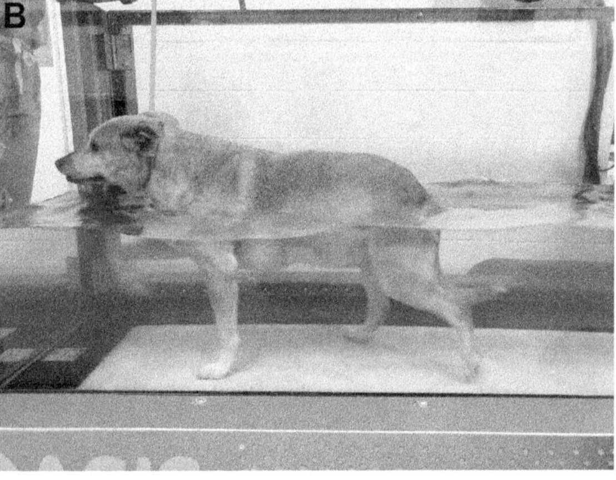

FIG. 4 An arthritic patient is exercised in an underwater treadmill at differing water depths. With insufficient buoyancy (**A**), the topline is sloping. With deeper water (**B**), the dog's posture is correct and comfort increases.

Decreased weight-bearing on joints and bones in a dog with OA allows for increased muscle contractions and reduced pain associated with OA during movement. Water temperature helps reduce muscle spasms, whereas adjusting water depth improves muscle weakness [31]. Using hydrostatic pressure to reduce edema and swelling can also result in decreased pain during exercise. Unloading painful joints during exercise allows for improved range of motion, increased muscular fatigue, and an improvement in endurance.

Research shows aquatic exercise provides benefits in pain, function, and quality of life in people with OA [30]. These benefits of aquatic exercise can transfer to small animals as well [1,31]. Nonsurgical management for dogs diagnosed with OA is centered on improving muscle strength, endurance, cardiac function, and coordination. It is recommended that dogs with OA participate in low-impact exercise, preferably throughout multiple shorter sessions instead of one long treatment session. Aquatic exercise helps achieve these goals in a dog with OA by applying the principles of hydrodynamics, similar to the human patient. Reducing the amount of weight that a dog must support during exercise allows for safe functional movement with a reduction in pain.

SWIMMING VERSUS WALKING

A common question that arises when addressing aquatic exercise for small animals is whether they should walk in an underwater treadmill or swim in an open pool. Besides the same hydrodynamic principles, there are different reasons behind prescribing swimming or walking in water. Swimming promotes the use of all limbs, improving muscle movement patterns [31]. Aquatic treadmill enhances cardiac endurance, improves muscle strength, reduces pain, and improves balance and range of motion [1,31]. Joint flexion in the canine is increased in both underwater treadmill walking and swimming compared with walking on ground; however, close to normal joint extension is observed walking in the underwater treadmill compared with swimming, where hip and knee joint extension is limited. Furthermore, walking or trotting in the underwater treadmill encourages a more normal gait pattern in the dog, compared with swimming. Deciding between the 2 forms of therapeutic exercise depends on your goals for treatment.

SUMMARY

Although there is little evidence specific to dogs regarding strengthening exercises for the management of OA, there is a substantial body of evidence in the human literature that consistently supports the value of strength training for the treatment of OA. Regular exercise should be considered a core treatment strategy for the management of OA in dogs. The improved muscular strength from resistance, aerobic, and aquatic therapy can help protect an arthritic joint and improve pain and function in the short and long term. It is imperative that owner education focuses on the importance of exercise for management of all animals suffering from OA, even for the management of early and mild cases of OA.

CLINICS CARE POINTS

- Exercise can help control the pain of osteoarthritis and improve functional scores, regardless of the type of exercise.
- Benefits from strengthening exercise can be seen in the short term (3 months) and long term (12 months) after completion of an exercise program.
- Positive effects from exercise may require a long duration of exercise program (>35 weeks) before improvement may be apparent, but exercise can have long-lasting benefits.
- Aquatic exercise may be initially easier than land exercise for an arthritic patient, but targeted strengthening exercises on dry land are also important to control pain and improve function.

REFERENCES

[1] Johnston SA. Osteoarthritis. Joint anatomy, physiology, and pathobiology. Vet Clin North Am Small Anim Pract 1997;27:699–723.

[2] Bannuru RR, Osani MC, Vaysbrot EE, et al. OARSI guidelines for the non-surgical management of knee, hip, and polyarticular osteoarthritis. Osteoarthritis Cartilage 2019;27:1578–89.

[3] Pettitt RG, German AJ. Investigation and management of canine osteoarthritis. In Pract 2015;37:1–8.

[4] McAlindon TE, Bannuru RR, Sullivan MC, et al. OARSI guidelines for the non-surgical management of knee osteoarthritis. Osteoarthritis Cartilage 2014;22:363–88.

[5] McLean H, Millis D, Levine D. Surface electromyography of the vastus lateralis, biceps femoris, and gluteus medius in dogs during stance, walking, trotting, and selected therapeutic exercises. Front Vet Sci 2019;6:211.

[6] Ellis RG, Rankin JW, Hutchinson JR. Limb kinematics, kinetics and muscle dynamics during the sit-to-stand

transition in greyhounds. Front Bioeng Biotechnol 2018; 6:162.

[7] Bockstahler B, Krautler C, Holler P, et al. Pelvic limb kinematics and surface electromyography of the vastus lateralis, biceps femoris, and gluteus medius muscle in dogs with hip osteoarthritis. Vet Surg 2012;41:54–62.

[8] Jansen MJ, Viechtbauer W, Lenssen AF, et al. Strength training alone, exercise therapy alone, and exercise therapy with passive manual mobilisation each reduce pain and disability in people with knee osteoarthritis: a systematic review. J Physiother 2011;57:11–20.

[9] Fransen M, McConnell S, Harmer AR, et al. Exercise for osteoarthritis of the knee: a cochrane systematic review. Br J Sports Med 2015;49:1554–7.

[10] Hurley M, Dickson K, Hallett R, et al. Exercise interventions and patient beliefs for people with hip, knee or hip and knee osteoarthritis: a mixed methods review. Cochrane Database Syst Rev 2018;4:CD010842.

[11] Arendt-Nielsen L, Nie H, Laursen MB, et al. Sensitization in patients with painful knee osteoarthritis. Pain 2010; 149:573–81.

[12] Belshaw Z, Dean R, Asher L. Slower, shorter, sadder: a qualitative study exploring how dog walks change when the canine participant develops osteoarthritis. BMC Vet Res 2020;16:85.

[13] Greene LM, Marcellin-Little DJ, Lascelles BD. Associations among exercise duration, lameness severity, and hip joint range of motion in labrador retrievers with hip dysplasia. J Am Vet Med Assoc 2013;242:1528–33.

[14] Topp R, Woolley S, Hornyak J 3rd, et al. The effect of dynamic versus isometric resistance training on pain and functioning among adults with osteoarthritis of the knee. Arch Phys Med Rehabil 2002;83:1187–95.

[15] Perez-Huerta BD, Diaz-Pulido B, Pecos-Martin D, et al. Effectiveness of a program combining strengthening, stretching, and aerobic training exercises in a standing versus a sitting position in overweight subjects with knee osteoarthritis: a randomized controlled trial. J Clin Med 2020;9:4113.

[16] Tanaka R, Ozawa J, Kito N, et al. Efficacy of strengthening or aerobic exercise on pain relief in people with knee osteoarthritis: a systematic review and meta-analysis of randomized controlled trials. Clin Rehabil 2013;27: 1059–71.

[17] Latham N, Liu CJ. Strength training in older adults: the benefits for osteoarthritis. Clin Geriatr Med 2010;26: 445–59.

[18] Jan MH, Lin JJ, Liau JJ, et al. Investigation of clinical effects of high- and low-resistance training for patients with knee osteoarthritis: a randomized controlled trial. Phys Ther 2008;88:427–36.

[19] Zacharias A, Green RA, Semciw AI, et al. Efficacy of rehabilitation programs for improving muscle strength in people with hip or knee osteoarthritis: a systematic review with meta-analysis. Osteoarthritis Cartilage 2014; 22:1752–73.

[20] Bennell KL, Hunt MA, Wrigley TV, et al. Hip strengthening reduces symptoms but not knee load in people with medial knee osteoarthritis and varus malalignment: a randomised controlled trial. Osteoarthritis Cartilage 2010;18:621–8.

[21] Souza ANA, Escobar ASA, Germano B, et al. Kinetic and kinematic analysis of dogs suffering from hip osteoarthritis and healthy dogs across different physical activities. Vet Comp Orthop Traumatol 2019;32:104–11.

[22] Bockstahler BA, Prickler B, Lewy E, et al. Hind limb kinematics during therapeutic exercises in dogs with osteoarthritis of the hip joints. Am J Vet Res 2012;73:1371–6.

[23] Feeney LC, Lin CF, Marcellin-Little DJ, et al. Validation of two-dimensional kinematic analysis of walk and sit-to-stand motions in dogs. Am J Vet Res 2007;68:277–82.

[24] Kim SE, Jones SC, Lewis DD, et al. In-vivo three-dimensional knee kinematics during daily activities in dogs. J Orthop Res 2015;33:1603–10.

[25] Bennett RL, DeCamp CE, Flo GL, et al. Kinematic gait analysis in dogs with hip dysplasia. Am J Vet Res 1996; 57:966–71.

[26] DeCamp CE. Kinetic and kinematic gait analysis and the assessment of lameness in the dog. Vet Clin North Am Small Anim Pract 1997;27:825–40.

[27] Alcalde GE, Fonseca AC, Boscoa TF, et al. Effect of aquatic physical therapy on pain perception, functional capacity and quality of life in older people with knee osteoarthritis: study protocol for a randomized controlled trial. Trials 2017;18:317.

[28] Wang TJ, Belza B, Elaine Thompson F, et al. Effects of aquatic exercise on flexibility, strength and aerobic fitness in adults with osteoarthritis of the hip or knee. J Adv Nurs 2007;57:141–52.

[29] Rahmann AE. Exercise for people with hip or knee osteoarthritis: a comparison of land-based and aquatic interventions. Open Access J Sports Med 2010;1:123–35.

[30] Mattos F, Leite N, Pitta A, et al. Effects of aquatic exercise on muscle strength and functional performance of individuals with osteoarthritis: a systematic review. Rev Bras Reumatol Engl Ed 2016;56:530–42.

[31] Dycus DL, Levine D, Marcellin-Little DJ. Physical rehabilitation for the management of canine hip dysplasia. Vet Clin North Am Small Anim Pract 2017;47:823–50.

Emergency and Critical Care

Advances in Small Animal Care 2 (2021) 39–48
ADVANCES IN SMALL ANIMAL CARE

Crystalloids versus Colloids

Same Controversy, New Information

Christopher G. Byers, DVM, DACVECC, DACVIM (SAIM), CVJ
CriticalCareDVM.com

KEYWORDS

- Balanced electrolyte solution • Endothelial glycocalyx • Albumin • Acute kidney injury • Coagulopathy
- Hyperchloremic metabolic acidosis • Immunologic reaction

KEY POINTS

- Veterinarians should understand the unique properties of individual fluids to help them select the most appropriate one for a given condition to maximize the likelihood of a positive outcome.
- Balanced electrolyte solutions may be preferable over normal (0.9%) saline for both fluid resuscitation, replacement, and daily physiologic requirements and to reduce the incidence of hyperchloremic metabolic acidosis.
- Synthetic colloids are used most commonly in cats and dogs for intravascular volume resuscitation and support of colloid osmotic pressure, but properties of specific hydroxyethyl starches may increase the risk of acute kidney injury and mortality in certain patient populations.

INTRODUCTION

Veterinarians frequently prescribe intravenous (IV) fluids to their patients for a variety of reasons, notably to restore tissue perfusion, prevent organ dysfunction, and maintain homeostasis. Veterinarians have myriad fluid choices available to them, including crystalloids and colloids. Various human and veterinary studies have investigated potential adverse events like acute kidney injury (AKI), coagulopathies, and immunologic reactions with IV crystalloid and/or colloid administration.

SIGNIFICANCE

Total body water comprises 60% of body weight [1]. The 2 main fluid compartments in the body are intracellular fluid (ICF) and extracellular fluid (ECF). The ECF compartment comprises approximately 60% of total body water, and the ECF compartment makes up the other 40% [1]. ICF is in osmotic equilibrium with the ECF. The ECF compartment is divided into the interstitial space, intravascular space, and potential third spaces [1]. The interstitial compartment is the fluid space that surrounds cells and allows movement of ions, proteins, and nutrients across cell membranes. Fluid does not accumulate in third spaces in nondiseased states [1].

Crystalloids are fluids that contain variable amounts of electrolytes, water, buffers, and dextrose. They are characterized by tonicity and their effect on acid-base status. Crystalloids may be described as replacement fluids or maintenance fluids. The latter term should not be confused or used interchangeably with a rate of fluid administration. Replacement crystalloids are designed to replace existing fluid deficits and to restore both water and electrolyte balance. Approximately one-third of administered isotonic replacement fluid remains in the intravascular space and two-thirds enter the interstitial space. Common examples of replacement crystalloids are 0.9% sodium chloride (NaCl),

E-mail address: CriticalCareDVM@gmail.com
Twitter: CriticalCareDVM.com (C.G.B.)

https://doi.org/10.1016/j.yasa.2021.06.002
2666-450X/21/ © 2021 Elsevier Inc. All rights reserved.

pHyLyte, Normosol-R, PlasmaLyte-A, and lactated Ringer solution. In contrast, maintenance crystalloids are formulated to meet a patient's ongoing sensible and insensible fluid losses. In cats and dogs, these losses primarily are water with a lesser degree of electrolyte loss. Examples of maintenance crystalloids are Plasma-Lyte 56, 0.45% NaCl with dextrose, and Normosol-M. Maintenance fluids do not stay in the intravascular space and do not meaningfully expand intravascular blood volume. Accordingly, they never should be used for volume resuscitation. Hypertonic saline may be used for temporary rapid intravascular volume expansion. The optimal fluid type depends on serum electrolyte and acid-base status and concurrent administration of drugs and blood products.

Colloids are large molecules that remain in the intravascular space due to the Gibbs-Donnan equilibrium. Smaller volumes of a colloid are needed compared with crystalloids to achieve intravascular expansion. Colloids are less likely to induce hemodilution, hypoproteinemia, edema, and fluid overload [2]. Colloids may be synthetic (eg, hydroxyethyl starches [HESs], dextrans, and gelatins) or natural (eg, albumin and plasma). Synthetic colloids contain high-molecular-weight particles that increase plasma colloid osmotic pressure (COP). Synthetic colloids vary based on concentration, mean molecular weight, molar substitution, and site of substitution on the initial glucose molecule (ie, C2:C6 ratio). Fresh frozen plasma (FFP) is collected and spun within 6 hours and frozen (ideally at −70°C) for up to 1 year. This fluid contains stable clotting factors (eg, II, VII, IX, and X), labile clotting factors (eg, V and VIII), von Willebrand factor, fibrinogen, and albumin. FFP does not contain red blood cells or platelets. Frozen plasma (FP) is collected similarly to FFP but is stored for longer than 1 year. FP contains stable clotting factors, fibrinogen and albumin, but does not contain red blood cells, platelets, or labile clotting factors. Both human serum albumin (HSA) and canine serum albumin are available for administration to cats and dogs.

Endothelial Glycocalyx

The endothelial glycocalyx (EG) is a carbohydrate-rich layer that lines the vascular endothelium. This structure is composed of membrane-bound proteoglycans and glycoproteins as well as adsorbed plasma components that are in a dynamic equilibrium with the blood. The composition of the EG is not static, but rather there is a unique balance between component synthesis and shedding [3]. Proteoglycans and glycoproteins are the backbones of the EG, because they are bound mainly to the endothelial cell surface. Proteoglycans are composed of a core protein and glycosaminoglycan (GAG) chains. Each core protein has different GAGs. Common proteoglycans are syndecans, glypicans, mimecans, perlecans, and biglycans. The major GAGs are heparin sulfate, chondroitin sulfate, dermatan sulfate, keratan sulfate, and hyaluronan. Glycoproteins are relatively small, consisting of 2 to 15 sugar residues. The major glycoproteins are selectins, integrins, the immunoglobulin superfamily, and hemostatic proteins.

The EG has 3 major functions: endothelial gatekeeper, microenvironment control center, and mechanotransducer [3–7]. In contrast to Dr Ernest Starling's original hypothesis about fluid dynamics, the EG is the vital semipermeable membrane for microvascular fluid exchange with an oncotic pressure gradient between the plasma compartment and the sub-EG space. The interstitial oncotic pressure exerts minimal effect on microvascular fluid exchange. Net outward movement is opposed but is not reversed by the oncotic gradient. The EG has a net negative charge due to sulfation of GAGs and is able to limit access of certain molecules to the endothelial cell membrane. This structure shields vascular walls from direct exposure to blood flow, mediating shear stress–dependent production of nitric oxide. Heparin sulfate and hyaluronan are major mechanotransducers and help retain vascular protective enzymes and coagulation inhibition factors. The EG also helps modulate the inflammatory response by preventing leukocyte adhesion and binding of chemokines, cytokines, and growth factors.

Volume-Sparing Effects

Crystalloids have a superior short-term effect on plasma volume compared with colloids, but 50% of the volume infused is gone within 20 minutes [8]. In nondiseased states, smaller volumes of colloids generally are needed to induce intravascular expansion compared with crystalloids. A prospective canine study that investigated changes in blood volume in response to rapid fluid administration of 0.9% saline, 7.5% saline, dextran-70, and HES showed administration of saline induced the largest immediate increase in blood volume, but this change was transient due to rapid redistribution of the fluid. Hypertonic saline caused the smallest increase in blood volume post-infusion. Both synthetic colloids investigated increased the blood volume by an amount greater than that infused, and the effect was sustained for a longer period of time compared with crystalloid administration [9].

Inflammation, hyperglycemia, infection, ischemia/reperfusion injury, and increased natriuretic peptide readily compromise the integrity of the EG [10–14]. Albumin uptake and permeability are increased with neutralization of the EG. Physical disruption of the EG leads to loss of the permeability function barrier, leading to the development of edema. Inflammatory cells release a variety of reactive species and enzymes that contribute to damage. Neutrophils produce and release reactive oxygen species, reactive nitrogen species, and proteases (eg, matrix metalloproteinases, neutrophil elastase, plasmin, tryptase, and cathepsin B) that degrade hyaluronan, heparin sulfate, and chondroitin sulfate [14]. Shedding also may be due to exposure to oxidized low density lipoprotein, tumor necrosis factor-α, and bacterial lipopolysaccharide [13]. Damage via thinning and/or shedding can be associated with myriad pathophysiologic consequences, including loss of vascular responsiveness, local hypercoagulability, global heparinization, impaired microcirculation, increased leukocyte-endothelium interaction, increased capillary permeability, and increased platelet aggregation. With damage to the EG, infusion of colloids may not reliably or superiorly expand plasma volume compared with crystalloids [15].

Rapid administration of crystalloid or colloids to treat hemorrhagic shock may cause EG shedding and subsequently increase inflammation because shedding of the EG precedes leukocyte activation and adherence. A randomized controlled trial of human patients who received fluid resuscitation for acute hypovolemia showed colloid infusion resulted in a significant reduction in 90-day mortality as well as more vasopressor-free and ventilator-free days by day 28, compared with crystalloids [16]. A retrospective case-control study documented an increased risk of fluid overload in critically ill dogs that was associated significantly with illness severity and mortality compared with healthy stable postoperative dogs [17]. An experimental canine hemorrhagic shock study measured plasma hyaluronan, multiple interleukins, tumor necrosis factor-α, monocyte chemoattractant protein-1, keratinocyte chemokine-like, and atrial natriuretic peptide at various time points following infusion of either fresh whole blood, HES 130/0.4, 4% succinylated gelatin, or isotonic crystalloid. Rapid large-volume crystalloid infusion was associated with increased hyaluronan and a greater inflammatory response compared with the other fluids [18]. Thus, colloid administration during the fluid resuscitation for hypovolemia may help reduce total volume of crystalloids, reduce inflammation, and prevent fluid overload.

Normal Saline Versus Balanced Electrolyte Solutions

Previous experiments have shown erythrocytes do not lyse when placed in 0.9% saline, leading to a conclusion the "blood of man was isotonic with a NaCl solution of 0.9%" [19]. This was an incorrect conclusion because human plasma, as well as that of cats and dogs, is 0.6% NaCl. The sodium and chloride concentrations of 0.9% saline are higher than that of plasma. Balanced electrolyte solutions are crystalloids with electrolyte compositions similar to ECF due to inclusion of potassium, calcium, lactate, and/or acetate. No balanced electrolyte solution completely replicates ECF composition and should not be considered truly physiologic. Lactated Ringer and Hartmann solutions are slightly hypotonic, and thus lower blood osmolality, increase brain water content, and temporarily raise intracranial pressure [20,21]. They have less of an adverse effect on acid-base equilibrium than normal 0.9% saline, which can induce hypernatremia and hyperchloremic acidosis when infused in large volumes. Hyperchloremia may lead to AKI, higher risk of in-hospital mortality, and increased systemic inflammation [22–28].

A study comparing the effects of PlasmaLyte A with 0.9% saline in human trauma patients showed initial PlasmaLyte A resuscitation caused a more rapid improvement in acid-base status and less hyperchloremia than saline [29]. In-hospital mortality rate was lower among patients who received a balanced electrolyte solution compared with those who received only saline [24]. A recent study showed patients treated with balanced electrolyte solutions had lower composite outcome of death, new need for renal-replacement therapy, and sustained renal dysfunction compared with those patients who received saline [30]. Data in septic human patients also indicate balanced electrolyte solutions may be superior to 0.9% saline for fluid resuscitation [25]. The SMART clinical trial showed used of balanced crystalloids in human patients with sepsis was associated with a lower 30-day in-hospital mortality compared with use of saline [31]. Another study of critically ill adults with sepsis showed resuscitation with balanced fluids was associated with a lower risk of in-hospital mortality [24]. A retrospective cohort study of human patients with severe sepsis documented that coadministration of balanced crystalloids was associated with lower in-hospital mortality when compared to exclusive administration of isotonic saline [24].

In contrast, a study of noncritically ill adults, there was no difference in hospital-free days between treatment with balanced crystalloids or treatment with saline [32]. Similarly, there was no clinically significant difference in in-hospital mortality or postoperative renal, respiratory, infectious, or hemorrhagic complications associated with lactated Ringer solution or 0.9% saline in patients undergoing elective orthopedic and colorectal surgeries [33]. A recent meta-analysis of critically ill human patients receiving crystalloid fluid therapy documented that use of balanced electrolyte solutions did not reduce risk of mortality, AKI, or use of renal replacement therapies [34].

Comparable studies in veterinary medicine are limited. In a rat model of sepsis, 0.9% saline infusion was associated with significantly worse kidney function compared with PlasmaLyte-A infusion (83% vs 28%, respectively) [35]. The effects of lactated Ringer solution and 0.9% saline were investigated in severely decompensated cats with experimental-induced urethral obstruction. Patients treated with 0.9% saline had significantly lower pH, base excess, and bicarbonate concentrations at various time points compared with those who received lactated Ringer solution. Absolute serum potassium and chloride concentrations did not significantly differ between groups at any time [36]. In a randomized prospective clinical trial in cats with naturally occurring urethral obstruction, the effects of normal saline and Normosol-R on blood electrolytes and acid-base status were evaluated. Baseline values were similar between groups [37]. Both fluids resulted in similar rates of potassium normalization, but those who received Normosol-R experienced a significantly more rapid correction of acid-base status within the first 12 hours of fluid therapy [37].

Acute Kidney Injury and Colloids

Human medical research has repeatedly documented synthetic colloids can AKI. Although the exact mechanisms have not been fully elucidated, the development of AKI is thought to be multifactorial [38–42]. Morphologic abnormalities of proximal tubular cells and osmotic nephrosis have been documented after infusion of HESs and low-molecular-weight dextrans. In the proximal tubule, lesions reflect lysosomal accumulation and pinocytosis of exogenous osmotic solutes (eg, colloids) that induce cellular swelling [43,44]. Phagocytosed intracellular HESs can persist for up to 18 days in the canine kidney, depending on the dose received [45]. Renal function also is impaired by reduced renal filtration pressure induced by the oncotic force of the colloids [40].

HESs vary according to several characteristics, including concentration, mean molecular weight, molar substitution, and C2:C6 ratio. Molar substitution refers to the modification of the original substance by the addition of hydroxyethyl groups. The higher the degree of molar substitution, the greater the resistance to degradation; consequently, the fluid remains in the intravascular space longer. A value of 0.7 indicates the HES preparation has an average of 7 hydroxyethyl residues per 10 glucose subunits. Starches with this level of substitution are called hetastarches, and similar names are applied to describe other levels of substitution (0.4—tetrastarch; 0.5—pentastarch; and 0.6—hexastarch).

Three generations of HESs exist, and the most recent generation have both lower molecular weights and degree of substitution [46]. In multiple populations of hospitalized human patients, first-generation and second-generation HESs induced AKI [47–50]. Third-generation HESs have molecular weights less than 200 kDa and degree of molar substitution less than 0.5. These characteristics may reduce renal tubular colloid accumulation and subsequent toxicity. Various human clinical trials have documented an increased risk of AKI and death in critically ill patients treated with HESs compared with crystalloids [47,51,52]. In contrast, studies in cats and dogs showed inconsistent results regarding the development of AKI or increased mortality associated with administration of HESs compared with crystalloid infusion.

One study investigated a model of hemorrhagic shock and subsequent fluid resuscitation on renal function in dogs. Following removal of approximately 40% blood volume to achieve a mean arterial pressure of 40 mm Hg, patients received either lactated Ringer solution, 6% HES, 7.5% hypertonic saline, and 7.5% hypertonic saline with 6% dextran-70. Renal blood flow and glomerular filtration rate were higher in the dogs that received lactated Ringer solution at 60 minutes but returned to baseline values in all groups at 120 minutes. There were no differences in renal variables 120 minutes after treatment among all groups [53]. A prospective study of septic dogs undergoing emergency laparotomy showed those that received HESs had significantly higher urinary neutrophil gelatinase–associated lipocalin (NGAL) across all time points compared with those that did not. This result suggested HES infusion induced renal epithelial injury [54]. A cohort study of critically ill dogs showed a higher incidence of AKI and nonsurvival to discharge with administration of 10% HES-250/0.5/5:1 compared with a control group [55]. A retrospective cohort study in canine patients showed those treated with HES-130/0.4 were not more prone to develop AKI compared with those who did not receive HES. The number of HES days was significantly associated, however, with an increase in AKI grade within 10 days of HES administration [56]. A case report of a golden retriever with ascites who received 6% HES-130/0.4 to increase plasma osmolality revealed that the patient had documented mild azotemia prior to HES administration and had a rapid deterioration of kidney function HES administration. Cumulative clinical and histopathologic data of AKI provided support of the nephrotoxic effects of HES [57]. An experimental interventional study of former racing greyhounds investigated the association between administration of synthetic colloids and biomarkers of AKI following induction of hemorrhagic shock. Following hemorrhage, dogs were volume resuscitated with fresh whole blood, 6% HES-130/.0.4, 4% succinylated gelatin, or isotonic crystalloid. Concentrations of AKI biomarkers were measured at baseline and at multiple time points posthemorrhage. Resuscitation with 4% succinylated gelatin was associated with greater magnitude increases in both urinary biomarkers of AKI and tubular microvesiculation compared with the other groups [58].

In contrast, a retrospective case series of 201 dogs admitted to the intensive care unit investigated the effects of HES infusion on plasma creatinine concentration. All dogs had normal initial plasma creatinine concentrations. During hospitalization, patients received either crystalloids alone or HES with or without crystalloids. HESs administration was not associated with increased creatinine concentrations compared with administration of only crystalloids [59]. A similar study in critically ill cats showed administration of HES did not result in a significantly greater increase in creatinine from values measured on admission or higher mortality compared with administration of crystalloids [60]. A retrospective cohort study of critically ill nonazotemic cats showed the short-term percent change in serum creatinine concentration and the development of AKI was not significantly different between those received 6% HES-130/0.4 and those who did not [61]. A crossover study on healthy English pointer dogs showed neither infusion of lactated Ringer solution nor 6% HES-130/0.4 caused AKI when used for volume resuscitation in experimental hemorrhage performed under anesthesia [62]. The results of all of these studies are challenging to interpret accurately because evidence of AKI was assessed via measurement of novel biomarkers of renal function, such as NGAL, and urinary NGAL:creatinine ratio is highly sensitive and specific for detection of early-stage AKI in dogs before serum creatinine and urinalysis parameters change. Researchers did not necessarily adhere to the canine AKI grading scheme developed and recommended by the International Renal Interest Society that biochemically categorizes AKI severity based on serum creatinine [63].

Coagulopathies and Colloids

Synthetic colloids have been associated with coagulopathies, and several mechanisms have been theorized (Box 1) [64,65].

Fluids with lower molecular weights and molar substitution are degraded and eliminated more rapidly, and these characteristics appear to reduce the likelihood of adverse events, including coagulopathies [64]. In contrast, high C2:C6 ratios have a more meaningful negative impact on hemostasis [66,67].

In vitro and in vivo canine and feline studies have documented inconsistent primary and secondary hemostatic effects following administration of synthetic colloids. A randomized blinded prospective study of adult mixed-breed hound dogs investigated the effects of 6% HES-600/0.75 and lactated Ringer solution anesthetized for orthopedic surgery. Dogs were randomly assigned to receive a 10-mL/kg IV bolus of either 6% HES-600/0.75 or lactated Ringer solution over 20 minutes followed by a maintenance infusion of lactated Ringer solution (10 mL/kg IV) during anesthesia. Packed cell volume, total protein concentration, prothrombin time, activated partial thromboplastin time, von Willebrand factor antigen concentration, factor VIII activity, platelet count, platelet aggregation, COP, and buccal mucosal bleeding time were measured. Although HES and lactated Ringer solution altered hemostatic variables, neither fluid was associated with increased clinical bleeding [66]. An in vitro experimental canine study investigated the effects of 0.9% saline, various hypertonic solutions, and synthetic colloids on coagulation. Results showed hypertonic solutions affected platelet function and whole blood coagulation to a greater extent than saline and HES. At high dilutions, HES significantly affected fibrinogen function and extrinsic thromboelastometry clotting time but to no greater extent than 0.9% saline at clinically relevant dilutions [68]. An experimental model of hemorrhagic shock in healthy greyhounds showed 6% HES-130/0.4 and 0.9% NaCl administration after induction of shock increased platelet closure time, indicating HES administration did not induce clinically relevant platelet dysfunction beyond hemodilution [69].

In contrast, McBride and colleagues [69] showed 1:3 dilution of blood samples from healthy dogs with 10% HES-200/0.5 significantly increased closure time

BOX 1
Proposed mechanisms of coagulopathy associated with colloid administration

- Inactivation of factor VIII and von Willebrand factor inhibiting fibrin network formation
- Glycoprotein IIb/IIIa inhibition preventing blood clot formation
- Impaired and inhibited binding of von Willebrand factor and fibrinogen to glycoprotein IIb/IIIa receptors
- Accelerated fibrin degradation

Data from Refs [63,64].

beyond the dilutional effect, suggesting IV administration of 10% HES-200/0.5 in dogs might cause platelet dysfunction. Another prospective randomized study of client-owned dogs undergoing anesthesia for arthroscopy or diagnostic imaging investigated the effects of 6% HES-130/0.42 mixed with a balanced electrolyte solution or 0.9% saline on platelet function and whole blood coagulation. A single bolus of 15-mL/kg 6% HES-130/0.42 induced a temporary significant prolongation of platelet closure time, increase in clot formation time, decrease in maximal clot firmness regardless of carrier solution [70]. A randomized, placebo-controlled, blinded study of healthy beagles investigated the effects of 0.9% NaCl and 6% HES-130/0.4 following administration of lipopolysaccharide or placebo. HESs bolus administration induced transient hypocoagulability characterized by a prolonged activated partial thromboplastin time, decreased clot formation speed and clot strength, and acquired type 1 von Willebrand disease [71]. An in vitro feline study investigated the effects of 6% HES-130/0.42 on whole-blood coagulation based on rotational thromboelastometry. Blood samples from healthy cats were collected by atraumatic jugular phlebotomy following intramuscular sedation. Analyses were performed at baseline and after dilution with either Ringer acetate or 6% HES-130/0.42 in a 1:6 dilution. A small but significant impairment of whole blood coagulation was documented with both fluids, and HES-130/0.42 led to a significantly greater effect on coagulation than Ringer acetate [72].

There are a variety of coagulation defects, including hyperfibrinolysis, that have been documented in veterinary patients with critical illness. A study of client-owned dogs with spontaneous hemoperitoneum documented evidence of hypocoagulability, protein C deficiency, and hyperfibrinolysis [73]. In this investigation, some dogs had coagulation defects despite not having received colloid or large-volume crystalloid infusions. Another study in experimentally hemorrhaged dogs showed HES-130/0.4 solution induced a transient dilutional coagulopathy similar to lactated Ringer solution but did not impair primary hemostasis. Furthermore, results indicated this effect could be avoided through infusion of smaller volumes of HES [74]. In another canine study using a hemorrhagic shock model, HES-130/0.4 and 4% succinylated gelatin induced coagulation abnormalities. Although shock alone produced some evidence of hypocoagulability, volume replacement with 4% succinylated gelatin caused mild platelet dysfunction, and HES was associated with hypocoagulability beyond effects of hemodilution [75]. Considered together, the results of these studies suggest synthetic colloids should be used cautiously and sparingly in canine patients with active hemorrhage and/or preexisting hemostatic disorders.

Albumin

Serum albumin is the main contributor to COP. Hypoalbuminemia is common in a variety of companion animal diseases, including liver dysfunction, gastroenteropathies, pancreatopathies, hypoadrenocorticism, protein-losing nephropathies, malnutrition, and sepsis. Human physicians frequently treat their patients with HSA more commonly than their veterinary colleagues. Data on efficacy and superiority to other fluids in various patient populations, however, have been inconclusive. A study of human patients in an intensive care unit showed use of 4% albumin was not superior to 0.9% saline for fluid resuscitation [76]. In another post hoc study of critically ill patients with traumatic brain injury, fluid resuscitation with albumin was associated with higher mortality rates than was resuscitation with saline [77]. One meta-analysis of 38 trials showed no evidence that albumin reduced mortality compared with alternatives like 0.9% saline in patients with hypovolemia or in patients with burns or hypoalbuminemia [78]. Similarly, another meta-analysis showed that although albumin infusion was safe, its use as part of fluid volume expansion and resuscitation for critically ill adults with sepsis of any severity did not reduce all-cause mortality [79]. Investigators have also shown albumin replacement in addition to crystalloids compared with crystalloids alone did not improve the rate of survival at 28 days and 90 days, respectively, in patients with severe sepsis [80]. A MEDLINE literature review did not find a definitive role of albumin in the resuscitation of patients with severe sepsis and sepsis; furthermore, crystalloids were the preferred solution for the resuscitation of emergency department patients with severe sepsis and septic shock [81]. Using an ovine model of septic shock, however, investigators showed kidney function and cumulative diuresis were preserved with 5% albumin and crystalloid resuscitation; however, creatinine clearance was diminished with 6% HES 130/0.4 6% infusion [82].

HSA has been used successfully in both dogs and cats. In 1 study, investigators concluded that administration of HSA significantly increased serum albumin, total protein concentration, and COP. The complications observed, however, were not related specifically to HSA administration and could have been present due to the confounding factors of critical illness [83]. Adverse immunologic reactions have been documented following HSA infusion. One study confirmed dogs have a marked immunoglobulin G response 4 weeks to 6 weeks after exposure to HSA [84]. Another report confirmed delayed immunologic reactions, including edema, facial swelling, vasculitis, and hemorrhage, in 2 critically ill dogs [85]. A recent case series documented death as a potential outcome in dogs receiving HSA [86]. In 1 relatively large veterinary study of critically ill cats and dogs, no severe hypersensitivity reactions were documented [87].

PRESENT RELEVANCE AND FUTURE AVENUES TO CONSIDER OR TO INVESTIGATE

The EG is a vital endovascular structure with a primary function of maintaining vascular permeability. Synthetic colloids may readily disrupt this structure. Nevertheless, HESs have been recommended for volume resuscitation given their ability to induce more rapid and lasting circulatory stabilization than crystalloids. In the past decade, the use of these synthetic colloids has been called into question given various adverse reactions. Clinical trials in human patients documented an increased risk of AKI and death in specific patient populations, but companion animal studies have shown inconsistent results. HESs may induce several coagulation abnormalities in cats and dogs. The clinical relevance of these studies is not yet known, and clinical prospective investigation is warranted HESs with lower molecular weights and molar substitution appear to be associated with fewer adverse events. Human serum and canine albumin infusion in cats and dogs have been associated with infrequent immunologic reactions in cats and dogs have been documented. Administration of HSA after more than 1 week from the initial dosing is not currently recommended due of the increased risk of foreign antigenicity. Research is needed regarding the EG to develop effective therapeutic strategies that maintain vascular permeability, reduce inappropriate fluid shifts, and restore and maintain tissue perfusion.

SUMMARY

Veterinarians should have a comprehensive knowledge of fluid dynamics and composition to understand fluid distribution throughout the body. Inappropriate IV fluid administration may contribute to disease morbidity (eg, pulmonary venous congestion, acid-base disturbances, AKI, coagulopathies, and increased hospitalization time) and mortality. HESs with lower molecular weights and molar substitution appear to be associated with fewer adverse events. Veterinarians should review data from human studies with caution until more relevant and comprehensive veterinary data are available.

CLINICS CARE POINTS

- Colloids have been linked to AKI, coagulopathies, and adverse immunologic reactions; these events largely appear to be product-dependent and dose-related.
- Development of AKI is multifactorial, and morphologic abnormalities includes proximal tubulopathies and osmotic nephrosis.
- Proposed mechanisms of coagulopathies induced by HESs are inhibition of both fibrin network formation and blood clot formation as well as accelerated fibrin degradation.
- Veterinarians should administer IV fluids in a manner that allows the team to accurately and serially assess patient response and monitor for any adverse reactions.

REFERENCES

[1] Kohn K, DiBartola S. Composition and distribution of body fluids in dogs and cats. In: DiBartola S, editor. Fluid therapy in small animal practice. 2nd edition. Philadelphia: WB Saunders; 2000. p. 6.

[2] Shoemaker WC, Schluchter M, Hopkins JA, et al. Comparison of the relative effectiveness of colloids and crystalloids in emergency resuscitation. Am J Surg 1981; 142(1):73–84.

[3] Reitsma S, Slaaf DW, Vink H, et al. The endothelial glycocalyx: composition, function, and visualization. Pflugers Arch 2007;454(3):345–59.

[4] Gouverneur M, Berg B, Nieuwdorp M, et al. Vasculoprotective properties of the endothelial glycocalyx: effects of fluid shear stress. J Intern Med 2006;259(4):393–400.

[5] Constantinescu AA, Vink H, Spaan JAE. Endothelial cell glycocalyx modulates immobilization of leukocytes at the endothelial surface. Arterioscler Thromb Vasc Biol 2003;23(9):1541–7.

[6] Becker BF, Chappell D, Bruegger D, et al. Therapeutic strategies targeting the endothelial glycocalyx: acute deficits, but great potential. Cardiovasc Res 2010;87(2):300–10.

[7] Becker BF, Chappell D, Jacob M. Endothelial glycocalyx and coronary vascular permeability: the fringe benefit. Basic Res Cardiol 2010;105(6):687–701.

[8] Hahn RG. Why crystalloids will do the job in the operating room. Anaesthesiol Intensive Ther 2014;46(5):342–9.

[9] Silverstein DC, Aldrich J, Haskins SC, et al. Assessment of changes in blood volume in response to resuscitative fluid administration in dogs. J Vet Emerg Crit Care 2005;15(3):185–92.

[10] Rehm M, Bruegger D, Christ F, et al. Shedding of the endothelial glycocalyx in patients undergoing major vascular surgery with global and regional ischemia. Circulation 2007;116:1896–906.

[11] Bruegger D, Jacob M, Rehm M, et al. Atrial natriuretic peptide induces shedding of endothelial glycocalyx in coronary vascular bed of guinea pig hearts. Am J Physiol Heart Circ Physiol 2005;289(5):H1993–9.

[12] Nieuwdorp M, van Haeften TW, Gouverneur MC, et al. Loss of endothelial glycocalyx during acute hyperglycemia coincides with endothelial dysfunction and coagulation in vivo. Diabetes 2006;55(2):480–6.

[13] Chappell D, Hofmann-Kiefer K, Jacob M, et al. TNF-α induced shedding of the endothelial glycocalyx is prevented by hydrocortisone and antithrombin. Basic Res Cardiol 2009;104(1):78–89.

[14] Van Golen RE, van Gulik TM, Heger M. Mechanistic overview of reactive species-induced degradation of the endothelial glycocalyx during hepatic ischemia/reperfusion injury. Free Radic Biol Med 2012;52(8):1382–402.

[15] Guidet B, Martinet O, Boulain T, et al. Assessment of hemodynamic efficacy and safety of 6% hydroxyethyl starch 130/0.4 vs. 0.9% NaCl fluid replacement in patients with severe sepsis: The CRYSTMAS study. Crit Care 2012;16(3):R94.

[16] Annane D, Siami S, Jaber S, et al. Effects of fluid resuscitation with colloids vs. crystalloids on mortality in critically ill patients presenting with hypovolemic shock: the CRISTAL randomized trial. J Am Med Assoc 2013; 310(17):1809–17.

[17] Cavanagh AA, Sullivan LA, Hansen BD. Retrospective evaluation of fluid overload and relationship to outcome in critically ill dogs. J Vet Emerg Crit Care 2016;26(4): 578–86.

[18] Smart L, Boyd CJ, Claus MA, et al. Large-volume crystalloid fluid is associated with increased hyaluronan shedding and inflammation in a canine hemorrhagic shock model. Inflammation 2018;41(4):155–1523.

[19] Awad S, Allison SP, Lobo DN. The history of 0.9% saline. Clin Nutr 2008;27(2):179–88.

[20] Tommasino C, Moore S, Todd MM. Cerebral effects of isovolemic hemodilution with crystalloid or colloid solutions. Crit Care Med 1988;16(9):862–8.

[21] Williams EL, Hildebrand KL, McCormick SA, et al. The effect of intravenous lactated Ringer's solution versus 0.9% sodium chloride solution on serum osmolality in human volunteers. Anesth Analg 1999;88(5):999–1003.

[22] Yunos NM, Bellomo R, Hegarty C, et al. Association between a chloride-liberal vs chloride-restrictive intravenous fluid administration strategy and kidney injury in critically ill adults. JAMA 2012;308(15):1566–72.

[23] Shaw AD, Raghunathan K, Peyerl FW, et al. Association between intravenous chloride load during resuscitation and in-hospital mortality among patients with SIRS. Intensive Care Med 2014;40(12):1897–905.

[24] Raghunathan K, Shaw A, Nathanson B, et al. Association between the choice of IV crystalloid and in-hospital mortality among critically ill adults with sepsis. Crit Care Med 2014;42(7):1585–91.

[25] Rochwerg B, Alhazzani W, Sindi A, et al. Fluid resuscitation in sepsis: a systematic review and network meta-analysis. Ann Intern Med 2014;161(5):347–55.

[26] Kellum JA, Song M, Almasri E. Hyperchloremic acidosis increases circulating inflammatory molecules in experimental sepsis. Chest 2006;130(4):962–7.

[27] Hansen PB, Jensen BL, Skott O. Chloride regulates afferent arteriolar contraction in response to depolarization. Hypertension 1998;32(6):1066–70.

[28] Chowdhury AH, Cox EF, Francis ST, et al. A randomized, double blind crossover study on the effects of 2-L infusions of 0.9% saline and plasmalyte 148 on renal blood flow velocity and renal cortical tissue perfusion in healthy volunteers. Ann Surg 2012;256(1):18–24.

[29] Young JB, Utter GH, Schermer CR, et al. Saline versus plasmalyte-A in initial resuscitation of trauma patients: a randomized trial. Ann Surg 2014;259(2):255–62.

[30] Semler MW, Self WH, Wanderer JP, et al. Balanced crystalloids versus saline in critically ill adults. N Engl J Med 2018;378(9):829–39.

[31] Brown RM, Wang L, Coston TD, et al. Balanced crystalloid versus saline in sepsis. A secondary analysis of the

SMART clinical trial. Am J Respir Crit Care Med 2019; 200(12):1487–95.
[32] Self WH, Semler MW, Wanderer JP, et al. Balanced crystalloids versus saline in noncritically ill adults. N Engl J Med 2018;378(9):819–28.
[33] Maheshwari K, Turan A, Makarova N, et al. Saline versus lactated Ringer's solution: The saline or lactated Ringer's (SOLAR) trial. Anesthesiology 2020;132(4):614–24.
[34] Liu C, Lu G, Wang D, et al. Balanced crystalloids versus normal saline for fluid resuscitation in critically ill patients: a systematic review and meta-analysis with trial sequential analysis. Am J Emerg Med 2019;37(11): 2072–8.
[35] Zhou F, Peng ZY, Bishop JV, et al. Effects of fluid resuscitation with 0.9% saline versus a balanced electrolyte solution on acute kidney injury in a rat model of sepsis. Crit Care Med 2014;42(4):e270–8.
[36] Cunha M, Freitas GC, Carregaro AB, et al. Renal and cardiorespiratory effects of treatment with lactated Ringer's solution or physiologic saline (0.9% NaCl) solution in cats with experimentally induced urethral obstruction. Am J Vet Res 2010;71(7):840–6.
[37] Drobatz KJ, Cole SG. The influence of crystalloid type on acid-base and electrolyte status of cats with urethral obstruction. J Vet Emerg Crit Care 2008;18(4):355–61.
[38] Hüter L, Simon T, Weinmann L, et al. Hydroxyethyl starch impairs renal function and induces interstitial proliferation, macrophage infiltration and tubular damage in an isolated renal perfusion model. Crit Care 2009; 13(1):R23.
[39] Janssen CW Jr. Osmotic nephrosis. A clinical and experimental investigation. Acta Chir Scand 1968;134(6): 481–7.
[40] Moran M, Kapsner C. Acute renal failure associated with elevated plasma oncotic pressure. N Engl J Med 1987; 317(3):150–3.
[41] Druml W, Polzleitner D, Laggner AN, et al. Dextran-40, acute renal failure, and elevated plasma oncotic pressure. N Engl J Med 1988;318:252–4.
[42] Moore FA, McKinley BA, Moore EE. The next generation in shock resuscitation. Lancet 2004;363(9425): 1988–96.
[43] Dickenmann M, Oettl T, Mihatsch MJ. Osmotic nephrosis: acute kidney injury with accumulation of proximal tubular lysosomes due to administration of exogenous solutes. Am J Kidney Dis 2008;51(3): 491–503.
[44] Wiedermann CJ, Joannidis M. Accumulation of hydroxyethyl starch in human and animal tissues: a systematic review. Intensive Care Med 2014;40:160–70.
[45] Thompson WL, Fukushima T, Rutherford RB, et al. Intravascular persistence, tissue storage, and excretion of hydroxyethyl starch. Surg Gynecol Obstet 1970;131(5): 965–72.
[46] Boldt J, Suttner S. Plasma substitutes. Minerva Anestesiol 2005;71(12):741–58.
[47] Brunkhorst FM, Engel C, Bloos F, et al. Intensive insulin therapy and pentastarch resuscitation in severe sepsis. N Engl J Med 2008;358(2):125–39.
[48] Cittanova ML, Leblanc I, Legendre C, et al. Effect of hydroxyethylstarch in brain-dead kidney donors on renal function in kidney-transplant recipients. Lancet 1996; 348(9042):1620–2.
[49] Schortgen F, Lacherade JC, Bruneel F, et al. Effects of hydroxyethylstarch and gelatin on renal function in severe sepsis: a multicentre randomised study. Lancet 2001; 357(9260):911–6.
[50] Winkelmayer WC, Glynn RJ, Levin R, et al. Hydroxyethyl starch and change in renal function in patients undergoing coronary artery bypass graft surgery. Kidney Int 2003; 64(3):1046–9.
[51] Myburgh JA, Finfer S, Bellomo R, et al. Hydroxyethyl starch or saline for fluid resuscitation in intensive care. N Engl J Med 2012;367:1901–11.
[52] Perner A, Haase N, Guttormsen AB, et al. Hydroxyethyl starch 130/0.42 versus Ringer's acetate in severe sepsis. N Engl J Med 2012;367:124–34.
[53] Nascimento P Jr, de Paiva Filho O, de Carvalho L, et al. Early hemodynamic and renal effects of hemorrhagic shock resuscitation with lactated Ringer's solution, hydroxyethyl starch, and hypertonic saline with or without 6% dextran-70. J Surg Res 2006;136(1):98–105.
[54] Cortellini S, Pelligand L, Syme H, et al. Neutrophil gelatinase-associated lipocalin in dogs with sepsis undergoing emergency laparotomy: a prospective case-control study. J Vet Intern Med 2015;29(6):1595–602.
[55] Hayes G, Benedicenti L, Mathews K. Retrospective cohort study on the incidence of acute kidney injury and death following hydroxyethyl starch (HES 10% 250/0.5/5:1) administration in dogs (2007-2010). J Vet Emerg Crit Care 2016;26(1):35–40.
[56] Sigrist NE, Kalin N, Dreyfus A. Changes in serum creatinine concentration and acute kidney injury (AKI) grade in dogs treated with hydroxyethyl starch 130/0.4 from 2013-2015. J Vet Intern Med 2017;31(2):434–41.
[57] Bae J, Soliman M, Kin H, et al. Rapid exacerbation of renal function after administration of hydroxyethyl starch in a dog. J Vet Med Sci 2017;79(9):1591–5.
[58] Boyd CJ, Claus MA, Raisis AL, et al. Evaluation of biomarkers of kidney injury following 4% succinylated gelatin and 6% hydroxyethyl starch 130/0.4 administration in a canine hemorrhagic shock model. J Vet Emerg Crit Care 2019;29(2):132–42.
[59] Yozova ID, Howard J, Adamik KN. Retrospective evaluation of the effects of administration of tetrastarch (hydroxyethyl starch 130/0.4) on plasma creatinine concentration in dogs (2010-2013): 201 dogs. J Vet Emerg Crit Care 2016;26(4):568–77.
[60] Yozova ID, Howard J, Adamik KN. Effect of tetrastarch (hydroxyethyl starch 130/0.4) on plasma creatinine concentration in cats: a retrospective analysis (2010-2015). J Feline Med Surg 2017;19(1):1073–9.

[61] Sigrist NE, Kalin N, Dreyfus A. Effects of hydroxyethyl-starch 130/0.4 on serum creatinine concentration and development of acute kidney injury in nonazotemic cats. J Vet Intern Med 2017;31(6):1748–56.
[62] Diniz MS, Teixeira-Neto FJ, Celeita-Redriguez N, et al. Effects of 6% tetrastarch and lactated Ringer's solution on extravascular lung water and markers of acute kidney injury in hemorrhaged isoflurane-anesthetized healthy dogs. J Vet Intern Med 2018;32(2):712–21.
[63] Cowgill L. Grading of acute kidney injury. International Renal Interest Society; 2016. Available at: http://www.iris-kidney.com/pdf/4_ldc-revised-grading-of-acute-kidney-injury.pdf. Accessed 21 February 2021.
[64] Fenger-Eriksen C, Tonnesen E, Ingerslev J, et al. Mechanisms of hydroxyethyl starch-induced dilutional coagulopathy. J Thromb Haemost 2009;7(7):1099–105.
[65] Toyoda D, Shinoda S, Kotake Y. Pros and cons of tetrastarch solution for critically ill patients. J Intensive Care 2014;2(1):23.
[66] Treib J, Haass A, Pindur G, et al. Influence of low and medium molecular weight hydroxyethyl starch on platelets during a long-term hemodilution in patients with cerebrovascular iseases. Arzneimittelforschung 1996; 46(11):1064–6.
[67] Chohan AS, Greene SA, Grubb TL, et al. Effects of 6% hetastarch (600/0.75) or lactated Ringer's solution on hemostatic variables and clinical bleeding in healthy dogs anesthetized for orthopedic surgery. Vet Anaesth Analg 2011;38(2):94–105.
[68] Wurlod VA, Howard J, Francey T, et al. Comparison of the in vitro effects of saline, hypertonic hydroxyethyl starch, hypertonic saline, and two forms of hydroxyethyl starch on whole blood coagulation and platelet function in dogs. J Vet Emerg Crit Care 2015;25(4):474–87.
[69] McBride D, Hosgood G, Raisis A, et al. Platelet closure time in anesthetized Greyhounds with hemorrhagic shock treated with hydroxyethyl starch 130/0.4 or 0.9% sodium chloride infusions. J Vet Emerg Crit Care 2016; 26(4):509–15.
[70] Reuteler A, Axiak-Flammer S, Howard J, et al. Comparison of the effects of a balanced crystalloid-based and a saline-based tetrastarch solution on canine whole blood coagulation and platelet function. J Vet Emerg Crit Care 2017;27(1):23–34.
[71] Gauthier V, Holowaychuk MK, Kerr CL, et al. Effect of synthetic colloid administration on coagulation in healthy dogs and dogs with systemic inflammation. J Vet Intern Med 2015;29(1):276–85.
[72] Albrecht NA, Howard J, Kovacevic A, et al. In vitro effects of 6% hydroxyethyl starch 130/0.42 solution on feline whole blood coagulation measured by rotational thromboelastometry. BMC Vet Res 2016;12(1):155.
[73] Fletcher DJ, Rozanski EA, Brainard BM, et al. Assessment of the relationships among coagulopathy, hyperfibrinolysis, plasma lactate, and protein C in dogs with spontaneous hemoperitoneum. J Vet Emerg Crit Care 2016;26(1):41–51.
[74] Diniz MS, Teixeira-Neto FJ, Goncalves DS, et al. Effects of 6% tetrastarch or lactated Ringer's solution on blood coagulation in hemorrhaged dogs. J Vet Intern Med 2018;32(6):1927–33.
[75] Boyd CJ, Claus MA, Raisis AL, et al. Hypocoagulability and platelet dysfunction are exacerbated by synthetic colloids in a canine hemorrhagic shock model. Front Vet Sci 2018;5:279.
[76] Finfer S, Bellomo R, Boyce N, et al. A comparison of albumin and saline for fluid resuscitation in the intensive care unit. N Engl J Med 2004;350(22):2247–56.
[77] SAFE Study Investigators, et al. Saline or albumin for fluid resuscitation in patients with traumatic brain injury. N Engl J Med 2007;357(9):874–84.
[78] Roberts I, Blackhall K, Alderson P, et al. Human albumin solution for resuscitation and volume expansion in critically ill patients. Cochrane Database Syst Rev 2011; 2011(11):CD001208.
[79] Patel A, Laffan MA, Waheed U, et al. Randomised trials of human albumin for adults with sepsis: systematic review and meta-analysis with trial sequential analysis of all-cause mortality. BMJ 2014;349:g4561.
[80] Caitroni P, Tognoni G, Masson S, et al. Albumin replacement in patients with severe sepsis or septic shock. N Engl J Med 2014;370(15):1412–21.
[81] Winters ME, Sherwin R, Vilke GM, et al. What is the preferred resuscitation fluid for patients with severe sepsis and septic shock? J Emerg Med 2017;53(6): 928–39.
[82] Kampmeier TG, Arnemann PH, Hessler M, et al. Effects of resuscitation with human albumin 5%, hydroxyethyl starch 130/0.4 6%, or crystalloid on kidney damage in an ovine model of septic shock. Br J Anaesth 2018; 121(3):581–7.
[83] Trow AV, Rozanski EA, De Laforcade AM, et al. Evaluation of use of human albumin in critically ill dogs: 73 cases (2003-2006). J Am Vet Med Assoc 2008;233(4): 607–12.
[84] Martin LG, Luther TY, Alperin DC, et al. Serum antibodies against human albumin in critically ill and healthy dogs. J Am Vet Med Assoc 2008;232(7):1004–9.
[85] Powell C, Thompson L, Murtaugh RJ. Type III hypersensitivity reaction with immune complex deposition in 2 critically ill dogs administered human serum albumin. J Vet Emerg Crit Care 2013;23(6):598–604.
[86] Mazzaferro EM, Balakrishnan A, Hackner SG, et al. Delayed Type III hypersensitivity reaction with acute kidney injury in two dogs following administration of concentrated human albumin during treatment for septic peritonitis. J Vet Emerg Crit Care 2020;30(5):574–80.
[87] Vigano F, Perissinotto L, Bosco VR. Administration of 5% human serum albumin in critically ill small animal patients with hypoalbuminemia: 418 dogs and 170 cats (1994-2008). J Vet Emerg Crit Care 2010;20(2):237–43.

Advances in Small Animal Care 2 (2021) 49–67
ADVANCES IN SMALL ANIMAL CARE

Current and Future Practice in the Diagnosis and Management of Sepsis and Septic Shock in Small Animals

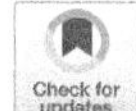

Thandeka R. Ngwenyama, DVM, DACVECC
Carlson College of Veterinary Medicine, Magruder Hall, 700 SW 30th St, Corvallis, OR 97331, USA

KEYWORDS

- Vasodilatory shock • Systemic inflammatory response syndrome (SIRS) • Organ dysfunction
- Multiple organ dysfunction (MODS) • Dysregulated immune system • Septic shock
- Sepsis-induced cardiomyopathy

KEY POINTS

- Early recognition and intervention are critical factors in the management of patients with sepsis and septic shock and are key to increasing the likelihood of a good outcome.
- Clinical perception is used to determine suspected infection in patients; especially those with undifferentiated disease, unexplained organ dysfunction, and/or hemodynamic instability.
- Empiric broad-spectrum antibiotics are initiated early until culture and sensitivity results guide more specific antibiotic selection.
- An individualized, physiologically guided, and judicious approach to fluid management is recommended. Early use of norepinephrine and/or a combination with other vasoactive drugs in patients with septic shock should be considered.
- Early and adequate source control after acute resuscitation and hemodynamic stabilization of septic patients is important to increase the likelihood of a good outcome.

INTRODUCTION

Sepsis is a serious life-threatening illness caused by a myriad of different infectious etiologies, host responses, and clinical contexts [1]. It is a prevailing cause of mortality in small animal patients, with a recent multicenter study showing a mortality rate of 70% in septic dogs that developed multiorgan dysfunction [2]. Understanding of the pathophysiology, diagnostic criteria, and management is incomplete and is continually evolving for this cryptic illness [1]. Sepsis is an enigmatic syndrome that does not aptly fit into a black-and-white diagnosis that can be neatly categorized and labeled. It is important to understand terminology and definitions associated with sepsis and the continuum to septic shock, to critically evaluate and interpret current literature and manage septic patients. In veterinary medicine, sepsis is defined as a systemic inflammatory response to an infectious etiology. *Systemic inflammatory response syndrome* (SIRS) is a clinical response to an infectious or noninfectious physiologic stressor; clinical criteria include abnormalities in temperature, respiratory rate, heart rate, and white blood cell count/morphology. Patients that have a suspected or confirmed infection and meet a minimum of two (in dogs) or three (in cats) out of a selection of four of the SIRS criteria have sepsis (Table 1) [3]. Limitations

The author has no disclosures to report.

E-mail address: tandi.ngwenyama@oregonstate.edu

https://doi.org/10.1016/j.yasa.2021.07.005
2666-450X/21/ © 2021 Elsevier Inc. All rights reserved.

TABLE 1
Veterinary Definitions and Diagnostic Criteria

Veterinary definitions:

Systemic inflammatory response syndrome (SIRS) is a clinical response to a physiologic stressor, which may or may not be infectious in etiology. Patients who are considered to have SIRS must meet at least 2 (dogs) or 3 (cats) of the following clinical criteria: tachycardia/bradycardia (cats), tachypnea, fever or hypothermia, and leukocytosis or leukopenia

SIRS Criteria	*Dogs*	*Cats*	*People*
Temperature	>39.2<37.2°C >102.6<99°F	<37.8>40.0°C >103.5<100°F	>38.0<36.0°C >100.4<96.8°F
Heart rate	>140 beats/min	>225, <140 beats/min	>140 beats/min
Respiratory rate	>30 breaths/min	>40 breaths/min	>20 breaths/min
White blood cell count	>19,000<6000	>19,500, <5000 >5% bands	>12,000<4000

- Sepsis = evidence of infection (suspected or confirmed) and the clinical picture of the systemic inflammatory response syndrome (SIRS + infection)
- Severe sepsis = sepsis complicated by acute organ dysfunction (tissue hypoperfusion or end organ dysfunction)
- Septic shock: despite adequate intravascular fluid resuscitation, persistent hypotension and acute circulatory failure
- Multiple organ dysfunction syndrome (MODS): physiologic derangements of at least 2 major organ systems associated with SIRS and due to a serious potentially life-threatening insult.

Data from Levy MM, Fink MP, Marshall JC, et al; International Sepsis Definitions Conference. 2001 SCCM/ESICM/ACCP/ATS/SIS International Sepsis Definitions Conference. *Intensive Care Med* 2003;29(4):530-538.

are that SIRS criteria lack specificity, and there are many false positives. In dogs, the sensitivity ranges from 77% to 97% while the specificity is between 64% and 77%; there are no corresponding studies in cats [4]. Severe sepsis is defined as SIRS with evidence of organ dysfunction, and septic shock is severe sepsis with persistent hypotension and acute circulatory failure despite adequate intravascular fluid resuscitation [3].

Definitions of sepsis and septic shock in human medicine were updated in 2016 with the release of the third international consensus definitions (Sepsis-3) [5] (Box 1). This third iteration of the Surviving Sepsis Campaign (SSC) now defines sepsis as a "life-threatening organ dysfunction caused by a dysregulated host response to infection" [5]. This new definition moves the focal point to the mortality caused by organ dysfunction. Conversely, in veterinary medicine, the definition has not been updated for nearly 2 decades and mirrors the Sepsis-2 definition. The Sepsis-3 definition removed the severe sepsis label, and septic shock is defined as "a subset of sepsis in which underlying circulatory and cellular metabolism abnormalities are profound enough to substantially increase mortality." Patients with septic shock can be identified by persistent hypotension requiring vasopressors to maintain mean arterial pressure (MAP) ≥65 mm Hg and a serum lactate level greater than 2 mmol/L despite adequate volume resuscitation [5].

Organ dysfunction is defined as an increase of 2 points or more in the Sequential Organ Failure Assessment (SOFA) score (see Box 1). The SOFA score has been validated and can be used in the human intensive care unit (ICU) patient population [6–10]. It is a clinical prediction tool to determine level of acuity and mortality risk by quantifying end organ dysfunction in septic patients. It can be used for quality assessment, as a research tool, and as a prognostic indicator. It is based on the degree of dysfunction of 6 organ systems: respiratory, cardiovascular, central nervous system, renal, hepatic, and coagulation. The score is calculated at the time of admission and every 24 hours until the time of discharge. Points are assigned and codified for a total score between 0 and 24. Mortality risk is then stratified based on initial, mean, and highest values [6]. In veterinary medicine, the SOFA score has not yet been validated in small animal patients, as such Sepsis-3 definitions are not yet applicable. In the emergency setting, a quick SOFA (qSOFA) score may identify

BOX 1
Human Definitions and Diagnostic Criteria

Sepsis-3.0 (SEP-3) definitions: This is the current recommendation but has had some difficulty in being adopted

- *Sepsis:* a life-threatening organ dysfunction caused by a dysregulated host response to infection.
- Clinically, a SOFA score+ (see below) increase of 2 or more points can be used to characterize organ dysfunction
- *Severe sepsis:* removed from the definition

ICU setting: organ dysfunction is defined as an increase of 2 points or more in the Sequential Organ Failure Assessment (SOFA) score.

The SOFA score has been validated and can be used in the ICU patient population. It is a clinical prediction tool to determine level of acuity and mortality risk by quantifying end organ dysfunction in septic patients. It can be used for quality assessment, as a research tool, and as a prognostic indicator. It is based on the degree of dysfunction of 6 organ systems:

1. Respiration (Pao_2/Fio_2, mm Hg)
2. Coagulation (platelet count $\times$ 10^3/mm^3)
3. Liver (bilirubin concentration mg/dL)
4. Cardiovascular (MAP mm Hg)
5. Central nervous system (Glasgow coma score)
6. Renal (creatinine mg/dL or urine output ml/kg/h).

The score is calculated on admission and every 24 hours until discharge. Points are assigned and tabulated for a total score between 0 and 24. Mortality risk is then stratified based on initial, mean, and highest values.

Emergency setting: $\geq$2 or more of the following criteria for the *quick SOFA (qSOFA)* score may identify high-risk patients with suspected infection outside the ICU with increased mortality:

1. Altered mental status
2. Respiratory rate $\geq$22 breaths per minutes
3. Systolic blood pressure of $\leq$100 mm Hg

- *Septic Shock:* a subset of sepsis in which particularly profound circulatory, cellular, and metabolic abnormalities are associated with a greater risk of mortality than with sepsis alone. Clinically identified by a serum lactate level greater than 2 mmol/L (>18 mg/dL) in the absence of hypovolemia or vasopressor requirement to maintain MAP of 65 mm Hg or greater.

Data from Refs. [5–14].

patients with increased mortality. The qSOFA was retrospectively acquired and internally validated inside and outside the ICU setting. If patients have two or more of the following criteria — altered mental status, respiratory rate $\geq$22 breaths per minutes, and/or systolic blood pressure of $\leq$100 mm Hg and have suspected infection — then they are at high risk of in-hospital mortality [11–14]. However, the publication of the new definitions and diagnostic criteria by the SSC has been contentious and has potential limitations.

SIGNIFICANCE (IN DEPTH ANALYSIS)

Surviving Sepsis Campaign Guidelines for Management of Sepsis and Septic Shock

The embryonic SSC guidelines for management of sepsis and septic shock in human medicine were first published in 2004 and then amended in 2008, 2012, and 2016. The current version is the third iteration based on updated scientific evidence assimilated into the evolving manuscript. A consensus committee of 55 international experts representing 25 international organizations was assembled in 2016 for this task [15]. The SSC guidelines are a resource document that can guide the clinician through different aspects of the management continuum and offers practical, evidence-based recommendations for the management of "prototypical" septic patient. It gives a narrative about the approach to treating a septic patient—starting with diagnosis, acute resuscitation, antimicrobial therapy, source control, and fluid/vasoactive therapy and then advancing through organ support and adjunctive therapy recommendations (refer Box 2 for a summary of key recommendations).

BOX 2
Summary and Highlights of the SSC Guidelines

1. *Initial resuscitation:* recommend at least 30 mL/kg crystalloid fluid in first 3 hours (no recommendations on 0.9% NaCl vs balanced solution), albumin infusion is recommended if patients require "substantial" fluids (weak)
   - Use dynamic resuscitation markers (eg, passive leg raise) to target an MAP of 65 mm Hg, reassess hemodynamic status to guide resuscitation, normalize lactate.
2. *Vasopressors:* (target MAP >65 mm Hg)
   a. Norepinephrine is first line vasopressor
   b. Epinephrine is second line vasopressor if not at target MAP or vasopressin to reduce norepinephrine requirement
   c. Avoid dopamine in most patients (tachyarrhythmia)
3. *Steroids:* only indicated for patients with septic shock refractory to adequate fluids and vasopressors (CIRCI)
4. *Antibiotics:* initial broad-spectrum antibiotics
   a. Against combined therapy (No double coverage for pseudomonas)
   b. May use procalcitonin to guide de-escalation
5. *Source control:* achieve as soon as medically and logically feasible
6. *Ventilator:* 6 mL/kg tidal volume, prone patients with severe ARDS (P/F <150)
7. SSC Bundle 2018 Update
   a. 2018 updates previous 3-h and 6-h bundles into one 1-h bundle
   b. Adequate resuscitation may take greater than 1 hr, but should be started immediately

Data from Rhodes A, Evans LE, Alhazzani W, et al. Surviving Sepsis Campaign: international guidelines for management of sepsis and septic shock: 2016. *Crit Care Med* 2017;45(3):486-552.

A conceptual approach for how to best interpret and constructively use the 2016 SSC guidelines for the management of sepsis and septic shock is by using the concentric circles model. An analogy to better explain this model is by evoking images of the ripples that radiate when a pebble is thrown into a lake. The inner or core concentric circle represents the collated existing scientific data which have been categorized into tables based on quality of evidence and magnitude of benefit or harm. The clinician scientist with a special interest in sepsis may use this resource to critically evaluate evidentiary tables and grading of that evidence to gain better insight into the logic used for the recommendations, especially if it differs from what is expected. One can also compare and contrast differences in the 2012 and 2016 guidelines, often referred to as Sepsis-2 and Sepsis-3, respectively. The next concentric circle symbolizes the tenets of sepsis management. A clinician who wants to gain a deeper understanding, to learn more about both the recommendations and the thought processes behind them (ie, the evidence and physiologic underpinnings), can review the new recommendations and corresponding rationale. The outermost concentric circle denotes the clinical practice recommendations for the essential management of sepsis. These have been abridged into a 7-page document that can be used immediately by the frontline clinician in their decision-making and patient management. These clinicians can review new recommendations and refer to the explanation for better clarity [16].

The significance of the strength of recommendations (weak or strong) in the SSC guidelines document is that they are actionable. A strong recommendation signifies that the intervention should be part of usual care in all or almost all cases. A weak recommendation, rather, may not be followed by some clinicians for certain patients in particular scenarios, but in most contexts, clinicians would want to adhere to the guidelines. While acknowledging the complexity and heterogeneity of patients with an array of pathologies and comorbidities, clinical reasoning may dictate that even a strong recommendation is not advisable for a patient. The most widely used framework called Grading of Recommendations, Assessment, Development, and Evaluations (GRADE) provides a systematic approach for making clinical practice recommendations. This is the tool used by the SSC for grading quality of evidence into 4 levels ranging from high to very low. Evidence from randomized controlled trials, for example, starts at a high-quality level. The certainty in evidence is shifted by many determinants, which either decrease the level (risk of bias, imprecision, inconsistency, indirectness, and publication bias) or increase it (large magnitude of effect, dose-response gradient) [17]. The best-practice statement recommendations are considered strong recommendations but are devoid of evidentiary literature because they are common sense [15,16].

Concerns that rigidly adhering to the guidelines will undermine individualized patient care, in essence practicing "cook-book" medicine, have been expressed by some in the medical community. There is apprehension about blindly following and using prescriptive medicine especially given the kaleidoscopic nature of sepsis. Advocates purport that those recommendations are there to aid the busy, time-pressured clinician and provide general treatment guidance; this does not preclude clinicians from using their own clinical acumen [16]. Controversy surrounds the recommendation for administration of antibiotics within the 1-hour timeframe of diagnosis of sepsis. This resistance is likely due to logistical barriers and harm from reflexive inappropriate antibiotic use that may promote multiple-drug-resistant bacteria and *Clostridium difficile* colitis [18]. Proponents of this mandate argue that this is an "aspirational recommendation" especially for the subset of patients with septic shock and represents best practices that the health care team should strive to operationalize. A sepsis care bundle refers to an amalgamation of interventions which, when instituted collectively, have a positive effect on outcome compared with when implemented alone [19]. Care bundles are considered the bedrock of quality improvement in the treatment of sepsis since they were started in 2005. The SSC in 2018 updated previous 3-hour and 6-hour bundles into one 1-hour bundle during which time lactate introduction, blood cultures before initiating antibiotics, broad-spectrum antibiotic administration, a rapid 30-mL/kg crystalloid fluid bolus, and starting vasopressors if the patient is hypotensive during or after fluid resuscitation are strongly recommended. Authors of the SSC guidelines acknowledge that adequate resuscitation may take more than 1 hour but that it should be started urgently [16].

The progenitor study for the inception of the SSC was the Early Goal-Directed Therapy (EGDT) trial [20]. This single-center, randomized, controlled trial in the emergency setting recommended an aggressive, goal-directed resuscitation strategy within 6 hours of presentation. The five key elements of this protocol targeted optimizing oxygen delivery to tissues using these end goals: central venous pressure (CVP) 8 to 12 mm Hg, MAP 65 to 90 mm Hg, urine output greater than 0.5 mL/kg/h, mixed venous oxygen saturation greater than 65%/central venous oxygen saturation (ScvO2) greater than 70%, and hematocrit greater than 30%. This landmark trial showed a 16% reduction in mortality [20]. These treatment goals were implemented into and were the foundation of the SSC. Subsequent randomized trials and literature have not been able to replicate the mortality benefit. The 3 most well-known trials are the ARISE, PROMISE, and PROCESS trials, based in Australia and New Zealand, United States, and UK, respectively, which have collectively shown no significant difference in mortality between EGDT versus usual care. Thus protocol-based care and invasive monitoring (central venous catheter hemodynamic monitoring and central venous oxygen saturation) may not be helpful, and some critics have warned of the potential harm of protocolized care for patients with severe sepsis and septic shock [21–23].

An alternative explanation for these findings may be that awareness of early recognition and initiation of resuscitation with endpoints has led to overall better care despite using a specific protocol. The components of the EGDT protocol have not endured, and subsequent studies have not reproduced corroborating results. In addition to the lack of repeatable results, the study has been criticized because of a conflict of interest that the primary investigator held a patent for the central catheter used to measure the mixed central venous saturation. Other limitations include nonblinding at a single-center hospital and above-average mortality rate in the control group (47%) [24].

PRESENT RELEVANCE AND FUTURE AVENUES TO CONSIDER OR TO INVESTIGATE

Clinicians in the ICU setting provide comprehensive care for patients with acute and chronic life-threatening conditions. Sepsis is the quintessential illness in critical care medicine as it is ubiquitous, potentially fatal, and treatable. Practitioners learn to recognize and respond to the complexity, uncertainty, and ambiguity ingrained in critical care medicine practice by performing patient-centered clinical assessment and establish a management plan. They elicit a history, perform a clinically relevant focused physical examination, select appropriate diagnostic testing, and interpret the results for the purpose of diagnosis and therapeutic management, disease prevention, and patient advocacy. Procedures or therapies are prioritized, taking into account clinical urgency and available resources.

Crucial clinical questions and use of evidence-based medicine and clinical reasoning are essential to guide patient management decisions. At present, there are no evidence-based veterinary guidelines or recommendations on management of sepsis and septic shock comparable to SSC. The development and implementation of specific, evidence-based clinical guidelines for management of sepsis are a requisite in veterinary medicine. A similar approach to that used for the Reassessment Campaign on Veterinary Resuscitation (RECOVER) CPR initiative could be used. The main aims would be to

1. Develop, publish, and revise evidence-based, consensus veterinary sepsis management guidelines through comprehensive review of the sepsis literature;
2. Identify knowledge gaps or areas of sepsis management that require further inquiry;
3. Implement guidelines and collect data for outcomes assessment.

DISCUSSION

Diagnosis

Clinical reasoning and diagnostic schema

Context serves as a framework for predicting which information might be useful to gather, which tests might be valuable, and which diagnostic procedures deserve further attention. When acquiring history from the owner, use the presenting complaint and clinical reasoning to direct questioning: (1) obtain a focused complete pertinent history in an organized fashion. Information on chronic underlying illnesses (chronic kidney disease, chronic degenerative valvular disease, neoplasia, hepatopathy), foreign body ingestion, current medications (steroids, nonsteroidal anti-inflammatory drugs, chemotherapeutic drugs), travel history (endemic infections), temporal association with current clinical signs (acute onset, progressive deterioration), trauma (bite wounds), and previous invasive procedures (recent surgeries, implants, invasive medical devices) is helpful to solicit from owners; (2) perform a clinically relevant thorough physical examination germane to the patient's presenting complaint. An ill-appearing patient with vomiting, dehydration, and abdominal pain ("praying position") with a penchant for chewing toys would prompt the clinician to consider acute abdomen differentials such as septic peritonitis; (3) interpret findings based on the clinical setting and how they increase or decrease likelihood of differentials; (4) develop a reasonable working differential diagnosis list for the patient's major problem(s) by critically evaluating the findings supporting the differential and identifying inconsistencies in physical examination or history; (5) organize and rank differentials based on most likely and cannot miss life-threatening causes such as sepsis, (6) recommend an appropriate prioritized diagnostic plan based on the patient's status, clinical reasoning, evidence-based medicine, situational awareness, cost awareness, and shared decision-making with the owner for testing decisions. This will help guide efficient, directed diagnostic workup. In the aforementioned example, the first tier of diagnostics consists of emergency blood work (PCV/TS, lactate, blood glucose, blood urea nitrogen, blood smear), Doppler blood pressure, point-of-care ultrasound of the abdomen, and abdominocentesis if there is any free fluid with cytology and/or biochemical analysis.

Dogs (clinical features)

In dogs, the gastrointestinal (GI) tract is the most common nidus of infection and, in one study, accounted for approximately 35% of cases of sepsis. The second-most common source was from pneumonia (20%), followed by trauma [25]. Gram-negative infections and specifically *Escherichia coli* was the most common organism isolated, followed by *Streptococcus* species. The clinical manifestations of sepsis are dynamic and vary across a wide acuity spectrum. This variation results from multiple factors such as focus of infection, causative pathogen, underlying immunologic status, chronic comorbidities, acute organ dysfunction, and temporal association with treatment intervention. On triage evaluation, patients often, but not always, appear ill, especially in the early stages of sepsis or in compensatory shock. They often have altered mental status (obtunded), are laterally recumbent, and are not interested in their environment.

Signs of SIRS and/or compensatory shock in dogs typically manifest as a hyperdynamic response that is typified by tachycardia, tachypnea, fever, hyperemic mucous membranes with rapid capillary refill time, and bounding pulses secondary to wide pulse pressure with proportionally lower diastolic blood pressure. The shock index (heart rate/systolic blood pressure) may be a helpful diagnostic tool to detect occult shock [26–29]. There is currently no prospective study validating the use of the shock index to guide resuscitation in veterinary patients with septic shock. Depending on the magnitude of hemodynamic instability, a low blood pressure may be recorded (<90 mm Hg systolic, <65 mm Hg MAP, narrow pulse pressure). Overt signs of end organ hypoperfusion manifest as prolonged CRT, low rectal temperature, hypokinetic pulses, and decreased urine production. Hyperlactatemia likely represents physiologic stress and mirrors levels of endogenous catecholamines and will be discussed in more detail later.

Bloodwork may reveal abnormalities in inflammatory indices such as leukocytosis, leukopenia, left shift, toxic neutrophil changes, and elevated neutrophil to lymphocyte ratio. Serum biochemistry shows a constellation of aberrations such as initial hyperglycemia (stress response) and then later hypoglycemia, hypoproteinemia, hypoalbuminemia, hyperbilirubinemia [30,31], elevated liver values, and azotemia [32]. Elevated liver enzyme activities have been associated with increased mortality in dogs with septic peritonitis. Acid-base and electrolyte abnormalities commonly consist of a metabolic acidosis with hyperlactatemia, hypocalcemia, hyperkalemia or hypokalemia, dysnatremias, and disturbances in the sodium-to-chloride ratio. Organ dysfunction variables to track are arterial hypoxemia (VQ mismatch), acute oliguria (urine output <0.5 mL/kg/h, elevated creatinine or increase of >0.3 mg/dL above baseline), coagulation abnormalities (elevated PT/PTT, thrombocytopenia, elevated D dimers and fibrin degradation products, low fibrinogen levels, decreased antithrombin levels, protein C deficiency) [25,33,34], GI dysmotility (gastroparesis, intestinal ileus), and hyperbilirubinemia. Hyperbilirubinemia has been reported in dogs and cats with gram-negative bacterial sepsis and septic shock [31]. Cause of hypocalcemia in sepsis has not been fully elucidated and is probably multifactorial. Proposed mechanisms are suppression of the parathyroid gland by cytokines resulting in decreased levels of parathyroid hormone, electrolyte derangements (hypomagnesemia), alkalosis, elevated procalcitonin concentrations, chelation with anions, and dysregulated calcium homeostasis (inadequate vitamin D concentrations and parathyroid hormone/vitamin D resistance) [35,36]. Urinalysis and urine culture and sensitivity may lead to the source of infection. Imaging studies such as radiography, contrast radiography, ultrasonography, computed tomography scan, and MRI can also aid in the identification of the source of infection.

Acute kidney injury

Acute kidney injury (AKI) is a clinical syndrome defined by alteration of renal homeostatic functions resulting in rapid decrease in renal excretory function and accumulation of the nitrogenous waste products creatinine and urea, dysregulation of volume balance, acid-base derangements manifested by metabolic acidosis, electrolyte abnormalities such as hyperkalemia and hyperphosphatemia, and changes in urine output. Kidney Disease Improving Global Outcomes (KDIGO), the international nephrology guideline organization, has established a consensus definition and staging criteria for AKI that have been validated and correlated with severity of illness, mortality rate, and length of hospitalization in human patients. It has replaced two other similar systems, the RIFLE criteria and AKIN system [37]. The Veterinary Acute Kidney Injury (VAKI) score is an AKI staging system that was retrospectively applied to 164 hospitalized dogs that were classified into stages 0 to 3 based on creatinine level increase from baseline. Patients in stage 1 to 3 were less likely to survive to discharge, and only 4 of 19 dogs in stage 1 had creatinine levels above the reference range [38]. AKI can be divided into three broad categories based on etiology, namely prerenal azotemia (hemodynamic), intrinsic renal failure, and postrenal azotemia (obstructive uropathy) [39]. AKI is documented to occur in 12% of dogs with septic peritonitis, with 14% of those surviving to discharge [2]. Causes include maldistribution of blood flow within the different regions of the kidney, proinflammatory response, oxidative stress (ischemia reperfusion injury, reactive oxygen species), epithelial dysfunction, tubular absorption dysfunction, disruption of tight junctions resulting in interstitial edema, and disruption of basement membrane adhesions resulting in sloughing of tubular cells causing obstruction and casts. Sublethal damage may result in tubulointerstitial fibrosis and chronic kidney disease [40].

Cat (clinical features)

There is significant individual variation, but often cats have a different clinical pattern or septic phenotype in contrast to dogs. Common clinical features in feline patients encompass tachypnea, bradycardia, hypothermia, lethargy, nonlocalizing abdominal pain (43% [41] and 62% [42] of septic peritonitis patients), vomiting (48%) [41], weak pulses, anemia, band neutrophilia, hypoalbuminemia, and icterus [43]. Unlike the changes observed in dogs with sepsis, cats display a hypodynamic state with bradycardia (16%–66%) [42], hypothermia, and hypotension. Clinical diagnoses included pyothorax, septic peritonitis, bacteremia secondary to GI tract disease, pneumonia, endocarditis, pyelonephritis, osteomyelitis, pyometra, and bite wounds [43].

Bradycardia and hypothermia are negative prognostic indicators and can be used in risk stratification [42,43]. It is postulated that bradycardic septic feline patients represent an advanced decompensatory stage of sepsis, as early clinical signs may go unnoticed by owners. Cats typically show an exuberant physiologic stress response in the hospital setting. Catecholamine stores may become depleted, or receptors desensitized in the context of severe acute injury or plausibly in patients with chronic underlying pathology and organ dysfunction. One may posit that the sickest cats develop an autonomic neuropathy due to loss of coordination between vagal and sympathetic activity. Anemia is a common laboratory finding, and the pathogenesis is assumably manifold from iatrogenic causes (hemodilution, frequent blood sampling), oxidative damage (decreased antioxidant stores, reactive sulfhydryl groups on the hemoglobin molecule), decreased production and dampened response to erythropoietin due to inflammatory mediators, blood loss (gastrointestinal bleeding), and hemolysis (mechanical and immune-mediated). Hypochloremia may be a negative prognostic indicator in cats with sepsis and SIRS [44], and hyperglycemia was greater in septic cats that did not survive [45].

A prospective, observational study evaluated a population of cats with a variety of underlying etiologies for sepsis and found a 63% survival rate. Pyothorax was the most common nidus of infection, followed by septic peritonitis and viral infection. Common clinical abnormalities included nonspecific signs such as dehydration, lethargy, anorexia, pale mucous membranes, and dullness. New laboratory findings included metarubricytosis, hypertriglyceridemia, and high circulating muscle enzyme activities. Coagulation abnormalities showed median activated partial thromboplastin time, plasma D-dimer concentrations were significantly higher, and total protein C and antithrombin activities were significantly lower, as compared to healthy controls [31]. In another population of cats with septic peritonitis, a retrospective study found an overall survival rate of 56%. Frequency of ionized hypocalcemia was 89% at the time of diagnosis and in 93% of cats at any time point during hospitalization. Failure to resolve their ionized hypocalcemia correlated to decreased survival [46].

Pathogenesis of vasodilation in septic shock

Normal response to hypotension is profound vasoconstriction through activation of neurohormonal mechanisms such as activation of the sympathetic nervous system, renin-angiotensin aldosterone system, and antidiuretic hormone. Vasodilatory shock is likely due to the imbalance of the numerous, interactive mechanisms involved in vasodilation and vasoconstriction. The three crucial mechanisms for the pathologic vasodilation and blunted response to endogenous vasopressors characteristic of septic shock are activation of ATP-sensitive potassium channels (K_{ATP}) in the plasma membrane of vascular smooth muscles, increased production of nitric oxide (NO) through activation of inducible nitric oxide synthase, and depletion of vasopressin [47]. This is the rationale for a fixed-dose vasopressin constant rate infusion (CRI) in the background of norepinephrine infusion in septic shock patients. In a prospective, observational study in dogs, NO breakdown products (nitrate/nitrite) were significantly greater in septic and noninfectious SIRS dogs than those in healthy controls [48]. Septic shock is characterized by vasoplegia of both the afferent (arterial) and efferent (venous) segments of the circulatory system. The venous vasculature, capacitance vessels, contains approximately 70% of blood volume at any one time. Venoconstriction shifts the unstressed volume to stressed volume and increases venous return. Arterial constriction increases the driving pressure (upstream pressure) and may improve perfusion. Degree and duration of hypotension correlate with outcome [49].

A practical systematic approach of sequentially assessing heart rate, volume status, cardiac performance, and systemic vascular resistance can narrow the differential and guide management. Frequent reassessment of septic patients to evaluate response to intervention and avoidance of underresuscitating or overresuscitating with fluids is important. A systematic assessment of the patient's heart rate and rhythm, effective circulating volume and venous return, myocardial function with focused echocardiography, and consideration of systemic vascular resistance in animals with disproportionately decreased diastolic pressure can help guide a clinician to improve hemodynamics and perfusion. A focused echocardiography can help identify the presence of pericardial effusion, heart chamber size, and whether contractility is normal.

Treatment

Resuscitation

Practices for initial hemodynamic resuscitation and management of sepsis and septic shock patients have changed with time. Fluid therapy has been the cornerstone for resuscitation in patients with evidence of septic shock. Often aliquots of isotonic crystalloid fluids are rapidly administered in patients deemed to be fluid-responsive until they are assessed to be volume replete. Then, aliquots of synthetic colloids are used in combination with crystalloids. If there is evidence of ongoing hypoperfusion then vasopressors are initiated until end goals of blood pressure and other end organ perfusion parameters are met. Steroids are added in patients that remain unresponsive to both fluids and vasopressors. This strategy involves escalating resuscitation over several hours resulting in the most severely affected patients remaining hypotensive for an extended time period. Recent evidence and practice provide rationale for the early use of vasopressors [49], conservative use of fluids [50] (smaller boluses over longer time period), avoidance of synthetic colloids [51], use of plasma or albumin [52] for resuscitation, and considerations for steroids [53].

An accelerated goal-directed resuscitation strategy may be beneficial in the sickest subset of patients so as to escalate multiple interventions simultaneously and quickly to achieve resuscitation goals. The primary goal is to achieve an MAP greater than 65 mm Hg as soon as possible by initiating an infusion of norepinephrine contemporaneously with intravenous fluid resuscitation. The author typically starts a norepinephrine CRI at a mid-range of 0.5 mcg/kg/min through a peripheral catheter. It can be titrated up or down depending on patient response. It is reasonable to consider a background fixed dose of vasopressin CRI as there is evidence of vasopressin deficiency in vasodilatory shock, and it may work synergistically with norepinephrine. Epinephrine may be considered early as a second-line vasopressor if blood pressure goals are not being met and to augment cardiac output [54]. Exceedingly ill patients with decompensatory shock that are inadequately responding to initial aggressive stabilization efforts may benefit from early steroids.

Early goal-directed therapy

A prospective observational veterinary study [55], using protocolized care (similar to EGDT) [20], to treat severe sepsis and septic shock dogs with pyometra evaluated the changes in ScvO2, lactate, and base deficit in response to goal-directed therapy and correlated these values with mortality. Overall mortality was 36%, with 12 of 13 patients in the septic shock group dying. Nonsurvivors had greater need for vasoactive drugs (dopamine) and crystalloids during the initial resuscitation period (<7.5 hours). Nonsurvivors also had lower ScvO2, higher base deficits, and higher lactate, but there was no significant effect of change in parameters on mortality. This study had no control cohort for comparison to the relatively homogenous population of dogs with pyometra [55]. Approach to patients with sepsis and septic shock should be individualized rather than based on rigid, inflexible protocols [56].

Lactate

Lactate has been used as a surrogate marker of hypoperfusion and to guide resuscitation efforts especially regarding fluid therapy. Traditional dogma dictates that in sepsis, impaired microcirculatory flow, tissue hypoxia, and resultant anaerobic metabolism cause elevation in lactate levels, which has directed tactics to increase oxygen delivery [57]. A newer paradigm is that lactate generation is due to physiologic stress and occurs aerobically in nearly all clinical conditions. In times of physiologic stress, release of compensatory catecholamines increases glycolysis by beta agonism to produce more pyruvate to enter the mitochondrial Tricarboxylic acid cycle for energy production. Excess pyruvate is converted to lactate by the enzyme lactate dehydrogenase because the Krebs cycle operates at a slower pace than the glycolytic influx and not because of an oxygen deficiency [58,59]. This phenomenon can be demonstrated by administering exogenous epinephrine which leads to elevated lactate levels. This stress hyperlactatemia is analogous to stress hyperglycemia or sinus tachycardia. Lactate is not harmful per se and has beneficial effects as a biofuel, facilitates carbon shuttling in vital organs such as the brain and heart, and may improve cardiac performance [60]. Elevated lactate levels may also reveal the presence of an occult catecholamine-dependent shock state which is being masked by relatively normal vitals [59]. Lactate is a better prognostic parameter; it likely represents ongoing physiologic stress and corresponds to severity of illness [61].

This misconception of using lactate to drive fluid resuscitation has been deeply ingrained in critical care practice especially as it pertains to septic patients. It is also embedded in the definition of septic shock by the SSC. The common practice of reflexively bolusing fluid in response to an elevated lactate may be detrimental in some situations. Lactate-guided resuscitation has been called into question especially after results of the ADROMEDA-SHOCK trial [62] which showed a trend toward potential harm. This study compared CRT-guided versus lactate-guided resuscitation strategy in human septic shock patients; the primary outcome was the 28-day mortality rate, which was 34.9% in the CRT group versus 43.4% in the lactate group, which was not statistically significantly different [62]. It is crucial that a clinician understand the underlying physiology of lactate to interpret this parameter appropriately. Treatment of hyperlactatemia should be aimed at identifying and addressing the underlying cause.

Lactate as a prognostic indicator in dogs is well documented in the literature; however, most studies have been retrospective with their inherent limitations. Association between high initial lactate and poorer outcomes in a variety of illnesses such as SIRS and sepsis, severe soft-tissue infection, shock, trauma, Gastric dilatation volvulus, and others has been described [63,64]. There is a dearth of feline lactate studies, and results are variable and less consistent than those for dogs. Admission lactate of >4 mmol/L has been associated with lower survival and increased length of hospitalization. In regard to lactate clearance, with a lactate greater than 4 mmol/L and a decrease of greater then 30% within 8 hours of admission resulted in higher survival than lactate clearance of less than 30% [41,42].

Fluid therapy

Hypovolemia is a very common contributing factor to shock in small animal patients. A septic patient is often systemically ill and decreases water intake because of nausea. They may also have increased GI losses due to vomiting and/or diarrhea or have third space losses (septic peritonitis) resulting in hypovolemia. Treatment for hypovolemic shock primarily includes volume resuscitation with intravenous (IV) fluids. It is reasonable to use pH-appropriate resuscitation fluids to avoid exacerbating underlying acid base and electrolyte abnormalities. In most scenarios, a balanced isotonic fluid such an lactated ringer solution or Plasmalyte-A would suffice. While intravenous fluid therapy may be an initial step in management of hypovolemia, vasopressors to increase vascular resistance also should be considered in the early treatment of sepsis.

The endothelial glycocalyx

Starling's original theory of capillary fluid dynamics has been updated, especially with a new perception of the integral role of the glycocalyx [65]. It has led to a better understanding of the mechanism of edema formation in critically ill patients with SIRS and sepsis [66]. Colloid osmotic pressure does not cause the bidirectional movement of fluid, as interstitial and intravascular colloid osmotic pressures are very similar. Extravasation of fluid from the capillaries is predominantly dependent on capillary hydrostatic pressure, and not on decreased intravascular colloid osmotic pressure as was previously thought [67]. Thus, it makes sense to minimize rapid increases in capillary hydrostatic pressure with administration of large rapid fluid boluses. This rationale has led to the use of small-volume crystalloid boluses and early use of alpha-agonists such as norepinephrine. Afferent arteriolar constriction dampens the increase in capillary hydrostatic pressures. Albumin is needed for the integrity of endothelial glycocalyx, and the use of albumin and plasma may be protective to the glycocalyx. Plasma is reasonable to consider as a resuscitation fluid because availability of albumin is unpredictable and may be cost-prohibitive. The lymphatics play a pivotal role in the prevention of edema formation by returning interstitial fluid to the venous circulation. They have calcium-dependent contractile collecting ducts that are inhibited by atrial natriuretic peptide [68]. In addition, this hormone denudes the glycocalyx which then results in increased permeability [69].

Fluid therapy requires careful management of a neutral fluid balance which involves clinical assessment of both interstitial hydration and intravascular volume status. A fluid prescription is a fluid treatment plan personalized for the specific patient, taking into consideration the indications, fluid choice, dose, duration, contraindications, and adverse effects. When selecting a fluid type, patient and fluid pH, osmolality, and distribution into compartments should be considered. The goal of acute resuscitation in hypotensive patients is to restore effective circulating volume and organ perfusion and then maintain intravascular volume homeostasis without fluid accumulation [70]. Repeated and frequent reassessment of fluid and electrolyte balance is used to direct appropriate changes in the treatment plan in response to the rapidly changing clinical situation.

Albumin

Hypoalbuminemia is common in sepsis and is caused by a composite of factors such as leakage from vasculature (eg, SIRS, wounds, peritonitis), inflammation (negative acute phase protein, denatured), decreased production (liver failure), and dilution with large-volume crystalloid infusions. In human patients with severe sepsis, hypoalbuminemia is associated with a higher risk of mortality [71]. The SSC suggests using a combination of albumin in addition to crystalloids for initial resuscitation of patients with sepsis and septic shock, when large volumes of crystalloids are required [15]. Albumin is needed for the integrity of the glycocalyx and the use of albumin and plasma as resuscitation fluids may be protective to the glycocalyx. The 2008 SAFE study [52] evaluated 4% albumin versus 0.9% NaCl during fluid resuscitation for human patients with septic shock. There was no difference between groups in terms of mortality but worse outcomes in patients with traumatic brain injury [72]. A post-hoc analysis of the 2014 ALBIOS study [73] revealed significant improvement in 90-day mortality in severe sepsis and septic shock patients receiving 20% albumin to maintain albumin >3 g/dL. Other advantages included faster hemodynamic stabilization and reduced requirement for vasopressors.

In a prospective randomized clinical trial, 5% canine-specific albumin was safely administered to treat hypoalbuminemia in a subset of dogs with septic peritonitis after surgical source control. The transfusion resulted in a significant increase in albumin, colloid osmotic pressure, and diastolic blood pressure 2 hours after administration; the increase in albumin persisted at 24 hours compared with the control group. One dog experienced tachypnea during infusion and died 120 hours later of unknown respiratory causes [74]. The use of 25% human albumin is controversial in veterinary medicine. Adverse reactions have been documented in healthy dogs, and the risk of anaphylactoid and severe delayed type III hypersensitivity reactions is high because of the production of antihuman albumin antibodies. It has been postulated that critically ill, immunocompromised patients are less likely to show an increase in hypersensitivity response to the foreign protein. However, a recent case report described severe type III hypersensitivity reactions in 2 canine patients with septic peritonitis receiving a transfusion of 25% human albumin which resulted in AKI and death [75]. Cryo-poor plasma infusion may be a viable option for treatment of hypoalbuminemia and to maintain effective circulating volume [76,77].

Vasopressors

Triggers for the initiation of vasopressor therapy comprise the following clinical parameters indicative of hypoperfusion: altered mental status in an ill-appearing patient, prolonged CRT, hyper/hypokinetic pulse quality, MAP less than 65 mm Hg, and urine output <1 mL/kg/h. There is no consensus on initiation of vasopressor therapy, either early with concurrent fluid administration or later when patient is volume replete and no longer fluid responsive. Optimal choice of vasopressor/s (norepinephrine, epinephrine, dopamine, vasopressin) is also contentious and dependent on factors such as hemodynamic profile, concomitant organ dysfunction, and patient response to intervention target parameters. As mentioned previously, these patients likely will have global reduction in their systemic vascular resistance (vasoplegia) with resultant hypotension. However, these patients often have concomitant hypovolemia and potentially myocardial dysfunction. The Sepsis-3 guidelines recommend initiating vasopressors to maintain a MAP greater than 65 mm Hg if a patient is hypotensive during or after fluid resuscitation.

Norepinephrine is considered the first-line vasopressor [15]. Norepinephrine is more potent than dopamine, and evidence demonstrates lower risk of tachyarrhythmias and mortality. The use of dopamine as an alternative in highly selected patients showed no benefit for renal protection. Either vasopressin or epinephrine can be added to norepinephrine to raise MAP to target or add vasopressin to decrease norepinephrine dose [15]. Dobutamine in patients who show persistent hypoperfusion despite adequate fluid loading and the use of vasopressor agents is recommended. In a veterinary study that investigated vasopressin therapy in dogs with dopamine-resistant hypotension and vasodilatory shock, MAP increased after vasopressin therapy in all dogs, indicating that vasopressin may prove useful in the treatment of vasodilatory shock [78].

Norepinephrine

Norepinephrine, or noradrenaline, is a potent alpha-adrenergic agonist and has some beta-adrenergic agonism. It is regarded as an efficacious intervention in undifferentiated shock and septic shock. Because there is risk of tissue necrosis if it extravasates, it is ideally administered via a central venous catheter, but it is reasonable to use in a peripheral line in the initial resuscitation phase. In septic cats, because endogenous concentrations of endogenous catecholamines are high, these high concentrations may also cause desensitization of receptors [78].

Typical dosing range: 0.1-2 mcg/kg/min.

Epinephrine

Epinephrine, or adrenaline, is a constitutively expressed agonist for the gamut of adrenergic receptors. It has a dose-dependent spectrum of activity. At low doses, beta-adrenergic receptors are predominately stimulated; beta 1 receptor agonism augments contractility and increases heart rate, and beta 2 receptor agonism promotes smooth muscle relaxation. At escalating doses, alpha adrenergic 1 agonism prevails, inducing vasoconstriction. This versatile inopressor may be useful in the context of a septic patient with vasodilatory shock and concomitant sepsis-induced cardiomyopathy with systolic dysfunction. Pitfalls are that the dose-dependent response may be variable and unpredictable, and increased lactate levels due to beta 2 agonism may confound some methods to measure perfusion.

Typical dosing range is 0.05-1 mcg/kg/min.

Dopamine

Dopamine is converted to norepinephrine and eventually epinephrine in the body. At low doses, it predominately has dopaminergic effects. At medium doses (5–10 mcg/kg/min), mostly beta 1 adrenergic agonism occurs, and at high doses (10–15 mcg/kg/min), alpha 1 effects dominate. It is similar to epinephrine, is multimodal, is an inopressor, and has a variable response. It is more likely to cause tachyarrhythmia in humans and, as such, has fallen out of favor.

Typical dosing range is 5 to 15 mcg/kg/min.

Dobutamine

Dobutamine is an inodilator that augments cardiac performance and causes vasodilation. It has more affinity for beta 1 receptors than for beta 2 receptors. It also has mild alpha-agonist activity. Adverse effects such as tachyarrhythmias and neurologic signs in cats have been reported.

Typical dosing range is 2 to 15 μg/kg/min.

Vasopressin

Deficiency of vasopressin is also implicated in the pathogenesis of vasodilatory shock in sepsis possibly due to the depletion of vasopressin stores in prolonged states of stimulation. Vasopressin is needed in very low concentrations for V-2 receptor activity in the kidney (via increase in cGMP in distal tubular cells and principal cells of collecting ducts in the kidneys). Several fold higher concentrations are needed for V-1-mediated effects. Vasopressin binding to V-1 receptors causes opening of voltage-gated calcium channels and closure of the K_{ATP} channels, resulting in vasoconstriction. Because of the large amount of vasopressin needed for V-1 activity, the hypothalamus and posterior pituitary deplete their stores quickly. Vasopressin activity is resistant to acidemia unlike catecholamines, has no vasoconstricting effects on the pulmonary vasculature, and has no direct myocardial effects.

Typical dosing range is 0.5-5 U/kg/min.

Antibiotics

Antimicrobial therapy is the cornerstone for treatment of sepsis. Empiric intravenous antimicrobial therapy should be started as soon as it is feasible after appropriate cultures have been procured. The SSC guidelines recommend that "blood cultures should be obtained before administering antibiotics when possible, but this should not delay administration of antibiotics." Ideally blood cultures from 2 different locations should be acquired; in addition, cultures should be obtained from other suspected sources of infection such as urine, wounds, effusion, cerebral spinal fluid, intra-abdominal drains, lungs, and indwelling devices where indicated.

The SSC also recommends starting broad-spectrum intravenous empirical antimicrobials within 1 hour of recognition of sepsis/septic shock or as soon as possible [15]. A widely cited retrospective study of human ICU patients with severe sepsis and septic shock showed a direct correlation between mortality and time to initiation of antibiotic therapy, with a linear 7.6% increase in mortality and risk of end organ damage for every hour from the time of first measured hypotension to administration of effective antibiotics [79]. Delay in administration of antibiotics by 6 hours had a 43% survival rate versus 79.9% survival if given within 1 hour [79,80]. The feasibility of administration of antibiotics within 1 hour depends on clinicians' ability to recognize septic patients early and also on numerous logistical considerations such as nursing staff, caseload, financial considerations, pharmacy, vascular access, and drug administration protocol.

The choice of antibiotics is determined by multiple factors including patient-specific, disease-related, and pharmacotherapeutic elements. Identification of the most likely source or focus of infection and most commonly associated pathogens will help guide selection of empiric antimicrobial therapy. The patient's underlying disease state, immunologic status, and risk factors for a multiple-drug-resistant organism are important individual patient characteristics to consider. *Risk factors for infection with multidrug-resistant organisms include contemporaneous hospitalization, recent course of antimicrobial(s), and prolonged invasive medical devices such as vascular access port/catheter, chest tube, indwelling urinary catheter, and abdominal drains.* Dogs treated with enrofloxacin for 21 days shed large numbers of multiple-drug-resistant (MDR) *E. coli* in their feces, providing a source for MDR infections in other patients [81]. Knowledge of the clinic's antibiograms (eg, local microbiology and sensitivity patterns) should also be used to influence local practices and to assist in the development of specific infectious disease treatment protocols.

As the specific infecting pathogen(s) and sensitivity pattern(s) are unknown at the time of presentation, broad-spectrum coverage with two or more antibiotics is recommended. Adjustment and potential de-escalation to the narrowest effective spectrum can be done when the specific pathogen(s) has been isolated, and thus, targeted or definitive therapy can be used. Patients with septic peritonitis often have polymicrobial infections, with *E. coli*, *Clostridium spp.*, and *Enterococcus spp.* being the common bacterial isolates. Empirical selection to start may include a beta-lactamase plus aminoglycoside or fluroquinolone; metronidazole may be considered for better anaerobic (bacteroides) coverage. An aminoglycoside may not be ideal, however, because of risk of AKI. Limitations of fluroquinolones are due to emerging resistance patterns. In human medicine, there is a growing trend toward single-agent therapy with a third-generation cephalosporin and potential addition of metronidazole to increase anaerobic spectrum. Abdominal surgery and use of an antibiotic within

30 days before septic peritonitis were significantly associated with inappropriate antibiotic selection but did not affect survival outcome. In dogs with septic peritonitis, third-generation cephalosporins such as cefotaxime (22 mg/kg, IV, q 8 hours) or ceftazidime (30 mg/kg, IV, q4-8h) should be considered [80], as an empiric multimodal antibiotic regimen was not associated with improved outcome nor increased likelihood of appropriate empirical antibiotic selection [82]. However, cats treated with appropriate antibiotics were 4.4 times more likely to survive [45].

An antibiotic protocol for septic peritonitis in small animal patients was developed based on the SSC recommendations and evidence of survival benefit for early antibiotic administration [83]. This protocol was implemented in the small animal Emergency room setting to facilitate early diagnosis, timely interventions, and early antibiotic therapy in this subset of septic and septic shock patients. Options for antibiotic drug selection with broad spectrum, combination therapy, and suggested doses were provided to guide the clinician. This study however showed no significant difference in survival in the preprotocol (6 hours to antibiotic administration) versus postprotocol group (1 hour to antibiotic administration) and did not affect intraoperative culture results [84]. This mirrors findings in the only randomized human trial (PHANTASi trial) [84] looking at early intervention with antibiotics group (prehospital in the ambulance) versus usual care group (admission into the emergency department); the average time difference for initial administration of antibiotics was 96 minutes between the intervention and usual care group. There was no mortality benefit from early administration of antibiotics [84]. Interestingly, the only prospective study to date looking at aggressive versus conservative initiation of antibiotics in critically ill human surgical patients with hospital-acquired infection showed a positive effect for the more judicious antimicrobial approach [85]. Timely administration of antibiotics is recommended without the artificial time constraints of 1 hour, and choice of antibiotics is contextual. In patients with septic shock, high acuity, and severity, immediate administration of antibiotics is recommended. In patients with suspected sepsis that are not showing signs of shock, a clinician can potentially take the time to gather more clinical data to confirm diagnosis [18].

There are no clear guidelines for duration of antimicrobial therapy for septic and septic shock in small animal patients. Septic peritonitis patients are often discharged with a 7- to 14-day course of antibiotics [86]. De-escalation of the antimicrobial regimen according to susceptibility results and/or clinical response is strongly encouraged. Concerns for the overuse of antibiotics and potential complications such as increased antibiotic resistance, *C. difficile* infections, disruption of the gut microbiome, and organ dysfunction in human medicine support that shorter duration of antibiotics (3–5 days with rapid clinical resolution) results in clinical outcomes comparable to those in patients treated longer. A duration of 7 to 10 days is recommended for most serious infections plus septic shock. Development of biomarkers may help guide length of treatment, for example, C-reactive protein used to guide treatment of pneumonia [87]. The biomarker procalcitonin is the most widely studied biomarker for sepsis and has a role in antibiotic stewardship. Measurement of procalcitonin can potentially be used to differentiate between infectious and noninfectious causes of SIRS, prognosticate for risk stratification, organ dysfunction, and outcome, as well as be used therapeutically to guide initial antibiotic prescription and prevent antimicrobial overuse. In addition to clinical assessment of the patient, procalcitonin may limit initiation, shorten duration, and guide de-escalation of antimicrobials in patients with bacterial sepsis. A recent trial showed significant decrease in mortality with procalcitonin-guided antimicrobial therapy [88].

Steroids

Critical illness-related corticosteroid insufficiency (CIRCI) is typified by perturbations of the hypothalamic-pituitary-adrenal axis, aberrant cortisol metabolism, and tissue resistance to glucocorticoids. CIRCI is defined as "inadequate cellular corticosteroid activity for a patient's critical illness, manifested by insufficient glucocorticoid-glucocorticoid receptor-mediated downregulation of proinflammatory transcription factors" [53,89]. It is recognized clinically by persistent hypotension in volume-replete patients who are unresponsive to vasopressor therapy. The amount of cortisol produced is inadequate for the degree of physiologic stress. Steroids improve cardiovascular stability by synergistically increasing catecholamine responsiveness of adrenergic receptors allowing de-escalation of vasopressors and decreasing duration of hypoperfusion. There is no clear stratification of which patients may or may not benefit from steroids; it is reasonable that patients at the severe end of the spectrum may benefit more from steroids than patients with milder sepsis. A systematic review and metanalysis looking at safety and efficacy of stress-dose corticosteroids in human septic shock patients did not find a mortality benefit but did find a reduced duration of vasopressor-dependent shock and did not see increased risk of superinfection [90]. There was no evidence in human medicine that serum cortisol level or ACTH stimulation testing is helpful with identifying which septic shock patients would benefit from steroids [90]. Interestingly, delta cortisol less than 3 mcg/dL after cosyntropin was associated with systemic hypotension and decreased survival in septic dogs [91]. There is no consensus in veterinary medicine regarding optimal protocol, and much has been extrapolated from human medicine.

A modified protocol was published in a retrospective study in dogs with septic shock and suspected CIRCI using hydrocortisone 1 mg/kg IV loading dose, followed by a CRI at 0.08 mg/kg/h (or 2 mg/kg/d) [92].

Source control

Localizing any anatomic source of infection after initial resuscitation or concurrently and intervening quickly are of paramount importance in the treatment of sepsis. Insufficient source control is a common reason for treatment failure and poor outcome, as all other interventions will be rendered ineffective. Examples involve debridement of devitalized and infected wounds, abscess drainage, removal of infected medical devices or hardware, decompression in obstructive nephrolithiasis with concurrent infection, and definitive control of ongoing source of microbial contamination. A thorough investigation usually with advanced imaging is undertaken to look for a nidus and determine the full extent of infection. An exemplar of source control in septic peritonitis is to perform a surgical exploratory laparotomy, lavage, and repair of obstructed and perforated GI tract. The most recurrent cause of GI leakage is surgical wound dehiscence in the dog [93–95]; one study found foreign body ingestion as the most frequent cause [96]. Typical causes of GI leakage in cats are neoplasia and trauma [41,45]. Time from admission to surgical intervention for dogs with septic peritonitis was analyzed on a linear basis and also categorically by classifying patients in 6- or 12-hour groups; neither analysis showed an association with survival outcome [97]. Peritoneal lavage with copious amounts (~200–300 mL/kg) of 0.9% sterile saline and removal of excess fluid is recommended. In a prospective observational study investigating bacterial growth, antimicrobial efficacy, and resistance patterns before and after lavage in dogs with septic peritonitis, 92.5% and 87.5% of dogs had bacterial growth before and after lavage, respectively. MDR organisms were commonly reported both before (33%) and after lavage (14.3%). New bacterial isolates were identified after lavage in half of the dogs. The authors postulated that contamination, uneven distribution of effusion, or biofilm may explain this finding. Overall survival was high in this population of dogs at 87.5% [98]. Selection criteria for method of peritoneal drainage are based on magnitude of the peritonitis, definitive source control, and surgeon judgment. There is no significant difference in survival outcome based on method of peritoneal drainage (ie, peritoneal closure without drain placement vs open peritoneal drainage vs vacuum-assisted closure vs closed-suction drainage) [93,98–101]. Vacuum-assisted peritoneal drainage reduced fluid losses and bandage changes but developed complications such as nosocomial infections and hypoproteinemia [102]. Dogs with closed suction drains had higher blood pressure than those with open drains likely because of differences in fluid losses [102].

Nutrition

The SSC strongly recommends early enteral nutrition. This is preferred to parenteral nutrition, either alone or in combination, if patient can tolerate enteral feedings. Enteral nutrition is physiologic and preserves the integrity of the GI mucosal barrier, villi, and GI immunologic function [103]. Early feeding (within 24 hours) and late feeding (after 24 hours) were both associated with an 81% survival, compared with 46% survival in patients with peritonitis who were not fed [103]. Dogs fed with intermittent bolus and constant infusion fed enterally had a significantly higher frequency of regurgitation and diarrhea than cats fed enterally [104,105]. Patients with sepsis should be fed resting energy requirement (RER) based on the allometric formula $RER = 70 \times kg^{0.75}$. The linear formula is $30 \times$ body weight + 70 and is acceptable for patients weighing between 3 and 25 kgs. Underweight and overweight patients should still be fed at their current weight. Patients that are significantly overweight (>25% ideal body weight) should have an adjusted "current weight" to be used to calculate RER [103].

Nursing care

Each patient undergoes a daily comprehensive evaluation with consideration of physiologic body systems including pulmonary; cardiovascular; neurologic (including pain and sedation management); renal, fluid, and electrolytes; GI, nutrition, and metabolic; hematologic, infection, and immunosuppression issues (Table 2). High-quality nursing care that is patient-centered, evidence-based, and goal-orientated is paramount to managing the septic patient. In addition, a team-based, multidisciplinary approach in an open collaborative ICU environment is

TABLE 2
Comprehensive Patient Evaluation

Physiologic Body System	Parameters
Respiratory	Airway patency, RR and character; oxygenation-SpO2, Pa_{O_2}, oxygen therapy, Fi_{O_2}; ventilation-PaCO2; arterial blood gas data
Cardiovascular	Hemodynamic status-BP, HR, rhythm (ECG), peripheral pulses, evidence of ischemia; interventions to adjust preload, contractility and afterload; antiarrhythmic therapy
Neurologic	Pain and anxiolytic management-type/route of medications, pain scale score, modified Glasgow Coma Score (MGCS), intracranial pressure, seizure control
Renal/fluid/electrolytes	Net fluid balance, urine output, weight, volume status, electrolytes, BUN/ creatinine, UA
Gastrointestinal/metabolic/nutrition	Metabolic-glycemic control; RER, nutrition-route/rate/composition of nutritional support; GI integrity-use of prokinetic or antiemetic agents, prophylaxis against GI bleeding
Hematologic	Bleeding risk-red cell count/coagulation parameters, transfusion requirements-cross-match/type, thrombotic risk and prophylaxis
Infectious/immunosuppression	Temperature, findings suggestive of infection on P.E., C&S results, infectious disease control, procedures to diagnose and/or control infection, antimicrobial regimen-escalation, de-escalation

Abbreviations: BP, blood pressure; BUN, blood urea nitrogen; ECG, electrocardiogram; FiO2, fraction of inspired oxygen; GI, gastrointestinal; PaO2, partial pressure of oxygen; PaCO2, partial pressure of carbon dioxide; SpO2, pulse oximetry; RER, resting energy requirement; RR, respiratory rate; UA, urinalysis.

crucial. Nurse expertise is needed in advanced monitoring (direct arterial blood pressure, telemetry, mechanical ventilation), management of invasive medical devices (central line, indwelling urinary catheters, tubes, drains), bandage changes, biosecurity, and overall patient comfort and well-being.

SUMMARY

Sepsis is the ultimate brain teaser and is one of the most difficult conundrums for clinicians. Sepsis is challenging to identify and can be veiled by related or unrelated conditions. A precise definition of sepsis has eluded us; the pathophysiology is still unclear; clinical manifestations, diagnostic criteria, and treatment options are ever evolving for this puzzling disorder. Sepsis remains important because it is a leading cause of morbidity and mortality in both human and veterinary medicine. Complex problem-solving involves domain-specific knowledge, deliberate practice, and collaboration within a diverse team. A clinician can aptly apply biomedical knowledge to clinical decision-making and prediction; they look for clusters of clinical features or clues to arrive at a diagnosis. The lack of consensus surrounding the priorities and goals during sepsis resuscitation is likely the crux of the problem. The ultimate outcomes are to preserve organ function and quality of life for long term, by avoiding complications such as renal failure, endothelial damage, and volume overload. Sepsis can be conceptualized as both an acute and chronic illness. Early identification and interventions, with an integrated approach to resuscitation and treatment, are vital. Early and empiric broad-spectrum antibiotics are used until culture and sensitivity results guide a more specific choice. A personalized, physiologically guided, and conversative approach to fluid management is recommended. Recent evidence and physiologic concepts support the rationale for the early use of norepinephrine and/or combination with other vasoactive drugs to treat septic shock. Steroids are a plausible option in high-acuity patients that are unresponsive to early resuscitation efforts. Early and sufficient source control after acute resuscitation and hemodynamic stabilization is recommended. High-quality supportive care in the ICU setting is patient-centered with high-intensity nursing, focused on physiologic systems, goal-oriented, and multidisciplinary with a team-based approach to patient care.

CLINICS CARE POINTS

Pearls:

- Focus on the value of alertness for life-threatening manifestations or complications especially in patients with significant comorbidities, immunosuppressed, and/or are ill-appearing.
- Aptly apply biomedical knowledge to clinical decision-making and prediction.
- Reassess patients frequently, gauge their response to treatment, and follow their trajectory of disease, escalate or deescalate accordingly.

Pitfalls:

- Delay in initiation of antibiotics, inappropriate antibiotic choice, not obtaining necessary samples for culture and sensitivity, and not practicing antibiotic stewardship.
- Insufficient or delayed source control and incomplete diagnostic investigation for source of infection.
- Excessive fluid administration resulting in damage to the endothelial glycocalyx and a positive fluid balance.
- Delayed initiation of vasopressor therapy until the patient receives full shock dose of fluids.

REFERENCES

[1] Angus DC, van der Poll T. Severe sepsis and septic shock. N Engl J Med 2013;369(9):840–51.

[2] Kenney EM, Rozanski EA, Rush JE, et al. Association between outcome and organ system dysfunction in dogs with sepsis: 114 cases (2003-2007). J Am Vet Med Assoc 2010;236(1):83–7.

[3] Levy MM, Fink MP, Marshall JC, et al. International Sepsis Definitions Conference. 2001 SCCM/ESICM/ACCP/ATS/SIS International Sepsis Definitions Conference. Intensive Care Med 2003;29(4):530–8.

[4] Hauptman JG, Walshaw R, Olivier NB. Evaluation of the sensitivity and specificity of diagnostic criteria for sepsis in dogs. Vet Surg 1997;26(5):393–7.

[5] Singer M, Deutschman CS, Seymour CW, et al. The Third International Consensus Definitions for Sepsis and Septic Shock (Sepsis-3). JAMA 2016;315(8):801–10.

[6] Vincent JL, Moreno R, Takala J, et al. The SOFA (Sepsis-related Organ Failure Assessment) score to describe organ dysfunction/failure. On behalf of the Working Group on Sepsis-Related Problems of the European Society of Intensive Care Medicine. Intensive Care Med 1996;22(7):707–10.

[7] Vincent JL, de Mendonça A, Cantraine F, et al. Use of the SOFA score to assess the incidence of organ dysfunction/failure in intensive care units: results of a multicenter, prospective study. Working group on "sepsis-related problems" of the European Society of Intensive Care Medicine. Crit Care Med 1998;26(11):1793–800.

[8] Ferreira FL, Bota DP, Bross A, et al. Serial evaluation of the SOFA score to predict outcome in critically ill patients. JAMA 2001;286(14):1754–8.

[9] Cárdenas-Turanzas M, Ensor J, Wakefield C, et al. Cross-validation of a Sequential Organ Failure Assessment score-based model to predict mortality in patients with cancer admitted to the intensive care unit. J Crit Care 2012;27(6):673–80.

[10] Lambden S, Laterre PF, Levy MM, et al. The SOFA score-development, utility and challenges of accurate assessment in clinical trials. Crit Care 2019;23(1):374.

[11] Seymour CW, Liu VX, Iwashyna TJ, et al. Assessment of Clinical Criteria for Sepsis: For the Third International Consensus Definitions for Sepsis and Septic Shock (Sepsis-3). JAMA 2016;315(8):762–74.

[12] Raith EP, Udy AA, Bailey M, et al. Prognostic Accuracy of the SOFA Score, SIRS Criteria, and qSOFA Score for In-Hospital Mortality Among Adults With Suspected Infection Admitted to the Intensive Care Unit. JAMA 2017;317(3):290–300.

[13] Shankar-Hari M, Phillips GS, Levy ML, et al. Developing a New Definition and Assessing New Clinical Criteria for Septic Shock: For the Third International Consensus Definitions for Sepsis and Septic Shock (Sepsis-3). JAMA 2016;315(8):775–87.

[14] Freund Y, Lemachatti N, Krastinova E, et al. Prognostic Accuracy of Sepsis-3 Criteria for In-Hospital Mortality Among Patients with Suspected Infection Presenting to the Emergency Department. JAMA 2017;317(3):301–8.

[15] Rhodes A, Evans LE, Alhazzani W, et al. Surviving Sepsis Campaign: international guidelines for management of sepsis and septic shock: 2016. Crit Care Med 2017;45(3):486–552.

[16] Dellinger RP, Schorr CA, Levy MM. A Users' Guide to the 2016 Surviving Sepsis Guidelines. Crit Care Med 2017;45(3):381–5.

[17] Guyatt GH, Oxman AD, Vist GE, et al. GRADE: an emerging consensus on rating quality of evidence and strength of recommendations. BMJ 2008;336(7650):924–6.

[18] Schinkel M, Nannan Panday RS, Wiersinga WJ, et al. Timeliness of antibiotics for patients with sepsis and septic shock. J Thorac Dis 2020;12(Suppl 1):S66–71.

[19] Cinel I, Dellinger RP. Guidelines for severe infections: are they useful? Curr Opin Crit Care 2006;12(5):483–8.

[20] Rivers E, Nguyen B, Havstad S, et al. Early Goal-Directed Therapy Collaborative Group. Early goal-directed therapy in the treatment of severe sepsis and septic shock. N Engl J Med 2001;345(19):1368–77.

[21] ARISE Investigators; ANZICS Clinical Trials Group, Peake SL, Delaney A, Bailey M, et al. Goal-directed

resuscitation for patients with early septic shock. N Engl J Med 2014;371(16):1496–506.

[22] ProCESS Investigators, Yealy DM, Kellum JA, et al. A randomized trial of protocol-based care for early septic shock. N Engl J Med 2014;370(18):1683–93.

[23] Mouncey PR, Osborn TM, Power GS, et al. Trial of early, goal-directed resuscitation for septic shock. N Engl J Med 2015;372(14):1301–11.

[24] Marik PE, Farkas JD, Spiegel R, et al. POINT: Should the Surviving Sepsis Campaign Guidelines Be Retired? Yes *Chest* 2019;155(1):12–4.

[25] de Laforcade AM, Freeman LM, Shaw SP, et al. Hemostatic Changes in Dogs with Naturally Occurring Sepsis. JVIM 2003;17(5):674–9.

[26] Kraenzlin MN, Cortes Y, Fettig PK, et al. Shock index is associated with mortality in canine vehicular trauma patients. J Vet Emerg Crit Care 2020;30(6):706–11.

[27] Peterson KL, Hardy BT, Hall K. Assessment of shock index in healthy dogs and dogs in hemorrhagic shock. J Vet Emerg Crit Care 2013;23(5):545–50.

[28] Zollo AM, Ayoob AL, Prittie JE, et al. Utility of admission lactate concentration, lactate variables, and shock index in outcome assessment in dogs diagnosed with shock. J Vet Emerg Crit Care 2019;29(5):505–13.

[29] Porter AE, Rozanski EA, Sharp CR, et al. Evaluation of the shock index in dogs presenting as emergencies. J Vet Emerg Crit Care 2013;23(5):538–44.

[30] Taboada J, Meyer DJ. Cholestasis Associated with Extrahepatic Bacterial Infection in Five Dogs. JVIM 1989; 3(4):216–21.

[31] Klainbart S, Agi L, Bdolah-Abram T, et al. Clinical, laboratory, and hemostatic findings in cats with naturally occurring sepsis. J Am Vet Med Assoc 2017;251(9): 1025–34.

[32] Winkler KP, Greenfield CL, Schaeffer DJ. Bacteremia and bacterial translocation in the naturally occurring canine gastric dilatation-volvulus patient. J Am Anim Hosp Assoc 2003;39(4):361–8.

[33] Bentley AM, Mayhew PD, Culp WT, et al. Alterations in the hemostatic profiles of dogs with naturally occurring septic peritonitis. J Vet Emerg Crit Care 2013;23(1):14–22.

[34] Li RH, Chan DL. Evaluation of platelet function using multiple electrode platelet aggregometry in dogs with septic peritonitis. J Vet Emerg Crit Care 2016;26(5): 630–8.

[35] Holowaychuk MK, Hansen BD, DeFrancesco TC, et al. Ionized hypocalcemia in critically ill dogs. J Vet Intern Med 2009;23(3):509–13.

[36] Luschini MA, Fletcher DJ, Schoeffler GL. Incidence of ionized hypocalcemia in septic dogs and its association with morbidity and mortality: 58 cases (2006-2007). J Vet Emerg Crit Care 2010;20(4):406–12.

[37] Kellum JA, Lameire N, Aspelin P, et al. Kidney disease: improving global outcomes (KDIGO) acute kidney injury working group. KDIGO clinical practice guideline for acute kidney injury. Kidney Int Suppl 2012; 2(1):1–138.

[38] Thoen ME, Kerl ME. Characterization of acute kidney injury in hospitalized dogs and evaluation of a veterinary acute kidney injury staging system. J Vet Emerg Crit Care 2011;21(6):648–57.

[39] Bellomo R, Ronco C, Kellum JA, et al. Acute renal failure—definition, outcome measures, animal models, fluid therapy and information technology needs: the Second International Consensus Conference of the Acute Dialysis Quality Initiative (ADQI) Group. Crit Care 2004;8(4):R204–12.

[40] Keir I, Kellum JA. Acute kidney injury in severe sepsis: Pathophysiology, diagnosis, and treatment recommendations. J Vet Emerg Crit Care 2015;25(2):200–9.

[41] Parsons KJ, Owen LJ, Lee K, et al. A retrospective study of surgically treated cases of septic peritonitis in the cat (2000-2007). J Small Anim Pract 2009;50(10):518–24.

[42] Costello MF, Drobatz KJ, Aronson LR, et al. Underlying cause, pathophysiologic abnormalities, and response to treatment in cats with septic peritonitis: 51 cases (1990-2001). J Am Vet Med Assoc 2004;225(6):897–902.

[43] Brady CA, Otto CM, Van Winkle TJ, et al. Severe sepsis in cats: 29 cases (1986-1998). J Am Vet Med Assoc 2000;217(4):531–5.

[44] DeClue AE, Osterbur K, Bigio A, et al. Evaluation of serum NT-pCNP as a diagnostic and prognostic biomarker for sepsis in dogs. J Vet Intern Med 2011; 25(3):453–9.

[45] Scotti KM, Koenigshof A, Sri-Jayantha LSH, et al. Prognostic indicators in cats with septic peritonitis (2002-2015): 83 cases. J Vet Emerg Crit Care 2019;29(6): 647–52.

[46] Kellett-Gregory LM, Mittleman Boller E, Brown DC, et al. Retrospective Study: Ionized calcium concentrations in cats with septic peritonitis: 55 cases (1990–2008). J Vet Emerg Crit Care 2010;20(4):398–405.

[47] Landry DW, Oliver JA. The pathogenesis of vasodilatory shock. N Engl J Med 2001;345(8):588–95.

[48] Osterbur K, Whitehead Z, Sharp CR, et al. Plasma nitrate/nitrite concentrations in dogs with naturally developing sepsis and non-infectious forms of the systemic inflammatory response syndrome. Vet Rec 2011; 169(21):554.

[49] Hamzaoui O, Shi R. Early norepinephrine use in septic shock. J Thorac Dis 2020;12(Suppl 1):S72–7.

[50] Marik PE, Byrne L, van Haren F. Fluid resuscitation in sepsis: the great 30 mL per kg hoax. J Thorac Dis 2020;12(Suppl 1):S37–47.

[51] Zarychanski R, Abou-Setta AM, Turgeon AF, et al. Association of Hydroxyethyl Starch Administration With Mortality and Acute Kidney Injury in Critically Ill Patients Requiring Volume Resuscitation: A Systematic Review and Meta-analysis. JAMA 2013;309(7):678–88.

[52] Finfer S, Bellomo R, Boyce N, et al. A comparison of albumin and saline for fluid resuscitation in the intensive care unit. N Engl J Med 2004;350(22):2247–56.

[53] Marik PE, Pastores SM, Annane D, et al. Recommendations for the diagnosis and management of

corticosteroid insufficiency in critically ill adult patients: consensus statements from an international task force by the American College of Critical Care Medicine. Crit Care Med 2008;36(6):1937–49.
[54] Myburgh JA, Higgins A, Jovanovska A, et al. A comparison of epinephrine and norepinephrine in critically ill patients. Intensive Care Med 2008;34(12): 2226–34.
[55] Conti-Patara A, de Araujo Caldeira J, de Mattos-Junior E, et al. Changes in tissue perfusion parameters in dogs with severe sepsis/septic shock in response to goal-directed hemodynamic optimization at admission to ICU and the relation to outcome. J Vet Emerg Crit Care 2012;22(4):409–18.
[56] Singer M. Sepsis: personalization v protocolization? Crit Care 2019;23(Suppl 1):127.
[57] Bone RC, Balk RA, Cerra FB, et al. Definitions for sepsis and organ failure and guidelines for the use of innovative therapies in sepsis. The ACCP/SCCM Consensus Conference Committee. American College of Chest Physicians/Society of Critical Care Medicine. Chest 1992;101(6):1644–55.
[58] Levy B, Gibot S, Franck P, et al. Relation between muscle Na+K+ ATPase activity and raised lactate concentrations in septic shock: a prospective study. Lancet 2005; 365(9462):871–5.
[59] Levy B, Desebbe O, Montemont C, et al. Increased aerobic glycolysis through beta2 stimulation is a common mechanism involved in lactate formation during shock states. Shock 2008;30(4):417–21.
[60] Nalos M, Leverve X, Huang S, et al. Half-molar sodium lactate infusion improves cardiac performance in acute heart failure: a pilot randomised controlled clinical trial. Crit Care 2014;18(2):R48.
[61] Trzeciak S, Dellinger RP, Chansky ME, et al. Serum lactate as a predictor of mortality in patients with infection. Intensive Care Med 2007;33:970–7.
[62] Hernández G, Ospina-Tascón GA, Damiani LP, et al. Effect of a Resuscitation Strategy Targeting Peripheral Perfusion Status vs Serum Lactate Levels on 28-Day Mortality Among Patients With Septic Shock: The ANDROMEDA-SHOCK Randomized Clinical Trial. JAMA 2019;321(7):654–64.
[63] Cortellini S, Seth M, Kellett-Gregory LM. Plasma lactate concentrations in septic peritonitis: A retrospective study of 83 dogs (2007-2012). J Vet Emerg Crit Care 2015;25(3):388–95.
[64] Oron LD, Klainbart S, Bruchim Y, et al. Comparison of saphenous and cephalic blood lactate concentrations in dogs with gastric dilatation and volvulus: 45 cases. Can J Vet Res 2018;82(4):271–7.
[65] Levick JR, Michel CC. Microvascular fluid exchange and the revised Starling principle. Cardiovasc Res 2010; 87(2):198–210.
[66] Lee WL, Slutsky AS. Sepsis and endothelial permeability. N Engl J Med 2010;363(7):689–91.
[67] Weinbaum S, Tarbell JM, Damiano ER. The structure and function of the endothelial glycocalyx layer. Annu Rev Biomed Eng 2007;9:121–67.
[68] Woodcock TE, Woodcock TM. Revised Starling equation and the glycocalyx model of transvascular fluid exchange: an improved paradigm for prescribing intravenous fluid therapy. Br J Anaesth 2012;108(3): 384–94.
[69] Hippensteel JA, Uchimido R, Tyler PD, et al. Intravenous fluid resuscitation is associated with septic endothelial glycocalyx degradation. Crit Care 2019;23(1): 259.
[70] Malbrain MLNG, Van Regenmortel N, Saugel B, et al. Principles of fluid management and stewardship in septic shock: it is time to consider the four D's and the four phases of fluid therapy. Ann Intensive Care 2018;8(1): 66.
[71] Cochrane Injuries Group Albumin Reviewers. Human albumin administration in critically ill patients: systematic review of randomised controlled trials. BMJ 1998; 317(7153):235–40.
[72] Myburgh J, Cooper DJ, Finfer S, et al. Saline or albumin for fluid resuscitation in patients with traumatic brain injury. N Engl J Med 2007;357(9):874–84.
[73] Caironi P, Tognoni G, Masson S, et al. Albumin replacement in patients with severe sepsis or septic shock. N Engl J Med 2014;370(15):1412–21.
[74] Craft EM, Powell LL. The use of canine-specific albumin in dogs with septic peritonitis. J Vet Emerg Crit Care 2012;22(6):631–9.
[75] Mazzaferro EM, Balakrishnan A, Hackner SG, et al. Delayed type III hypersensitivity reaction with acute kidney injury in two dogs following administration of concentrated human albumin during treatment for hypoalbuminemia secondary to septic peritonitis. J Vet Emerg Crit Care 2020;30(5):574–80.
[76] Ropski MK, Guillaumin J, Monnig AA, et al. Use of cryopoor plasma for albumin replacement and continuous antimicrobial infusion for treatment of septic peritonitis in a dog. J Vet Emerg Crit Care 2017;27(3): 348–56.
[77] Culler CA, Balakrishnan A, Yaxley PE, et al. Clinical use of cryopoor plasma continuous rate infusion in critically ill, hypoalbuminemic dogs. J Vet Emerg Crit Care 2019;29(3):314–20.
[78] Silverstein DC, Beer KA. Controversies regarding choice of vasopressor therapy for management of septic shock in animals. J Vet Emerg Crit Care 2015;25(1):48–54.
[79] Kumar A, Roberts D, Wood KE, et al. Duration of hypotension before initiation of effective antimicrobial therapy is the critical determinant of survival in human septic shock. Crit Care Med 2006;34:1589–96.
[80] Kalafut SR, Schwartz P, Currao RL, et al. Comparison of Initial and Postlavage Bacterial Culture Results of Septic Peritonitis in Dogs and Cats. J Am Anim Hosp Assoc 2018;54(5):257–66.

[81] Ogeer-Gyles J, Mathews KA, Sears W, et al. Development of antimicrobial drug resistance in rectal Escherichia coli isolates from dogs hospitalized in an intensive care unit. J Am Vet Med Assoc 2006;229(5):694–9.

[82] Dickinson AE, Summers JF, Wignal J, et al. Impact of appropriate empirical antimicrobial therapy on outcome of dogs with septic peritonitis. J Vet Emerg Crit Care 2015;25(1):152–9.

[83] Abelson AL, Buckley GJ, Rozanski EA. Positive impact of an emergency department protocol on time to antimicrobial administration in dogs with septic peritonitis. J Vet Emerg Crit Care 2013;23(5):551–6.

[84] Alam N, Oskam E, Stassen PM, et al. Prehospital antibiotics in the ambulance for sepsis: a multicentre, open label, randomised trial. Lancet Respir Med 2018;6(1): 40–50.

[85] Hranjec T, Rosenberger LH, Swenson B, et al. Aggressive versus conservative initiation of antimicrobial treatment in critically ill surgical patients with suspected intensive-care-unit-acquired infection: a quasi-experimental, before and after observation cohort study. Lancet Infect Dis 2012;12(10):774–80.

[86] Keir I, Dickinson AE. The role of antimicrobials in the treatment of sepsis and critical illness-related bacterial infections: examination of the evidence. J Vet Emerg Crit Care 2015;25(1):55–62.

[87] Viitanen SJ, Lappalainen AK, Christensen MB, et al. The Utility of Acute-Phase Proteins in the Assessment of Treatment Response in Dogs with Bacterial Pneumonia. J Vet Intern Med 2017;31(1):124–33.

[88] de Jong E, van Oers JA, Beishuizen A, et al. Procalcitonin to guide antibiotic stewardship in intensive care - Authors'reply. Lancet Infect Dis 2016;16(8):889–90.

[89] Annane D, Pastores SM, Arlt W, et al. Critical Illness-Related Corticosteroid Insufficiency (CIRCI): A Narrative Review from a Multispecialty Task Force of the Society of Critical Care Medicine (SCCM) and the European Society of Intensive Care Medicine (ESICM). Intensive Care Med 2017;43(12):1781–92.

[90] Sligl WI, Milner DA Jr, Sundar S, et al. Safety and efficacy of corticosteroids for the treatment of septic shock: A systematic review and meta-analysis. Clin Infect Dis 2009;49(1):93–101.

[91] Burkitt JM, Haskins SC, Nelson RW, et al. Relative adrenal insufficiency in dogs with sepsis. J Vet Intern Med 2007;21(2):226–31.

[92] Summers AM, Culler C, Yaxley PE, et al. Retrospective evaluation of the use of hydrocortisone for treatment of suspected critical illness–related corticosteroid insufficiency (CIRCI) in dogs with septic shock (2010–2017): 47 cases. J Vet Emerg Crit Care 2021;31(3): 371–9.

[93] Greenfield CL, Walshaw R. Open peritoneal drainage for treatment of contaminated peritoneal cavity and septic peritonitis in dogs and cats: 24 cases (1980-1986). J Am Vet Med Assoc 1987;191(1):100–5.

[94] Hosgood G, Salisbury SK, Cantwell HD, et al. Intraperitoneal circulation and drainage in the dog. Vet Surg 1989;18(4):261–8.

[95] Swann H, Hughes D. Diagnosis and management of peritonitis. Vet Clin North Am Small Anim Pract 2000;30(3):603–15.

[96] King LG. Postoperative complications and prognostic indicators in dogs and cats with septic peritonitis: 23 cases (1989-1992). J Am Vet Med Assoc 1994;204(3): 407–14.

[97] Bush M, Carno MA, St Germaine L, et al. The effect of time until surgical intervention on survival in dogs with secondary septic peritonitis. Can Vet J 2016; 57(12):1267–73.

[98] Marshall H, Sinnott-Stutzman V, Ewing P, et al. Effect of peritoneal lavage on bacterial isolates in 40 dogs with confirmed septic peritonitis. J Vet Emerg Crit Care 2019;29(6):635–42.

[99] Lanz OI, Ellison GW, Bellah JR, et al. Surgical treatment of septic peritonitis without abdominal drainage in 28 dogs. J Am Anim Hosp Assoc 2001;37(1):87–92.

[100] Staatz AJ, Monnet E, Seim HB 3rd. Open peritoneal drainage versus primary closure for the treatment of septic peritonitis in dogs and cats: 42 cases (1993-1999). Vet Surg 2002;31(2):174–80.

[101] Mueller MG, Ludwig LL, Barton LJ. Use of closed-suction drains to treat generalized peritonitis in dogs and cats: 40 cases (1997-1999). J Am Vet Med Assoc 2001;219(6):789–94.

[102] Cioffi KM, Schmiedt CW, Cornell KK, et al. Retrospective evaluation of vacuum-assisted peritoneal drainage for the treatment of septic peritonitis in dogs and cats: 8 cases (2003-2010). J Vet Emerg Crit Care 2012; 22(5):601–9.

[103] Chan DL, Freeman LM. Nutrition in critical illness. Vet Clin North Am Small Anim Pract 2006;36(6):1225–41, v–vi.

[104] Campbell JA, Jutkowitz LA, Santoro KA, et al. Continuous versus intermittent delivery of nutrition via nasoenteric feeding tubes in hospitalized canine and feline patients: 91 patients (2002-2007). J Vet Emerg Crit Care 2010;20(2):232–6.

[105] Holahan M, Abood S, Hauptman J, et al. Intermittent and continuous enteral nutrition in critically ill dogs: a prospective randomized trial. J Vet Intern Med 2010;24(3):520–6.

Advances in Small Animal Care 2 (2021) 69–83
ADVANCES IN SMALL ANIMAL CARE

Current Standards and Practices in Small Animal Mechanical Ventilation

Anusha Balakrishnan, BVSc, DACVECC
Triangle Veterinary Referral Hospital, 608 Morreene Road, Durham, NC 27705, USA

KEYWORDS

• Mechanical ventilation • Hypoxemia • Respiratory failure • Weaning • Ventilator associated pneumonia

KEY POINTS

- Mechanical ventilation is a lifesaving intervention that is used to manage a variety of conditions. Broad indications for mechanical ventilation include severe hypoxemia, severe hypercapnia, and increased work of breathing.
- The goals of ventilation are to:
  - Relieve respiratory distress
  - Improve gas exchange and oxygenation
  - Reduce hypercapnia and concomitant respiratory acidosis
  - Allow for interventions to resolve underlying disease
  - Reverse respiratory muscle fatigue.
- Mechanical ventilation, while lifesaving in some patients, can have serious complications impacting many organ systems. Intensive nursing care and monitoring can help mitigate several of these complications.
- If patients are prematurely weaned from the ventilator before they have adequate respiratory drive, muscle strength and pulmonary function, wean failure and respiratory fatigue may ensue.

Mechanical ventilation (MV) is a potentially life-saving intervention that is gaining more widespread application in small animal critical care medicine and plays a vital role in patient management for a variety of illnesses.

Indications for initiation of MV are variable (Table 1) but can be broadly classified into

- Hypoxemic respiratory failure with severe hypoxemia (Pao_2<60 mm Hg or SpO_2<90% despite an Fio_2>0.6); these comprise disease conditions that result in ventilation-perfusion mismatching, intrapulmonary shunting, and reduced functional residual capacity.
- Hypercapneic respiratory failure, as evidenced by a decrease in minute ventilation and subsequent severe hypercapnia ($Paco_2$>60 mm Hg), that cannot be readily reversed by treating the underlying disease.
- Increased work of breathing, with concern for impending respiratory fatigue; this is a much more subjective assessment and may be evidenced by markedly increased respiratory effort progressing to orthopnea, weakening chest wall excursions, and progressive hypercapnia (or even deceptively "normal" Pco_2 levels in animals that are visibly tachypneic with increased respiratory effort).
- Cardiovascular compromise such as in decompensated shock, where MV is used to offload energy requirements and oxygen consumption during spontaneous breathing.

The author does not have any disclosures to report.
E-mail address: anushabalakrish@gmail.com

https://doi.org/10.1016/j.yasa.2021.07.006
2666-450X/21/ © 2021 Elsevier Inc. All rights reserved.

TABLE 1
Common Causes of Hypoxemic and Hypercapneic Respiratory Failure

Common Causes of Hypoxemic Respiratory Failure	Common Causes of Hypercapneic Respiratory Failure
Bronchopneumonia Pulmonary thromboembolism Cardiogenic pulmonary edema Acute respiratory distress syndrome Interstitial lung disease Pulmonary contusion Smoke inhalation Pulmonary hemorrhage Pulmonary neoplasia	Central nervous system (CNS) disorders (reduced respiratory drive) • Cardiopulmonary arrest • Overdose with CNS depressants/toxins • Cerebrovascular accident • Traumatic brain injury • Intracranial neoplasia • Infectious/inflammatory CNS disease
	Neuromuscular dysfunction • Myasthenia gravis • Tetanus • Botulism • Polyradiculoneuritis • Electrolyte disorders (eg, hypokalemia) • Spinal cord injury
	Chest wall/pleural space diseases • Flail chest/rib fractures • Pneumothorax • Pleural effusion
	Conducting airway diseases • Lower airway inflammatory disease (eg, feline asthma)

MV allows for application of a positive pressure breath, the magnitude of which depends on the compliance and resistance of the respiratory system. The ultimate goals of ventilation are to relieve respiratory distress, improve gas exchange and thereby oxygenation, reduce hypercapnia and concomitant respiratory acidosis, allow for interventions targeted at resolution of underlying disease, and reverse respiratory muscle fatigue.

MV in small animals has been described well in the current literature [1–9]. In several studies that have evaluated outcomes in small animal patients undergoing MV for various reasons, between 30% and 62.5% of canine patients survived to discharge [1–4,9]. Feline patients have been shown to have considerably worse outcomes with between 15% and 42% of patients surviving to discharge, although a study evaluating mechanically ventilated cats with congestive heart failure showed a higher survival of 66% [3]. Overall improved survival has been found in patients treated for primary pulmonary parenchymal diseases, when compared to those treated for extrapulmonary disease or hypercapneic respiratory failure caused by hypoventilation [2]. This is likely a reflection of more readily treatable underlying diseases in the latter group. A notable exception to this general finding is the relatively high survival seen in patients ventilated for cardiogenic pulmonary edema, where ventilation is typically required for shorter durations of time when compared with other primary lung diseases [3].

INITIATING MECHANICAL VENTILATION

Once the decision is made to initiate MV for a patient, the clinician must consider the following:

- Mode of ventilation to be used and associated ventilator settings
- A sedation/anesthetic plan
- Patient monitoring and instrumentation

In order to make a decision regarding the most appropriate mode of ventilation for a given patient, clinicians must become familiar with basic terminology used in MV:

- Phase variable: These are variables that are responsible for each part of the MV breath and can be manipulated by the operator. These include,
    - Trigger variable: This is the variable that initiates inspiration. This is typically either a pressure or flow-based trigger value.
    - Limit variable: This is the variable that places a maximum value on the parameter chosen to be controlled during inspiration.
    - Cycle variable: This is the variable that causes a breath to end.
    - Baseline variable: This describes what is happening in the breath during expiration.
- Cycling mechanisms: These describe how a breath cycles between different phases (Table 2).
- Positive end-expiratory pressure (PEEP): application of constant positive pressure in the airways so that at end-expiration, pressure is never allowed to reach atmospheric pressure. PEEP is discussed in more detail in subsequent sections.
- Flow rate: This reflects the speed with which a given tidal volume is delivered.

TABLE 2
Variables and Cycling Mechanisms Used in Mechanical Ventilation

Cycling Mechanism	Control Variable	Dependent Variables (Depend on Compliance and Resistance of the Respiratory System)	Comments
Volume	Tidal volume (VT)	I-time, airway pressure	Two most commonly used cycling mechanisms
Pressure	Maximal airway pressure	I-time, VT	
Flow	Flow rate	VT, airway pressure	
Time	Inspiratory time (I-time)	VT, airway pressure	

- I:E ratio: Ratio of inspiratory time to expiratory time. Typically, the expiratory time is longer than the inspiratory time to allow for passive exhalation and mimic physiologic spontaneous breathing. However, in select circumstances, this ratio can be modified to increase the inspiratory time to be equal to, or rarely exceed, the expiratory time (reverse I:E ventilation) as a strategy to manage refractory hypoxemia. In general, longer inspiratory times will result in higher airway pressures and allow more time for the applied pressure to distribute more evenly across heterogenous areas of diseased lungs.
- Ventilator breath types:
  - Mandatory/controlled breaths: These breaths are triggered and/or cycled by the ventilator. All the work of breathing is performed by the ventilator.
  - Assisted breaths: These are triggered by the patient but cycled by the ventilator.
  - Supported breaths: These are triggered by the patient, and the ventilator provides some support in the form of positive airway pressure. Most of the work of breathing is performed by the patient.
  - Spontaneous breaths: The breath is triggered and completed by the patient with no support from the ventilator.

MODES OF VENTILATION

- Volume control modes (continuous mandatory ventilation [CMV] and intermittent mandatory ventilation [IMV]):
  - The clinician will set the respiratory rate, VT to be delivered, inspiratory flow pattern (either square or descending ramp, reflecting how rapidly the tidal volume is delivered), and peak inspiratory flow rate (this will then determine inspiratory time).
  - The ventilator will deliver the chosen VT at the chosen respiratory rate if the patient is apneic. Airway pressures reached are dependent on the patient's lung compliance.
  - If the patient triggers a breath, the ventilator will continue to deliver mandatory breaths as long as the patient's respiratory rate is higher than the set rate. Patient-triggered breaths will contribute to the total minute ventilation.
- Pressure control modes (CMV and IMV):
  - A preset airway pressure to be delivered is set by the clinician. The clinician also sets the respiratory rate and inspiratory time and, therefore, the I:E ratio (ratio of inspiratory to expiratory time).
  - The tidal volume delivered depends on the patient's lung compliance and resistance.
  - As patient effort and compliance improves, the overall VT delivered will improve, and as a result, minute ventilation will increase.

With both pressure and volume control modes, breaths can be either delivered as CMV or assist-control (AC) breaths or IMV. With the former, the machine will deliver the preset number of respiratory rates, but if the patient triggers a breath, the ventilator will deliver a full assisted breath with each patient trigger. With IMV modes, a set number of mandatory breaths is delivered between which spontaneous patient breathing can occur. In synchronized IMV (SIMV), the machine attempts to synchronize the patient's inspiratory effort with the mandatory breaths. This mode can be used for patients that are able to perform some work of breathing, whereas AC modes are chosen in patients with severe lung disease where respiratory muscle rest is desired, or those that have no respiratory drive.

- *Continuous positive airway pressure (CPAP):* This is an important mode of noninvasive ventilation where positive pressure is applied continuously throughout the airway cycle for a spontaneously breathing patient. This mode is a useful weaning mode for animals with a strong respiratory drive, as well as for intubated patients that are ventilating well on their own but may need some support (such as sedated patients intubated for upper airway obstructions).

- *Pressure support ventilation:* In this mode, the patient starts and ends the breath (spontaneous breath), and the size/VT of the breath is augmented with ventilator support. This can be used for patient support during the process of weaning or as a form of support for spontaneous breaths during with IMV.
- *Airway pressure release ventilation:* This is a specialized mode of bi-level ventilation available in newer ventilators. A high level of CPAP is applied, and the patient is allowed to breathe spontaneously. Each period of high airway pressure is interrupted by very short periods of low airway pressure that facilitates expiration, along with the application of PEEP. The ratio of time spent at high versus low airway pressures determines the rate of mandatory ventilation. This is a newer mode of ventilation that has been described in a veterinary case report [10]. There are other modes of bi-level ventilation available where the periods of high and low airway pressure are alternated for variable periods of time. These methods may minimize patient-ventilatory dyssynchrony because there is no restriction on the patient's ability to take spontaneous breaths.
- *High-frequency oscillatory ventilation:* This is a mode of ventilation where very small tidal volumes are applied at a very high rate. The theory behind this ventilatory mode is that delivery of small tidal volumes with frequent oscillations can avoid lung overdistension and further injury. This has not been reported in recent clinical veterinary studies but has been reported in older experimental canine studies [11]. This mode has been recently widely evaluated in humans with Acute Respiratory Distress Syndrome (ARDS) and has fallen out of favor because of negative outcomes in some studies [12].

APPLICATION OF POSITIVE END-EXPIRATORY PRESSURE

PEEP is a vital part of ventilator settings. PEEP has many beneficial effects, and a thorough understanding of the consequences of PEEP is imperative for clinicians managing ventilated patients. PEEP, when applied properly, can help splint open and "recruit" alveoli at the end of expiration and prevent airway collapse from atelectasis, thereby minimizing airway trauma and shear injury from cyclical opening and closing (atelectrauma).

In addition, PEEP can have complex effects on a patient's hemodynamic status and can increase intrathoracic pressure. PEEP can cause a reduction in right ventricular filling, a fall in the left ventricular stroke volume, and subsequently a decrease in cardiac output [13]. Therefore, while application of PEEP can play a crucial role in improving oxygenation and minimizing ongoing injury in severely diseased lungs, patients should be carefully monitored when high levels of PEEP are used. Relative contraindications for the use of PEEP include ongoing cardiovascular instability, unilateral lung disease, or hyperinflated lungs (such as with emphysema). PEEP should be used with caution in patients with elevated intracranial pressure where PEEP may impede cerebral venous return although some recent studies suggest that this effect may be minimal [14].

When selecting an optimal level of PEEP for a patient, care must be taken not to select a level too high which may result in lung overdistension. The pressure-volume loop, displayed on most ventilators for each patient, may be used as a guideline to select optimal PEEP levels. Ideally, the PEEP level chosen should be between the lower and upper inflection points (Fig. 1).

SUGGESTED INITIAL SETTINGS

While the appropriate ventilator modes and settings for each small animal patient may vary considerably based on their underlying primary disease process as well as other comorbidities, a general set of guidelines can be helpful to provide a starting point from which the settings can be further tailored to each patient (Table 3). The author typically uses the following settings as an initial starting point which is then customized further depending on the patient's needs:

- Fraction of inspired oxygen: 100%
- Mode: pressure/volume-controlled AC
- Target tidal volume: 8 to 12 mL/kg
- Pressure above PEEP: 10 to 15 cm H_2O
- PEEP: 3 to 7 cm H_2O
- I:E ratio: 1:2
- Inspiratory trigger: −1 to −2 cm H_2O (pressure trigger) or 0.5 to 2.0 L/min (flow trigger)

MONITORING THE MECHANICALLY VENTILATED PATIENT

Mechanically ventilated patients are among the most fragile of ICU patients and are heavily dependent on intensive nursing care with round-the-clock monitoring (Fig. 2). Appropriate nursing care is crucial in these

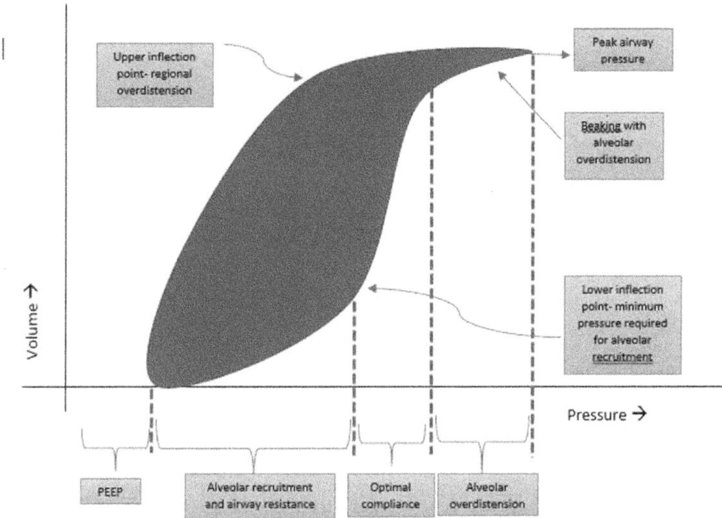

FIG. 1 Pressure-volume loop illustrating upper and lower inflection points for optimal PEEP selection.

patients to avoid or minimize ventilator-associated complications (which can be life-threatening) and to maximize chances of patient recovery and increase chances for a successful wean. Considerations for care of these patients include,

Equipment Care and Safety Checks

- Essential supplies should be kept close to the patient at all times and be easily accessible to the care team including an Ambu-bag, suction catheters (both sterile catheters to suction the endotracheal tube and catheters to suction the oropharynx), suction apparatus connected to a wall unit or portable suction, emergency reintubation supplies (endotracheal tubes, cuff syringe, and laryngoscope), drugs for rescue sedation (such as propofol), and an emergency drug sheet with doses of CPR drugs calculated for ease of reference.
- All ventilator and related equipment should be present and working well, and the ventilator should be connected to uninterrupted power supply. Ventilator safety alarms should be checked before each patient use. All medications and infusions should be checked for accuracy of dosage, composition, and infusion rates and be clearly labeled.

Patient Care

- Patient vitals should be monitored at least hourly. The "ABCs" should always be prioritized:
    - Airway: Is the endotracheal tube or tracheostomy tube patent and secure? Does the tube need suctioning or repositioning?
    - Breathing: Ensure adequate air movement and appropriate chest wall movement and assess mucous membrane color.
    - Circulation: The patient should have its heart rate, pulse quality, and mucous membrane color assessed closely. Continuous blood pressure monitoring, preferably directly through an arterial catheter, is recommended in these patients.
- Respiratory system care and monitoring:
    - Artificial airway:
        - Check for endotracheal tube or tracheostomy tube patency and secure tie.
        - The endotracheal tube cuff should be inflated, and overinflation or underinflation should be avoided. Overinflation may risk tracheal necrosis while underinflation may result in airway leaks and loss of tidal volume. The cuff should be deflated and repositioned before inflating the tube if readjustment of the tube is needed.
        - The ventilator tubing should be monitored for excessive condensation, kinks, or leaks.
    - The patient's respiratory rate (set rate and actual rate), tidal volume (set volume and actual volume), pulse oximetry, and capnography should be monitored continuously to ensure optimal oxygenation and ventilation.

TABLE 3
Various Commonly Used Mechanical Ventilation Modes with Their Indications, Advantages, and Disadvantages

Mode	Indications	Advantages	Disadvantages	Other Considerations
VC/AC	Normal respiratory drive but weak muscles WOB is too high	Allows patient control of rate with guaranteed minimal delivery of preset rate and volume	Patient cannot control volume or duration of breath. Respiratory alkalosis may ensue. Auto-PEEP may result. Disuse atrophy of muscles	Monitor: • PIP • Exhaled VT • Patient comfort • Acid-base status
VC/SIMV	Normal respiratory drive but weak muscles Patients can maintain their own RR/CO_2 WOB is too high. Weaning modality	Less risk of disuse atrophy and respiratory alkalosis Less hemodynamic impact since spontaneous breaths have a lower mean airway pressure and average pressure over time is less	WOB is still high for spontaneous breaths due to circuit resistance and lag time	Monitor: • PIP • Patient RR • Exhaled VT, especially of spontaneous breaths • Patient comfort
CPAP	During spontaneous breathing trials for weaning	Promotes alveolar stability and improves FRC. Obstructive airway disease	Caution to ensure apnea and low exhaled VT alarms are active	Monitor: • Patient RR, watch for signs of fatigue. • Exhaled VT • Patient comfort
PS	During spontaneous breathing trials for weaning Reduces WOB	Patient controls RR, I-time, and VT		• Inspiration ends when flow decreases to set limit (flow-cycled) • Ensure trigger sensitivity is set to allow for minimal patient work
PC/AC	Full vent support to patients with poor oxygenation	Can reduce PIP and subsequent barotrauma. Rapid initial pressure rise can open collapsed alveoli and splint them throughout inspiration (rise time). More even distribution of pressure within lung with laminar flow (decelerating flow wave pattern)	Increased mean airway pressure can reduce preload and cardiac output	Monitor: • Set RR • Exhaled VT and V_E • Hemodynamic status • I:E ratio

(*continued on next page*)

TABLE 3
(continued)

Mode	Indications	Advantages	Disadvantages	Other Considerations
PC/SIMV	Normal respiratory drive but weak muscles Patients can maintain their own. RR/CO_2 WOB is too high. Weaning modality	Guaranteed minimum V_E with each mandatory breath, patient can modify Vt of spontaneous breaths. Less hemodynamic impact than PC/AC		Monitor: • PIP • Patient RR • Exhaled VT, especially of spontaneous breaths • Patient comfort

Abbreviations: AC, assist-control; CPAP, continuous positive airway pressure; FRC, functional residual capacity; I:E ratio, inspiratory time-expiratory time ratio; PC, pressure control; PEEP, positive end-expiratory pressure; PIP, peak inspiratory pressure; PS, pressure support; RR, respiratory rate; SIMV, synchronized intermittent mandatory ventilation; VC, volume control; V_E, minute ventilation; VT, tidal volume; WOB, work of breathing.

- Arterial blood gas analysis should be performed at least every 6 to 12 hours to assess the effectiveness of ventilation and how well the patient is oxygenating.

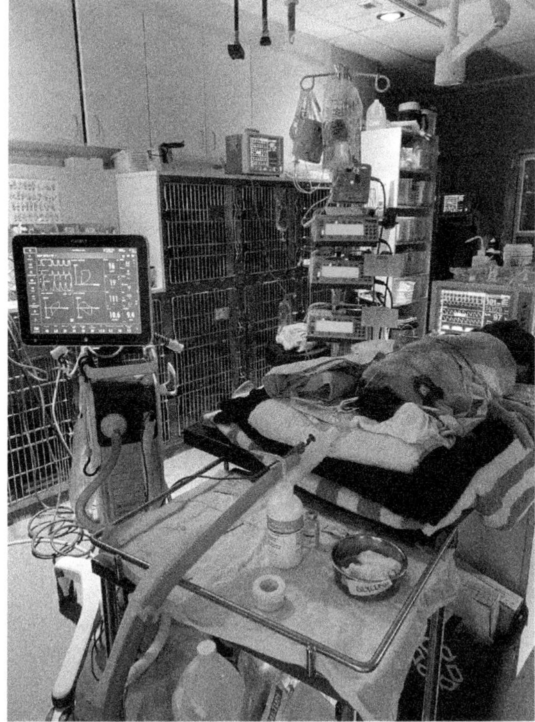

FIG. 2 A mechanically ventilated dog with complete monitoring in the ICU including continuous ECG, direct arterial blood pressure, pulse oximetry, and capnography.

- Ventilator settings and patient parameters should be recorded on a ventilator flow sheet at least hourly or after any changes.
- Airway secretions should be closely watched. Suctioning is vital to maintain a patent airway and can be used to obtain airway samples for cytology and culture. Patients should be preoxygenated with 100% oxygen before suctioning, and an aseptic technique should be used. Airway humidification is crucial and allows for protection of the airway epithelial lining and keeps secretions from thickening and drying out. Humidifier units can be attached to the patient circuit or alternatively, heat-moisture exchanging filters can be used to provide humidification. In-line suction catheters are also available for use in patients when disconnecting from the ventilator to suction them can result in a precipitous loss of alveolar recruitment and hypoxemia (Fig. 3).
- Rapid patient desaturation can occur occasionally for a variety of reasons, and this can be assessed using the useful "DOPES" acronym [15].
  - *D*isplacement/*D*islodgement: If the capnograph waveform is lost or decreases dramatically in magnitude, the patient should be evaluated immediately to ensure that they are not at risk for imminent cardiopulmonary arrest. Then they should be assessed for displacement or dislodgement of the endotracheal tube or circuit or a leak in the circuit.
  - *O*cclusion/*O*bstruction of the endotracheal tube or airways: the endotracheal tube should be checked for mucus plugs or secretions. Bronchospasms or an acute pneumothorax

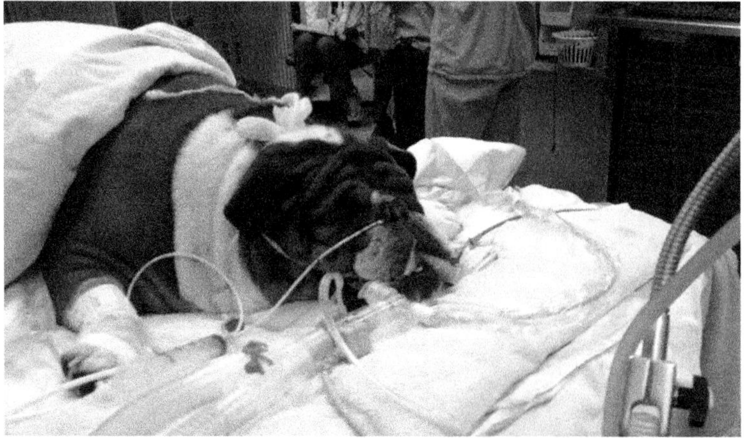

FIG. 3 In-line suction unit attached to the endotracheal tube and ventilator circuit to avoid disconnecting the patient from the ventilator during suctioning of the endotracheal tube.

can also result in acute desaturation. This should especially be a consideration if there is unexpected resistance encountered while bagging a patient.

- *P*neumothorax/*P*ulmonary thromboembolism/*P*ulmonary edema: the patient should be evaluated using point-of-care ultrasound to assess cardiac size and function evaluate for B-lines indicating new or worsening pulmonary edema, and thoracic radiographs should be considered.
- *E*quipment failure: If the patient's SpO_2 rises rapidly once they are disconnected from the ventilator and bagged manually, this may indicate an issue with the ventilator/equipment, and this should be assessed carefully.
- *S*tacked breaths: If the patient's desired respiratory rate is significantly different from the set rate, or if the expiratory time set is insufficient to allow for complete exhalation, breath stacking may occur resulting in patient-ventilatory dyssynchrony and hypoxemia.

- Cardiovascular system care:
  - The patient's heart rate and rhythm should be monitored via continuous electrocardiogram or telemetry.
  - Direct blood pressure measurements are ideal in these patients, although indirect measurements can be used if an arterial catheter is not able to be placed.
- Oral and ocular care:
  - Oral complications of MV include decreased swallowing of saliva and ranula formation (Fig. 4), oral ulceration, glossal edema, and increased bacterial colonization in the oropharynx.
  - Stringent oral care is vital in ventilated patients and has been shown to be associated with a significant decrease in the risk of ventilator-associated pneumonia (VAP) [16–18]. Human studies have evaluated various techniques for oral care including a combination of antiseptics such as chlorhexidine and using toothbrushes as well as total gastric decontamination with antibiotics to prevent VAP [17]. The prevalence of VAP in veterinary medicine is still unclear; there is only one published study evaluating this in dogs which revealed that 46.2% of ventilated patients developed VAP (defined as new-onset pneumonia/new bacterial isolate detected more than 48 hours after initiation of MV) [19]. The author recommends the use of dilute chlorhexidine (0.2%–2%) for oral care at least every 4 hours in mechanically ventilated dogs and cats. Patients should be watched closely for development of VAP, and early, appropriate antimicrobial therapy should be initiated if VAP is suspected.
  - Glycerin can be used to help prevent desiccation of the oral mucosa in ventilated dogs and cats. The tongue can be wrapped in saline- or glycerin-moistened gauze that is changed every 4 hours or sooner if soiled.
  - Ocular care: Eyes should be lubricated at least every 4 hours to prevent corneal ulceration.
- Gastrointestinal Care:
  - Nutritional support for the ventilated patient is a crucial aspect of their care in the ICU. Early

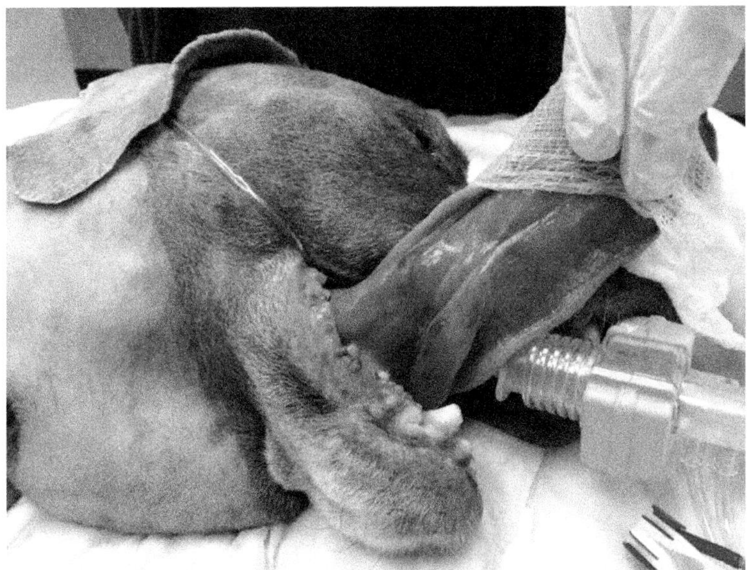

FIG. 4 Ranula formation in a mechanically ventilated dog.

nutritional support can help reduce catabolism, attenuate muscle wasting, and maintain nutritional status [20]. Enteral nutritional support can also modulate the immune response and reduce oxidative stress and infections by limiting bacterial translocation via the gut [20,21]. While nutritional support in mechanically ventilated small animals has not been reviewed specifically in the veterinary literature, it has been heavily studied in human patients. Lower mortality and more ventilator-free days have been reported in septic patients with severe pneumonia reaching higher protein and caloric intake earlier in their ICU stay [22]. It is also important to remember that nonnutritional calories (through infusions of dextrose or propofol) can also contribute to the caloric intake for individual patients.

- Patients should be evaluated for the presence of ileus via auscultation for borborygmi, and ultrasonographic evaluation of the gastrointestinal (GI) tract should be performed to look for evidence of peristalsis or dilation of the stomach/bowel loops.
- Nasogastric tubes can be placed to keep the stomach decompressed in patients with significant ileus to minimize the risk of regurgitation and aspiration of gastric contents.
- The frequency and character of bowel movements should be noted.
- The route of delivery of nutritional support has been heavily debated in human medicine, with recent evidence skewing in favor of enteral nutrition over parenteral nutrition in most patients. Enteral nutrition can be delivered in dogs and cats via nasogastric, gastric, or postpyloric (such as jejunal) routes.
- Patients should be monitored closely for signs of enteral feeding intolerance which may include high gastric residual volumes, regurgitation, and diarrhea. Recent data in humans have questioned the validity and utility of frequent measuring of gastric residual volumes [23]; however, repeated incidence of enteral feeding intolerance over multiple days has been found to be associated with a worse clinical outcome [24].
- Enteral feeding for critically ill patients receiving vasopressors has also been studied extensively in humans, but little data exist in mechanically ventilated dogs and cats. A recent study evaluating the use of enteral and parental nutrition in ventilated cats and dogs revealed that only 31% of patients received nutritional support, with a majority (88.9%) receiving parenteral nutrition. The study also found that animals with absent caloric intake for more than 72 hours had poor implementation of nutritional support [25]. The Society of Critical Care Medicine and American Society for Parenteral and Enteral

Nutrition clinical practice guidelines [26] suggest delaying enteral nutrition during uncontrolled shock, periods of hypotension, active resuscitation, or while administering high-dose vasopressors but recommend initiating nutrition as soon as shock is controlled or when pressor doses are low and stable. These patients should be watched closely for signs of GI intolerance including abdominal distension, lactic acidosis, dilated bowel loops, markedly worse nasogastric tube residual volumes, and worsening hemodynamic status (potentially indicating gut ischemia).

- Metabolic care and monitoring:
  - Patients should have regular monitoring of acid-base status, electrolytes, blood glucose, lactate, and complete blood count and chemistry profiles as needed.
  - Body temperature should be monitored continuously, and an indwelling rectal temperature probe may be used in these patients to detect hypothermia or hyperthermia/pyrexia. Hyperthermia may occur in patients with significant patient-ventilator dyssynchrony or during weaning trials, if the patient has excessive respiratory effort, and must be differentiated from pyrexia, which may be indicative of infection (such as VAP, or a different septic focus such as urosepsis or septic peritonitis) or inflammation (such as acute pancreatitis).
- Renal/urinary care:
  - Serial monitoring of renal values and urine output is recommended to monitor renal function.
  - Placement of a urinary catheter with a closed collection system in place is essential to prevent patient soiling, maintain hygiene, and quantify urinary output, as well as guide fluid therapy.
  - Urine output should be measured at least every 4 hours, and urine-specific gravity should be monitored as well. Strict aseptic precautions should be applied when handling the urinary catheter and collection system.
  - Mechanically ventilated patients have been known to develop hyponatremia and syndrome of inappropriate antidiuretic hormone secretion (SIADH), likely from nonosmotic stimulation of ADH secretion, as pulmonary venous baroreceptors respond to a reduction in effective blood volume (due to decreased left atrial pressure from increased pulmonary vascular resistance, or due to increased compression from hyperinflated lungs) [27]. In addition, opioid therapy may also trigger ADH secretion because of stimulation of opioid receptors in the hypothalamus [28]. Hypoxemia can also be a direct stimulus for ADH release by hypothalamic stimulation or arterial baroreceptor activation. There are no published studies documenting SIADH in ventilated dogs and cats, but the author has anecdotally noted oliguria to be a frequent occurrence in ventilated small animals. A single case report in a bulldog with aspiration pneumonia documents the development of SIADH, likely due to a combination of hypoxemia and decreased left atrial tension, although this dog was not mechanically ventilated [29]. Low-dose furosemide administration is often helpful in managing oliguria in these patients; the author typically uses a dose of 0.5 to 1.0 mg/kg IV every 6 to 8 hours as needed or a low-dose furosemide continuous infusion at a rate of 0.1 to 0.2 mg/kg/h.
- Neurologic care and monitoring:
  - Most ventilated small animals are maintained in a state of total intravenous anesthesia (TIVA), but animals that are maintained with tracheostomy tubes instead of endotracheal tubes may be able to remain much less sedate and more awake.
  - Sedative infusion protocols are typically a combination of 2 or more drug infusions and commonly include opioids (including pure mu agonists such as fentanyl or a mixed agonist-antagonist such as butorphanol), benzodiazepines, lidocaine, ketamine, dexmedetomidine, and propofol. The combination and infusion rates selected should ensure an adequate sedation plane such that the patient tolerates the endotracheal tube, and patient-ventilator dyssynchrony is avoided, particularly in the early stages of initiating ventilation. These infusions may also result in cardiovascular changes including hypotension, and doses may need to be adjusted in patients experiencing these effects. Inhalant anesthetics may be used as well, but this is less common.
    - Sedation protocols should be chosen based on a patient's underlying disease process, anticipated duration of ventilation, comorbidities, cost and availability considerations, and clinician comfort levels.
    - Commonly used drugs and infusion rates include,

  - Fentanyl: 2 to 15 mcg/kg/h
  - Butorphanol: 0.1 to 1.0 mg/kg/h
  - Midazolam (or diazepam): 0.1 to 1.0 mg/kg/h
  - Lidocaine: 25 to 60 mcg/kg/min
  - Dexmedetomidine: 0.1 to 1.0 mcg/kg/h
  - Ketamine: 0.05 to 0.5 mg/kg/h
  - Propofol: 0.05 to 0.5 mg/kg/min
  - Alfaxalone: 4 to 8 mg/kg/h
- Sedation interruption or "sedation vacation" has been extensively studied in human patients that are mechanically ventilated. The rationale behind sedation interruption is that prolonged continuous infusion of sedative drugs can cause bioaccumulation of these medications and potential adverse effects. The goal of sedation interruption (stopping or lowering sedation doses for a set period each day) is to minimize tissue drug accumulation and potentially allow for faster clearance which may facilitate more successful weaning when the patient is ready. Despite these benefits, recent studies have not documented a definitive survival benefit with this approach [30,31]. In general, the author recommends lowering sedation doses each day to the minimum effective dose to avoid excessive drug accumulation; a useful strategy is to lower sedation doses during night hours or other times when the ICU is likely to be quieter, to avoid causing stress and agitation in a patient on lower sedation doses.
- Neuromuscular blockade (NMB) and the use of paralytic agents during MV can be considered in patients to reduce patient-ventilator dyssynchrony and work of breathing [32]. Nondepolarizing NMBs such as atracurium and cisatracurium are most commonly used but should be used with great caution by intensive care clinicians experienced with their use. The recommended dose of atracurium is an initial bolus dose of 0.1 to 0.5 mg/kg IV, followed by a continuous infusion at a rate of 3 to 9 mcg/kg/min [33]. Risks of NMB include muscle weakness and atrophy with protracted use and failure to completely reverse paralytic effects. Seizures have also been reported in ventilated dogs receiving atracurium infusions [34]. *These drugs should not be routinely used to paralyze a dyssynchronous patient until underlying causes of patient-ventilator dyssynchrony have been thoroughly evaluated and addressed.*

- Integument and musculoskeletal care:
  - Recumbent sedated patients on MV remain at risk for development of decubital ulcers or pressure sores and can also develop atelectasis.
  - The patient's recumbency should be noted, and they should be turned at least every 4 hours to prevent pressure sore development. Patients should be well cushioned with adequate bedding (Fig. 5).
  - Passive range of motion exercises can be performed every 4 hours to prevent limb muscle atrophy from disuse, and massage and physical therapy exercises can also improve peripheral circulation and lymphatic flow, thereby helping to improve edema formation.
  - Intravenous catheter sites should be inspected several times every day, and catheters should be rewrapped frequently to minimize limb swelling and thrombophlebitis, as well as minimize the risk of catheter-related infections.

COMPLICATIONS OF MECHANICAL VENTILATION

MV, while lifesaving in critically ill patients, can have serious complications impacting a variety of organ systems. Intensive nursing care and monitoring can help mitigate several of these complications. These are summarized in Table 4.

WEANING FROM MECHANICAL VENTILATION

Weaning is the process of liberating the patient from the support of MV and from the endotracheal tube [37]. For a successful wean, the following criteria should be met:

- The patient should have adequate respiratory drive.
- The patient should have adequate neuromuscular function to take breaths of appropriate tidal volume.
- The patient's pulmonary function should be adequate to ensure that oxygenation can occur without ventilatory support.
- Ideally, the underlying disease that precipitated the need for MV should be addressed and should be either improving or resolved.

There are a multitude of different approaches to weaning patients, and each approach involves making small, single, incremental changes at a time to assess the impact of each change on the patient. As the patient's underlying disease improves or resolves, ventilatory support can be gradually reduced (such as reducing the magnitude of applied inspiratory pressure or PEEP) or allowing the patient to perform more of the work of

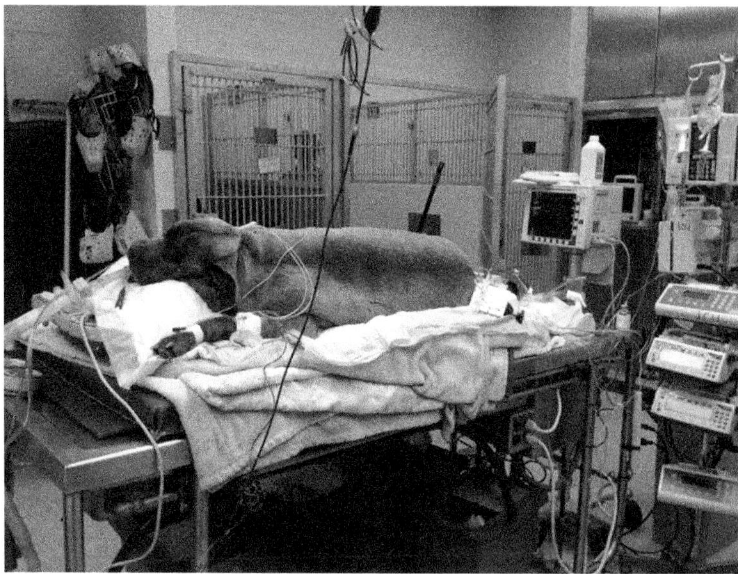

FIG. 5 Adequate padding and bedding should be ensured, especially in larger patients, to prevent formation of decubital ulcers with prolonged recumbency during mechanical ventilation.

breathing through modes such as SIMV or CPAP with pressure support. Each time such a change is made, the patient should be watched closely for signs of decompensation including desaturation and hypoxemia, hypercapnia and respiratory acidosis, tachypnea, tachycardia, hyperthermia, agitation/patient distress, hypotension, or patient-ventilator dyssynchrony and increased respiratory effort. If these occur, weaning efforts should be halted, and the patient should be placed back on the previous level (or higher if needed) of ventilatory support. Spontaneous breathing trials that assess the patient's ability to breathe spontaneously with minimal ventilator support are a crucial aspect of the weaning process.

The author recommends initially reducing the patient's FiO_2 from 100% down to at least 60% or lower during the first 24 to 48 hours of ventilation, if possible, to minimize the risk of oxygen toxicity. Subsequent weaning efforts will depend on how well the patient's underlying disease is improving. It is also important to plan for weaning attempts when assessing patient readiness by gradually titrating down doses of sedative infusions 12 to 24 hours ahead of time (particularly if long-acting medications such as barbiturates have been used for sedation) so that patients have adequate respiratory drive and are not excessively sedate during weaning attempts. Controlling patient anxiety and agitation as they are weaned is helpful to increase chances of success; the author typically uses low doses of acepromazine (0.003–0.01 mg/kg IV) administered 30 to 60 minutes before the patient is weaned to facilitate a calmer recovery. Rectal administration of trazodone has been recently described in dogs and may be a useful adjunct when weaning a patient off MV and discontinuing TIVA [38]. The author has had anecdotal success with rectal administration of trazodone (3–10 mg/kg) administered 30 to 60 minutes before discontinuing TIVA and weaning the patient.

It is important to remember that weaning a patient off MV is as much an art as it is a science, and there is a great deal of trial and error, coupled with close patient monitoring, involved. Weaning attempts will either succeed, in which case patients may be extubated ultimately, or fail, in which case patients may need to be reintubated and placed back on MV. Weaning failure in human patients is typically defined as failure of a spontaneous breathing trial or the need for reintubation within 48 hours of a prior extubation [39]. There are currently no accepted or established definitions for weaning failure in dogs and cats. Ultimately, if patients are prematurely weaned before they have adequate respiratory drive, muscle strength, and pulmonary function, wean failure and respiratory fatigue may ensue. If a patient is able to be successfully weaned off ventilatory support but fails extubation, consideration should be given to upper airway obstruction or excessive respiratory secretions that cannot be managed by the patient.

TABLE 4
Complications of Mechanical Ventilation

Hemodynamic effects	• High intrathoracic pressure can negatively impact right ventricular afterload and function due to increased pulmonary vascular resistance. • Increased intrathoracic pressure can also reduce venous return to the right side of the heart. • Increased right ventricular afterload may cause bulging of the interventricular septum toward the left ventricle resulting in decreased left ventricular size, volume, compliance, and ultimately cardiac output. • Hypotensive effects of sedative drugs via vasodilation, negative inotropy, or central mechanisms.
Respiratory complications	• Ventilator-associated pneumonia (VAP) • Respiratory muscle and diaphragmatic weakness • Ventilator-associated lung injury (VALI) [35]: Components of ventilator-associated lung injury include, ○ Volutrauma: Damage caused by overdistension of lungs with excessive tidal volumes. ○ Atelectotrauma: Lung injury associated with shear forces from repeated alveolar recruitment and collapse may be prevented by using a level of PEEP greater than the lower inflection point of the pressure volume curve. ○ Biotrauma: Pulmonary and systemic inflammation caused by the release of proinflammatory mediators/cytokines from lungs subjected to injurious mechanical ventilation. ○ Oxygen toxicity: Damage caused by a high concentration of inspired oxygen (typically FiO_2>60% for protracted periods of time). Consequences include reabsorption atelectasis, decreased parasympathetic tone, vasoconstrictive effects on cerebral and coronary perfusion, free-radical production. ○ Barotrauma: High pressure induced lung damage. This can result in pneumothorax, pulmonary interstitial emphysema, pneumomediastinum, pneumoperitoneum, pneumoretroperitoneum, and subcutaneous emphysema.
Renal effects	• Reduced renal blood flow due to reduced cardiac output can cause a "relative hypovolemia" and stimulation of the renin-angiotensin-aldosterone system leading to sodium and water retention. • SIADH in mechanically ventilated patients can cause decreased urine production.
Hepatic effects	• Downward movement of the diaphragm from positive pressure ventilation can increase portal venous pressure and impairment of bile and hepatic venous flow.
GI effects	• Functional ileus due to compromised splanchnic blood flow and reduced cardiac output. • GI bleeding from stress ulceration; this has been documented in humans [36] but has not definitively been established in ventilated small animal patients.
Complications related to operation of the ventilator	• Inaccurate or inappropriate ventilator settings. • Failure to set or address ventilator alarms. • Accidental loss of electrical power or disconnection of patient from the ventilator • Ventilator malfunction or failure (electrical, pneumatic, or microprocessor).

RECOVERY FROM MECHANICAL VENTILATION

Human patients that recover from MV have been documented to have a variety of long-term consequences that impact their quality of life and functional status. In veterinary medicine, this subject has not been explored in depth, likely because of a different patient population and comparatively shorter periods of time spent on the ventilator. However, a recent survey of pet owners whose pets survived MV revealed that cats and dogs are generally likely to recover well with minimal adverse effects on their quality of life [40]. In this study, owners of pets with neurologic diseases, particularly lower motor neuron diseases, reported poor quality of life for their pets. This is valuable information that may help critical care veterinarians when discussing the risks and benefits of MV with pet owners as part of a multipronged approach to clinical decision-making for these patients.

In conclusion, MV, when used appropriately, is a vital aspect of managing increasing numbers of critically ill small animals. As the use of MV in companion animal critical care grows, future research will be helpful in establishing guidelines and standards of care similar to those found in human medicine.

CLINICS CARE POINTS

- Once the decision is made to initiate MV for a patient, the clinician must consider the following:
  - Mode of ventilation to be used and associated ventilator settings
  - A sedation/anesthetic plan
  - Patient monitoring and instrumentation
- PEEP, when applied properly, can help splint open and "recruit" alveoli at the end of expiration and prevent airway collapse from atelectasis, thereby minimizing airway trauma and shear injury from cyclical opening and closing (atelectrauma). Judicious use of PEEP can be extremely beneficial for patients with diseased lungs, but care should be taken to monitor for its deleterious effects, including hemodynamic compromise and alveolar overdistension.
- As the patient's underlying disease improves or resolves, ventilatory support can be gradually reduced (such as reducing the magnitude of applied inspiratory pressure or PEEP or allowing the patient to perform more of the work of breathing through modes such as SIMV or CPAP with pressure support to facilitate weaning).

REFERENCES

[1] Bruchim Y, Aroch I, Sisso A, et al. A retrospective study of positive pressure ventilation in 58 dogs: indications, prognostic factors and outcome. J Small Anim Prac 2014;55(6):314–9.

[2] Hopper K, Haskins SC, Kass PH, et al. Indications, management, and outcome of long-term positive pressure ventilation in dogs and cats: 148 cases (1990-2001). J Am Vet Med Assoc 2007;230:64–75.

[3] Edwards TH, Coleman AE, Brainard BM, et al. Outcome of positive-pressure ventilation in dogs and cats with congestive heart failure: 16 cases (1992-2012). J Vet Emerg Crit Care 2014;24(5):586–93.

[4] King LG, Hendricks JC. Use of positive-pressure ventilation in dogs and cats: 41 cases (1990-1992). J Am Vet Med Assoc 1994;204(7):1045–52.

[5] Lee JA, Drobatz KJ, Koch MW, et al. Indications for and outcome of positive-pressure ventilation in cats: 53 cases (1993-2002). J Am Vet Med Assoc 2005;226(6):924–31.

[6] Hoareau GL, Mellema MS, Silverstein DC. Indication, management and outcome of brachycephalic dogs requiring mechanical ventilation. J Vet Emerg Crit Care 2011;21(3):226–35.

[7] Rutter CR, Rozanski EA, Sharp CR, et al. Outcome and medical management in dogs with lower motor neuron disease undergoing mechanical ventilation: 14 cases (2003-2009). J Vet Emerg Crit Care 2011;21(3):226–35.

[8] Webster RA, Mills PC, Morton JM. Indications, durations and outcomes of mechanical ventilation in dogs and cats with tick paralysis caused by Ixodes holocyclus: 61 cases (2008-2011). Aust Vet J 2013;91(6):233–9.

[9] Campbell VL, King LG. Pulmonary function, ventilator management and outcome of dogs with thoracic trauma and pulmonary contusions: 10 cases (1994-1998). J Am Vet Med Assoc 2000;217(10):1505–9.

[10] Sabino CV, Holowaychuk M, Bateman S. Management of acute respiratory distress syndrome in a French bulldog using airway pressure release ventilation. J Vet Emerg Crit Care 2013;23(4):447–54.

[11] Armengol J, Jones RL, King EG. Alveolar pressures and lung volumes during high frequency oscillatory ventilation in dogs. Crit Care Med 1985;13(8):632–6.

[12] Angriman F, Ferreyro BL, Donaldson L, et al. The harm of high-frequency oscillatory ventilation (HFOV) in ARDS is not related to a high baseline risk of acute cor pulmonale or short-term changes in hemodynamics. Intensive Care Med 2020;46(1):132–4.

[13] Luecke T, Pelosi P. Clinical review: Positive end-expiratory pressure and cardiac output. Crit Care 2005; 9(6):607–21.

[14] Boone MD, Jinadasa SP, Mueller A, et al. The effect of positive end-expiratory pressure on intracranial pressure and cerebral hemodynamics. Neurocrit Care 2017; 26(2):174–81.

[15] Hickey SM, Giwa AO. Mechanical ventilation. In: StatPearls. Treasure Island (FL): StatPearls Publishing; 2020.

[16] Hunter JD. Ventilator associated pneumonia. Br Med J 2012;344:e3325.

[17] Zhao T, Wu X, Zhang Q, et al. Oral hygiene care for critically ill patients to prevent ventilator-associated pneumonia. Cochrane Database Syst Rev 2020;(12): CD008367.

[18] Zand F, Zahed L, Mansouri P, et al. The effects of oral rinse with 0.2% and 2% chlorhexidine on oropharyngeal colonization and ventilator associated pneumonia in adults' intensive care units. J Crit Care 2017;40(1): 318–22.

[19] Fox C, Daly M, Bellis T. Identification of ventilator-associated pneumonia in dogs and evaluation of empiric antimicrobial therapy: 13 cases (2012–2016). J Vet Emerg Crit Care 2021;31(1):66–73.

[20] Bear DE, Wandrag L, Merriweather JL, et al. The role of nutritional support in the physical and functional recovery of critically ill patients: a narrative review. Crit Care 2017;21(1):226.

[21] Preiser JC, van Zanten AR, Berger MM, et al. Metabolic and nutritional support of critically ill patients: consensus and controversies. Crit Care 2015;19(1):35.

[22] Elke G, Wang M, Weiler N, et al. Close to recommended caloric and protein intake by enteral nutrition is associated with better clinical outcome of critically ill septic patients: secondary analysis of a large international nutrition database. Crit Care 2014;18(1):R29.

[23] Reignier J, Mercier E, Le Gouge A, et al. Effect of not monitoring residual gastric volume on risk of ventilator-associated pneumonia in adults receiving mechanical ventilation and early enteral feeding: a randomized controlled trial. JAMA 2013;309(3):249–56.

[24] Heyland DK, Ortiz A, Stoppe C, et al. Incidence, risk factors, and clinical consequence of enteral feeding intolerance in the mechanically ventilated critically Ill: an analysis of a multicenter, multiyear database. Crit Care Med 2021;49(1):49–59.

[25] Greensmith TD, Chan DL. Audit of the provision of nutritional support to mechanically ventilated dogs and cats. J Vet Emerg Crit Care 2021;31:387–95.

[26] Taylor BE, McClave SA, Martindale RG, et al. Guidelines for the provision and assessment of nutrition support therapy in the adult critically Ill patient: society of critical care medicine (SCCM) and American Society for Parenteral and Enteral Nutrition (A.S.P.E.N.). Crit Care Med 2016;44(2):390–438.

[27] Jones DP. Syndrome of inappropriate secretion of antidiuretic hormone and hyponatremia. Pediatr Rev 2018; 39(1):27–35.

[28] Karahan S, Karagöz H, Erden A, et al. Codeine-induced syndrome of inappropriate antidiuretic hormone: case report. Balkan Med J 2014;31(1):107–9.

[29] Bowles KD, Brainard BM, Coleman KD. Syndrome of inappropriate antidiuretic hormone in a bulldog with aspiration pneumonia. J Vet Intern Med 2015;29(3): 972–6.

[30] Olsen HT, Nedergaard HK, Strøm T, et al. Nonsedation or light sedation in critically ill, mechanically ventilated patients. N Engl J Med 2020;382(12):1103–11.

[31] Burry L, Rose L, McCullagh IJ, et al. Daily sedation interruption versus no daily sedation interruption for critically ill adult patients requiring invasive mechanical ventilation. Cochrane Database Syst Rev 2014;7: CD009176.

[32] National Heart, Lung, and Blood Institute PETAL Clinical Trials Network. Early neuromuscular blockade in the acute respiratory distress syndrome. N Engl J Med 2019;380(21):1997–2008.

[33] Plumb DC. Plumb's veterinary drug handbook. 8th edition. Ames, IA: Wiley Blackwell; 2015. p. 124–6.

[34] Donaldson RE, Cortellini S, Humm K. Seizure activity following atracurium continuous rate infusion in three mechanically ventilated juvenile dogs. J Vet Emerg Crit Care 2020;30(5):592–6.

[35] Pinhu L, Whitehead T, Evans T, et al. Ventilator-associated lung injury. Lancet 2003;361(9354):332–40.

[36] Cook D, Heyland D, Griffith L, et al, Canadian Critical Care Trials Group. Risk factors for clinically important upper gastrointestinal bleeding in patients requiring mechanical ventilation. Crit Care Med 1999;27(12):2812–7.

[37] Mellema MS, Haskins SC. Weaning from mechanical ventilation. Clin Tech Small Anim Pract 2000;15(3): 157–64.

[38] O'Donnell EM, Press SA, Karriker MJ, et al. Pharmacokinetics and efficacy of trazodone following rectal administration of a single dose to healthy dogs. Am J Vet Res 2020;81(9):739–46.

[39] Esteban A, Frutos F, Tobin MJ, et al. A comparison of four methods of weaning patients from mechanical ventilation. Spanish Lung Failure Collaborative Group. N Engl J Med 1995;332(6):345–50.

[40] Donaldson RE, Barfield D. Quality of life following mechanical ventilation in dogs and cats. J Vet Emerg Crit Care 2020;30(6):718–21.

Advances in Small Animal Care 2 (2021) 85–100
ADVANCES IN SMALL ANIMAL CARE

Medical and Surgical Management of Ureteral Obstructions

Dana L. Clarke, VMD, DACVECC
Interventional Radiology & Critical Care, Department of Clinical Sciences and Advanced Medicine, University of Pennsylvania School of Veterinary Medicine, 3900 Spruce Street, Philadelphia, PA 19104, USA

KEYWORDS

- Ureteral obstruction • Ureterolith • Ureteral surgery • Interventional radiology • Ureteral stenting
- Subcutaneous ureteral bypass (SUB)

KEY POINTS

- Ureteral obstructions are becoming an increasingly recognized cause of acute and chronic azotemia in small animal patients.
- The most common cause of ureteral obstructions in dogs and cats is ureterolithiasis.
- Although medical management is needed in most cases of ureteral obstruction, the vast majority of cases require surgical or interventional treatments to resolve the obstruction and preserve renal function.
- Interventional techniques are becoming more widely available for veterinary patients with ureteral obstructions, including ureteral stenting and subcutaneous ureteral bypass.

INTRODUCTION

Ureteral obstruction is an important differential in any azotemic patient and requires prompt diagnosis, treatment, and possible intervention, for successful management and preservation of renal function. Many animals with ureteral obstruction are critically ill at the time of emergency evaluation, especially if there is dysfunction of the contralateral kidney. Because historical information and clinical signs are often nonspecific, diagnostic testing, including blood work and imaging, is essential for confirming and characterizing the nature of the obstruction. Depending on the etiology, patient stability, and concurrent medical conditions, medical, surgical, and interventional options may be considered to relieve the obstruction. Controversy exists as to the ideal approach for treating ureteral obstructions in veterinary medicine. Factors such as cause and location of the obstruction, clinician experience, and client preference and finances will continue to guide much of the decision-making until a consensus on best practices for ureteral obstructions is reached.

ETIOLOGY

Although ureterolithiasis is the most common cause of ureteral obstructions, there are a variety of other causes, including strictures, congenital stenosis, solidified blood calculi, retroperitoneal fibrosis, circumcaval ureter, ureteral ectopia, iatrogenic ureteral ligation, obstructive pyonephrosis, and neoplasia (intraluminal obstruction, trigonal, and extraluminal compression) [1–25]. In addition to the primary pathology that causes the ureteral obstruction, chronicity and function of the contralateral kidney are other important factors

E-mail address: clarked@vet.upenn.edu

https://doi.org/10.1016/j.yasa.2021.07.009
2666-450X/21/ © 2021 Elsevier Inc. All rights reserved.

that impact the degree of illness and clinical decision-making. For all causes of ureteral obstruction, the pathophysiology that results in obstructive nephropathy is similar. Renal blood flow and glomerular filtration rate (GFR) are decreased owing to increased pressure within the ureter and renal pelvis, causing obstruction of urine flow. The reduced GFR causes tubular inflammation and injury that is dependent on not only the severity and duration of the obstruction but also the degree of underlying renal disease, such as chronic tubular interstitial nephritis. If the obstruction persists, the acute inflammation will contribute to nephron loss and fibrosis, resulting in a small, irregular kidney [26–31].

DIAGNOSTIC APPROACH

Clinical signs associated with ureteral obstructions are often nonspecific and associated with uremia. In dogs and cats with acute ureteral obstruction, halitosis, hypersalivation, vomiting, anorexia, lethargy, polyuria and polydipsia, and abdominal pain may be present. For more chronic obstructions, weight loss may also be noted [2,17,23–25,32]. Lower urinary tract signs such as hematuria, stranguria, pollakiuria, incontinence, and inappropriate urination may also be present and have been described in up to 25% of cats and 60% of dogs [2,10,17,23–25,32].

Physical examination findings are generally nonspecific in dogs and cats with ureteral obstructions: depression, dehydration, loss of muscle mass, abdominal pain (particularly on renal palpation), nausea, uremic ulcers, renomegaly, and/or decreased kidney size with or without irregular borders [2,10,17,23–25,32]. Two retrospective studies on cats undergoing ureteral stenting noted heart murmurs in 48% to 54% of cats, which could be due to concurrent anemia, cardiac dysfunction secondary to uremia, or underlying structural heart disease [23,24].

Because history and physical examination findings are rarely diagnostic for a ureteral obstruction, additional diagnostics, including blood work and imaging, are necessary in cases of suspected ureteral disease. First-line clinicopathologic diagnostics are complete blood count (CBC), serum chemistry, acid–base assessment, urinalysis, and urine culture. In anemic patients, or those for whom surgical intervention is being considered, blood type and cross-match (in cats) should be performed. In addition, coagulation testing should be performed in patients for whom surgery is anticipated or if there are concerns for coagulation derangements secondary to urosepsis.

Diagnostic imaging is essential for confirming a diagnosis of ureteral disease. Abdominal radiographs are useful to evaluate for radio-opaque calculi along the urinary tract, renomegaly, and loss of peritoneal and retroperitoneal detail. Abdominal radiographs have been shown to have 100% specificity and 66% sensitivity in cats [1,2] and 88% in dogs for detecting ureteral obstruction [25]. The lack of high sensitivity in cats may be due to radiolucent ureteroliths, obstruction by dried solidified blood stones, overlapping colonic contents, obscured visualization by vertebrae, and obstructive ureteroliths below the radiographic limit of detection (2 mm), as the internal diameter of feline ureter is 0.4 mm [33,34]. Larger stones are generally located in the proximal ureter in cats, with 44% of feline ureteroliths in the proximal ureter, 41% in the midureter, and 15% at the ureterovesicular junction (UVJ) [35].

Ultrasound has improved sensitivity (98%) and specificity (96%) for detection of ureteroliths in cats [36]. Like radiographs, ultrasonography cannot detect dried solidified blood stones within the ureter; therefore, it is important to keep this in mind in cases of suspected feline ureteral obstruction without a definitive cause of obstruction visualized intraluminally on sonography [4,9,36–38]. Ultrasound has the additional benefit of allowing assessment of renal pelvic and ureteral dilation, ureteral and renal inflammation, retroperitoneal and peritoneal effusion, ureteral stricture, extraluminal compressions, and urinary tract neoplasia [2,10,15,16,36–38]. While renal pelvic dilation and ureteral dilation can be identified with nonobstructive urinary tract diseases, such as pyelonephritis and pyonephrosis, dilation of the renal pelvis of greater than 13 mm was 100% sensitive for the diagnosis of a ureteral obstruction [37]. However, there is growing evidence and clinical experience supporting the idea that ureteral obstructions can occur with minimal, if any, dilation of the renal pelvis and/or ureter, especially in acute cases and obstructions at the ureteropelvic junction. In cats with pyelography confirmed ureteral obstruction at the time of placement of subcutaneous ureteral bypass (SUB), 35% of cats had less than 4 mm of pelvic dilation [39]. Therefore, lack of significant pelvic or ureteral dilation should not exclude the diagnosis of a ureteral obstruction, especially in cats. Ultrasound-guided aspiration of urine from the renal pelvis can be used for culture and sensitivity, which is more sensitive for detecting bacterial infection secondary to pyelonephritis than samples from the urinary bladder [40,41]. It can also be used for antegrade pyelography under digital radiography or fluoroscopy to confirm and localize the source of ureteral obstruction (Fig. 1). Complications of antegrade pyelography include contrast leakage precluding a diagnostic study, hemorrhage, renal pelvic laceration, and uroabomen/uroretroperitoneum [40,41]. If performed in the face of obstruction, capabilities for resolution of the obstruction surgically or interventionally need to be readily available, as urine leakage can occur from the site of renal puncture [40,41]. During cystoscopic procedures, aspiration of urine directly from the renal pelvis via retrograde ureteral catheterization is also feasible for culture and sensitivity testing [17]. The technique for antegrade pyelography used during ureteral stent or bypass placement is described later in discussion.

Because heart murmurs are diagnosed in approximately 50% of feline ureteral obstruction patients, and urosepsis secondary to ureteral obstruction is common in dogs which could result in cardiac dysfunction, echocardiographs and electrocardiogram (ECG) should also be considered in patients with suspected ureteral obstructions to guide fluid therapy, analgesic, and anesthetic choices [23,24].

MEDICAL MANAGEMENT

Management of interstitial and intravascular fluid imbalances, electrolyte derangements, complications of uremia, bacterial infection, and pain are important in patients with ureteral obstructions. The need for supportive care, as well as medical attempts at stone expulsion, and treatment of other causes of ureteral obstruction including pyonephrosis and ureteritis must be balanced with concerns for irreversible nephron loss that occurs with ongoing obstruction. In 52 cats, ureterolith passage into the bladder with medical management alone was successful in 9 cats (17%) [3]. Additionally, cats treated medically had a 66% one- and 2-year survival rate compared with 91% and 88% in cats managed with surgical intervention, respectively [3,40]. Given the impact on long-term survival, less than 20% success rate of medically induced ureterolith passage in cats, and complications with fluid overload and systemic inflammatory response syndrome (SIRS) and sepsis in patients with obstructive pyonephrosis, only short durations (1–3 days) of medical therapy as the sole treatment for ureteral obstructions are generally recommended before pursuing more definitive resolution if medical management is unsuccessful.

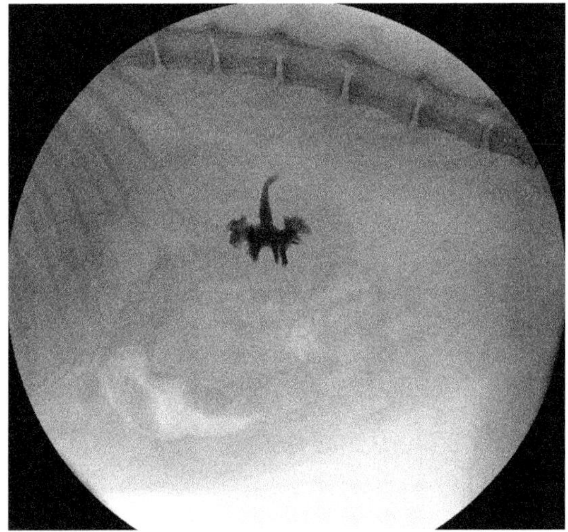

FIG. 1 Fluoroscopic image obtained after percutaneous pyelogram showing marked proximal ureteral narrowing distal to the renal pelvis consistent with a ureteral stricture.

Fluid therapy to correct hypovolemia and treat interstitial hydration is accomplished with isotonic replacement crystalloids. When hypernatremia secondary to free water deficit is present, hypotonic crystalloids may also be considered after correction of intravascular volume depletion. Regardless of the crystalloid used, avoidance of overhydration is appropriate. Careful monitoring of body weight, urine output, skin turgor, and mucous membranes should be done and trended closely for weight gain of more than 10%, chemosis, increased respiratory rate and effort, harsh lung sounds, and gelatinous feel to the skin and subcutaneous tissue [42]. Cage-side ultrasound to assess the left atrial-to-aortic root ratios (L_a:A_O) can also be helpful to assess intravascular volume expansion and monitor for volume overload with increase in the ratio. In dogs, the normal La:Ao ratio is 1.3, whereas the ratio is 1.5 in cats [43,44].

Hyperkalemia is a life-threatening complication of ureteral obstructions and decreased urine output. Intravenous fluid therapy, 25% dextrose (0.5 - 1 g/kg IV diluted, over 3–5 minutes), regular insulin/25% dextrose (0.5 - 1 U/kg IV and 1–2 g/kg IV diluted, over 3–5 minutes), beta-agonist therapy (0.01 mg/kg terbutaline IV), and sodium bicarbonate therapy [0.3 × weight (kg) × base deficit; diluted to make isotonic to the patient's pH and given in 1/3–1/2 dose increments while monitoring acid–base status and sodium] may be necessary to treat severe hyperkalemia (K>8.0 mEq/L) and prevent cardiac dysrhythmias secondary to hyperkalemia. When dysrhythmias are present, 10% calcium gluconate (0.5–1.5 mL/kg IV slowly over 5–10 min with continuous ECG evaluation) can be given to help restore cardiac myocyte electrochemical gradients that cause dysrhythmias but will not treat the hyperkalemia. Should the patient's hyperkalemia become refractory to medical intervention, intermittent hemodialysis (IHD) and continuous renal replacement therapy (CRRT) can provide the potassium stabilization needed until definitive relief of the obstruction occurs. Extracorporeal therapies may also be considered for patients who are anuric, critically ill from uremia, and are fluid overloaded. Limited availability, cost, dialysis disequilibrium syndrome, and complications associated with placement of large bore central catheters, anticoagulation, removal of large volumes of total vascular volume, and transfusion needs (especially in small patients) can limit the utility of this treatment modality patients with ureteral obstructions [45]. Extracorporeal therapies do not address the pathophysiology and renal injury caused by obstructive nephropathy, and therefore even in the face of improved azotemia, electrolyte disturbances, and fluid balance, renal injury continues.

Additional medications used in patients with ureteral obstructions include osmotic diuretics, alpha-receptor antagonists, ureteral smooth-muscle relaxants, and antibiotic therapy (Table 1). Broad-spectrum bactericidal antibiotics, preferably those that concentrate well in urine, are indicated in ureteral obstructions as up to 54% of dogs and 32% of cats have concurrent urinary tract infections [23–25,46]. Osmotic diuretics such as mannitol increase urine volume in effort to "push" stones and debris down the ureter. They are exclusively renally excreted and must therefore be used with caution in patients at risk for volume overload, especially with cardiac disease or decreased urine output. Limited data are available to support the efficacy of ureteral relaxation with alpha-reception antagonists such as prazosin and tamsulosin or ureteral smooth-muscle relaxation with glucagon or amitriptyline, though these medications may be considered in patients with obstructive ureteral calculi [20].

SURGICAL MANAGEMENT

Surgical management is the traditional mainstay of veterinary ureteral obstruction management, especially in cases of obstructive ureterolithiasis. Detailed discussion of these techniques is beyond the scope of this text, and consultation of veterinary surgical texts and surgeons experienced in these techniques is strongly advised given the challenging nature of veterinary ureteral surgery, especially in cats. Intraoperative magnification (8–15×), microsurgical instrumentation, and fine

TABLE 1
Medical Therapy Used in Conjunction with Fluid Therapy to Induce Ureterolith Passage

Drug	Mechanism of Action	Dose in Dogs	Dose in Cats
Amitriptyline	Ureteral smooth-muscle relaxation by opening of potassium-dependent voltage channels	0.25–4.4 mg/kg PO q12–24 h while on fluids	0.5–2 mg/kg PO q24 h or 10 mg per cat PO q12-24 h while on fluids
Glucagon	Ureteral smooth-muscle relaxation	0.05-0.1 mg/kg every 12 hours for up to 4 doses	0.05-0.1 mg/kg every 12 hours for up to 4 doses
Prazosin	Alpha-1 antagonist for ureteral smooth-muscle relaxation	1–2 mg per dog PO q8–12 h	0.25–0.5 mg per cat PO q12–24 h
Tamsulosin	Alpha-1 antagonist for ureteral smooth-muscle relaxation	0.004–0.006 mg/kg PO q12–24 h (Extralabel use and dose) May take 3 d to be effective	Safety, efficacy, and dose have not been studied in cats
Mannitol	Osmotic diuretic to increase flow of urine in the ureter	0.25-1 g/kg IV over 30 min; repeat q4–6 h × 3 if needed, CRI of 60–120 mg/kg/h can also be considered	0.25-1 g/kg IV over 30 min; repeat q4–6 h × 3 if needed, CRI of 60–120 mg/kg/h can also be considered
Amlodipine	Smooth-muscle relaxation via blockade of calcium channels	0.1–0.4 mg/kg PO q24 h	0.625–1.25 mg PO per cat q24 h

From Degner D, Clarke D. Chapter 21: Urinary Obstruction: Ureteral Obstruction. In: Aronson, LR, ed. Small Animal Surgical Emergencies. 1st ed. John Wiley & Sons, Ltd. 2016:224-236.

polypropylene or nylon suture (5–0 to 10–0) are needed for successful ureteral surgery.

A single ureterotomy, or in some cases, multiple ureterotomies, is one of the most common surgical techniques used for removal of obstructive ureteroliths. A longitudinal incision is made into the ureter proximal to the stone, being careful not to displace the stone cranially or damage the delicate ureteral blood supply during manipulation. After stone removal, the ureterotomy is closed in a simple interrupted pattern. If there is extensive damage to the ureter due to prolonged obstruction, or in cases of ureteral stricture or focal neoplasia, ureteral resection and anastomosis may be considered. Preservation of the ureteral fat and blood supply is important to promote healing of the anastomotic site. Spatulation of the proximal and distal ureteral segments is used to facilitate closure of the anastomosis using full-thickness circumferential simple interrupted sutures.

For ureteral obstructions located in the midureter to distal ureter, neoureterocystostomy (ureteral reimplantation) is another surgical technique commonly used for ureteral diseases, including ureterolithiasis and strictures. The ureter is ligated at its distal insertion into the bladder and transected proximal to the obstructive lesion after transmural positioning in the apex of the bladder. There are two techniques for reimplantation: the intravesicular technique that requires bladder eversion and the extravesicular technique that does not involve bladder herniation and therefore requires a smaller incision (Fig. 2). Regardless of the technique chosen, it is essential to ensure precise apposition of ureteral mucosa to bladder mucosa to facilitate healing, prevent urine leakage, and ensure that a secondary stricture at the reimplantation site does not form. If there is tension on the surgical site when the bladder is decompressed and retracted into its normal position in the caudal abdomen, a renal descensus, which involves dissection of the kidney from its retroperitoneal attachments for increased caudal mobility, and cystopexy are techniques for tension relief described in conjunction with ureteral surgery [3]. It is important to minimize tissue handling and trauma as much as possible to avoid inflammation and edema of the mucosa, which can result in obstruction of the site and has been reported to occur in 6% to 9% of cases and may delay resolution of azotemia [3,40]. Urine leakage or uroabdomen has been reported in 2% to 30% of cases undergoing ureterotomy or ureteral resection and anastomosis [3,21,24,47]. Other postoperative considerations for animals undergoing ureteral surgery include stone recurrence, stricture formation, and migration of nephroliths. Major postoperative complications are reported in up to 31% of cats, and mortality rates in this population may be as high as 21% [1,3,21,24,25,33,34,47,48].

Another surgical technique that has been described for a cat with a proximal ureteral stricture confirmed on antegrade pyelography and secondary obstruction was the use of a modified Boari flap [49]. The Boari flap is described for use in human patients requiring ureteral reconstruction after hysterectomy, difficult ureterotomy, ureteral strictures, and retroperitoneal fibrosis. To create the Boari flap, a tube is made from an apical portion of bladder that extends to and is attached to the ureteral orifice [50,51]. In the feline case report, the flap was created from the ventral bladder and attached to the ureter after transection proximal to the location of the obstruction. Closure was performed with a circumferential simple interrupted pattern, and there was no tension on the ureteroneocystotomy site requiring renal descensus or cystopexy. The diversion technique resolved the patient's azotemia and ultrasonographic evidence of obstruction, with the cat continuing to do well 7 months postoperatively [49].

Given the challenges surrounding ureteral surgery, especially in cats, as well as the complications and associated mortality, exploration into alternative techniques for urinary diversion has gained traction in veterinary medicine over the past 15 years.

INTERVENTIONAL MANAGEMENT

With growing experience in minimally invasive technology in veterinary medicine, adaptations of techniques previously reserved for human ureteral obstruction patients has become feasible and more widely available. Intraoperative imaging technology, such as fluoroscopy and cystoscopy, a variety of interventional equipment, including stents, guidewires, catheters, and access needles, as well as specialized training are needed to perform these procedures. As clinician experience and the body of literature regarding complications, outcomes, and techniques continues to expand, it is very likely that the widespread availability of veterinarians comfortable performing these procedures will expand as well.

Nephrostomy tubes can provide rapid, temporary decompression of the renal pelvis in patients with ureteral obstructions. They may also provide a preliminary indication of remaining renal function on relief of the obstructive process. However, renal recovery after

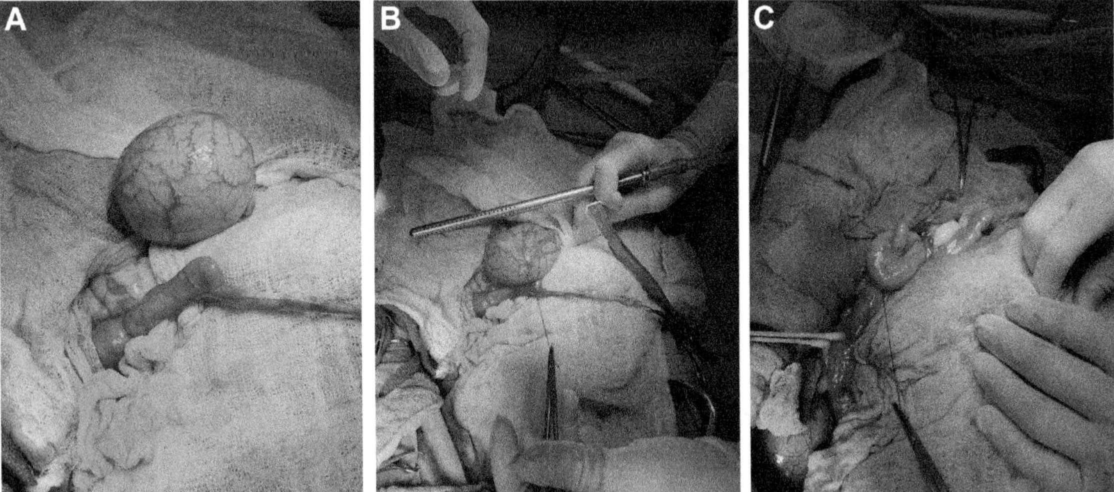

FIG. 2 (**A**) Intraoperative image of a dog with a markedly dilated ureter to the level of the midureter and narrowed ureter distally. The distal ureter has been transected in preparation for ureteral reimplantation. (**B**) Bladder positioning to confirm that the apex of the bladder can contact the dilated segment for an intravesicular technique for reimplantation. (**C**) Transected ureter has been pulled into the bladder lumen, which is everted, before suturing using an intravesicular technique.

obstruction can take up to 4 months in canine ureteral obstruction models, which are performed in dogs with normal renal function [26,52]. It is imperative to keep in mind that severity of obstruction (complete vs partial), duration, and prior underlying renal disease will contribute to the degree of recovery of renal function in clinical veterinary patients; therefore, a short-term lack of resolution of azotemia may not correlate with an inability to recover in the weeks to months that follow relief of the obstruction. Locking loop pig-tail catheters are recommended for nephrostomy tubes because their locking mechanism helps secure the catheter into the renal pelvis. Placement is achieved using ultrasound guidance and fluoroscopy. Percutaneous placement is feasible in dogs and cats, but surgical placement with nephropexy is recommended in cats owing to the mobility of their kidneys and increased risk of tube dislodgement with movement [3,22,34,53].

Ureteral stenting in veterinary patients has been described for the management ureterolithiasis, dried solidified blood stones, ureteral strictures, intraluminal bypass to facilitate healing after ureteral surgery or trauma, prevention of ureteral spasm after sclerotherapy for renal hematuria, drainage of obstructive pyonephrosis, passive ureteral dilation and stone fragment passage after extracorporeal shockwave lithotripsy (ESWL), and neoplasia [10,12,17,20,23–25,32,38,47,53–59]. Both temporary and long-term ureteral stent usages are described in dogs and cats, which is in contrast to most uses in human patients. In human urology, ureteral stents are generally left in place for only short periods of time before exchange or removal. Stents are removed because of concerns for infection and encrustation, as well as the discomfort people experience with ureteral stents [60,61].

There are a variety of techniques for placement of ureteral stents in veterinary patients, including antegrade and retrograde placement via laparotomy, cystoscopic placement using both rigid and flexible endoscopy, percutaneous antegrade placement, and using a percutaneous transvesicular scope–assisted technique described for urolith retrieval [62]. The technique for a given patient is determined by patient signalment, the nature of the ureteral obstruction, equipment and expertise availability, and if other concurrent abdominal procedures are necessary for the patient. Fluoroscopy is the preferred intraoperative imaging modality for ureteral stent placement and positioning, although it is possible repeated digital radiographs could be used in straightforward cases of surgical ureteral stent placement to visualize guidewire placement and stent positioning. However, radiographs not advised given concerns for inadvertent perforation of the ureteral wall or renal pelvis with the wire during manipulation if performed with only intermittent visualization. Rigid cystoscopy is preferred for minimally invasive ureteral stent placement owing to the challenges associated with wire manipulation, lack of angled visualization (0-degree scope), and the amount of scope support needed for retrograde cannulation of the UVJ using flexible cystoscopy. To avoid the challenges of flexible cystoscopy and ureteral stent placement in male dogs, a perineal access technique to facilitate rigid cystoscopy in male dogs has been described for endourologic treatment of obstructive ureterolithiasis, ectopic ureters, and idiopathic renal hematuria [63].

There are multiple benefits of ureteral stents, including passive ureteral dilation to facilitate stone or stone fragment passage and relief of obstruction, support for ureteral healing after surgery, drainage of inspissated and obstructive purulent material from the renal pelvis, prevention of ureteral spasm after chemical cauterization (sclerotherapy) for renal hematuria, and intraluminal decompression secondary to urinary tract neoplasia without surgical manipulation of the urinary tract [12,17,20,23,24,47,53,54,58,59,64,65]. Ureteral stents can also be removed or exchanged if there is excessive patient discomfort, migration, recurrent infections, or resolution of the obstruction.

Ureteral stents are available in a variety of different diameters and lengths, as well as different materials. Stents manufactured for human urology can often be used in medium to large dogs, but are too large for feline ureteral use given the small size (0.4 mm internal diameter) of the feline ureter [21,33]. Ureteral stents specifically designed for veterinary patients, including cats and canine malignant ureteral obstructions, are commercially available. Stents designed specifically for use with canine trigonal neoplasia do not have fenestrations on the portion of the stent positioned within the bladder to minimize tumor ingrowth into the stent. Ureteral stents designed for cats have a 2+ French diameter, which is just less than 1 mm diameter (3 Fr = 1 mm) and are available in 12-, 14-, and 16-cm lengths (Infiniti Medical, LLC). Ureteral stent sizes used in small dogs may range from 2+ to 3.7 Fr, 3.7 to 4.7 Fr in medium dogs, and 6 to 7 Fr in large dogs or those with marked ureteral dilation [48]. The diameter of the pig-tail coil varies with stent size and manufacturer. Ureteral stent length available for dogs varies on diameter and whether or not the stent is designed for dogs or human urology use. Stent length is described as the distance between both pig-tail coils, also known as the shaft length. Ureteral stent length is based on the distance from the renal pelvis to the UVJ in the bladder. Preoperative radiographs with a marker of known size for calibration, an intraoperative sterile ruler for direct ureteral length measurement, a marker catheter in the colon, or direct measurement of wire and/or ureteral catheter length can be used to determine ureteral stent length needed. In addition to the length needed to traverse the ureter, an additional short length (2–4 cm) is added to the measured distance to decide on the final stent size, for the stent to curve away from the trigone and toward the bladder apex to minimize trigonal irritation (Fig. 3). Deciding on stent length can be challenging with markedly tortuous ureters, in which case a longer stent should be selected to ensure it is positioned properly through the turn of the ureter.

For cystoscopic ureteral stenting via rigid cystoscopy in female dogs and rarely in female cats, and percutaneous perineal access in male dogs, dorsal patient positioning is preferred for ease of access to the ureteral openings. After diagnostic cystoscopy, the UVJ of the affected ureter is visualized using the cystoscope. Based on patient size, and anticipated ureteral stent diameter to be placed, the corresponding diameter angled hydrophilic wire is passed through the working channel of the scope and into the ureteral opening by an assistant. Once cannulated with the wire, fluoroscopy is used to visualize wire passage into the distal ureter. Because the distal ureter has a characteristic "J" shape, passage of the wire across this turn can be challenging. Positioning of the scope just at the UVJ to facilitate wire passage into the distal ureter provides stability while turning and directing the angled tip of the wire. Once the wire in positioned within the distal ureter, the "J"-shaped turn will straighten, making subsequent catheter and wire passage less difficult. An open-ended ureteral catheter is passed over the wire (within the working channel of the scope) into the distal ureter under fluoroscopic visualization and the wire subsequently removed. A 50:50 dilution of iodinated contrast agent is injected into the ureteral catheter to facilitate under fluoroscopy for retrograde ureteropyelography to determine the location(s) of the ureteral obstruction(s). Care must be taken not to overdistend the renal pelvis to prevent rupture of the pelvis. The wire is replaced and gently advanced into the renal pelvis under constant fluoroscopic visualization, again being sure not to puncture the ureter or renal pelvis with the end of the wire. Once the wire is curled within the renal pelvis, the ureteral catheter can be advanced over the wire and into the pelvis for sample collection (cytology, culture, and sensitivity) and lavage, which may be necessary in cases of obstructive pyonephrosis [17]. Once the appropriate stent length is determined, the ureteral stent is advanced over the wire. A "pusher" is also packaged with ureteral stents to facilitate advancement of

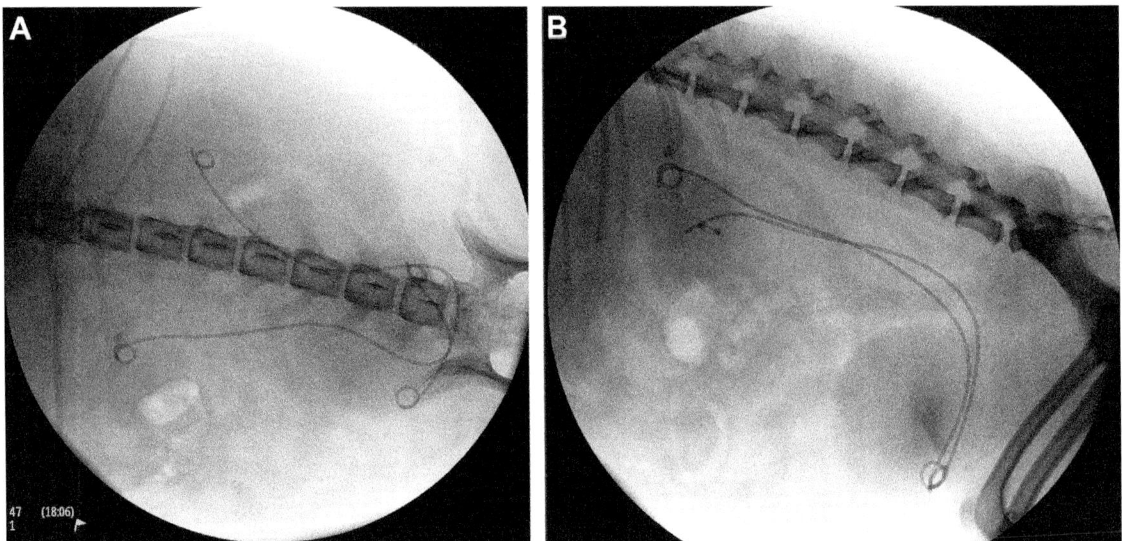

FIG. 3 (A) Ventrodorsal projection of bilateral cystoscopically placed ureteral stents in a dog. (B) Lateral projection of bilateral ureteral stents.

the stent into the ureter once the stent length is contained within the working channel of the scope and therefore no longer accessible for manual advancement. Once the stent is coiled within the renal pelvis, the wire is retracted into the end of the stent and the remaining length of the stent is "pushed" into the bladder using the pusher over the wire in the scope working channel. Ureteral stents are marked with a black line on the shaft at one end of the stent. For cystoscopic placement, it is essential that this line is placed within the bladder, as it is the indicator that the stent is near its end when visualized via the cystoscope.

Surgical retrograde ureteral stenting is performed similarly to retrograde cystoscopic stenting, via laparotomy and ventral cystotomy. The pusher is not needed because direct access to the bladder, and therefore the ability to manually position the stent, is possible during laparotomy as compared with cystoscopically. In cases of ureteral stenosis or stricture, dilation with the tapered end of the pusher/dilator may be necessary. In diseased, narrowed, or inflamed ureter(s), the need for careful tissue handling to prevent damage to the ureteral blood supply and trauma to the ureter cannot be overstated. When significant tortuosity to the ureter is present, wire and stent placement must be performed carefully and the use of silastic tubing on the proximal and distal ureter can be helpful to provide traction without excessive ureteral handling to straighten the ureter incrementally to allow wire passage. When wire passage proximal to an obstructive ureterolith is not possible, a ureterotomy for stone removal before completion of stenting may be necessary [23,24,47].

In cats, the preferred technique for ureteral stent placement is using access to the renal pelvis via parenchymal puncture, antegrade wire placement, and antegrade advancement and positioning of the stent. This technique can also be performed in dogs, especially for neoplastic ureteral obstruction patients for whom percutaneous access to the renal pelvis was not possible (see later discussion). After gently removing the retroperitoneal fat from the greater curvature of the kidney, without disrupting the capsular blood supply, a 22-g. over-the-needle catheter is passed through the parenchyma into the renal pelvis. Avoidance of vascular regions of parenchyma is preferred to decrease the risk of hemorrhage during catheter positioning and the creation of a blood clot in the renal pelvis. Urine should be collected for urine culture and sensitivity and urinalysis if indicated. Iodinated contrast agent mixed with saline is injected into the renal pelvis under constant fluoroscopic visualization, being careful not to overdistend the pelvis and create excessive pelvic and ureteral pressures which could exceed the obstructive pressure and cause urine to flow down the urine, complicating the assessment of the location or nature of the obstruction. A short hydrophilic wire (0.018″ × 50 cm) designed specifically for feline ureteral stenting is very helpful to minimize the amount of wire that must be handled in small patients during surgical stenting (Infiniti Medical, LLC). The wire is advanced out of the renal pelvis and antegrade down the ureter under fluoroscopic visualization, exercising care not to perforate the pelvis or ureter during wire advancement. Digital wire manipulation, as well as delicate cranial and caudal retraction of the ureter, can facilitate wire passage, especially past the obstruction and across any segment of nondilated ureter. Once the wire is passed out of the UVJ and contained within the bladder, a distal ventral cystotomy is performed to allow grasping of the wire with hemostats. Hemostats should also be placed on the wire at the site of renal parenchymal access to prevent inadvertent wire malpositioning during stent positioning. Once the ureteral stent length is chosen, the dilator packaged with the stent can be used to dilate the ureter as needed, from an antegrade and/or normograde approach as indicated based on the nature and location of the obstruction. After dilation (if needed), the stent is loaded onto the hydrophilic wire from the kidney to antegrade placement. The wire is passed out a fenestration in the stent shaft just below the kidney coil of the ureteral stent to allow the coil to self-form once in the renal pelvis. Once each coil is within the renal pelvis and bladder and positioned appropriately, the wire is removed and the bladder closed routinely. Closure of the renal pelvis puncture site is not needed.

For percutaneous antegrade ureteral stenting, the patient is positioned in lateral recumbency, such that the ureter to be stented is up. Ultrasound is used to visualize the renal pelvis and trajectory of the ureter at the UPJ. A small skin nick is made in the desired entry site with a #11 scalpel blade. Using an 18-gauge over-the-needle catheter, or preferably, a Teflon access needle/trocar, ultrasound and fluoroscopic guidance are used to cannulate the renal pelvis. Urine should be collected for urinalysis, cytology, and culture/sensitivity as indicated before injection of a 50:50 dilution of iodinated contrast agent under fluoroscopy. The resultant ureteropylogram highlights the trajectory of the often tortuous ureter. Using a stiff shaft angled tip hydrophilic wire, the wire is advanced down the ureter to the level of the obstructed UVJ. Passage of the wire across the UVJ can be very challenging owing to the obstructive mass, requiring passage of a 4-French Berenstein catheter over the wire down the ureter to help pass the wire into the bladder. Once wire access to the bladder is achieved, the wire is directed to the trigone and ultimately out the urethra. The wire should be secured externally with a hemostat at the percutaneous access site such that it is not inadvertently pulled into the kidney. A vascular access sheath is advanced over the wire from the urethra, into the trigone, and across the obstruction mass at the level of the UVJ. A second wire (angled hydrophilic standard shaft stiffness) is passed through the hemostasis valve on the vascular access sheath and up the distal ureter into the renal pelvis under fluoroscopic guidance. Pending the size of the stent and vascular access sheath used, it may be necessary to remove the vascular access sheath off the first wire and replace it retrograde over the second wire only to allow the stent to be passed through the sheath. A stent of appropriate length is passed up into the renal pelvis using the *second* (retrograde) placed wire, using a stent pusher in a similar fashion to that used for cystoscopic stenting. Once the stent is coiled within the pelvis, the second wire is retracted into the end of the stent, the vascular access sheath is retracted into the trigone, and the stent is pushed through the vascular sheath with the pusher to position it within the bladder, in a similar fashion to cystoscopic ureteral stenting. The original percutaneously placed wire is removed, and the small skin incision closed with a single cruciate or interrupted suture. Percutaneous stenting is often challenging and requires two skilled operators given the amount of wire and catheter manipulations needed. If percutaneous access is not possible or if attempts to access the renal pelvis with ultrasound guidance have failed, laparotomy access to the greater curvature of the kidney can facilitate direct puncture of the renal pelvis. Once access to the pelvis is obtained, the procedure is performed in the same fashion as when described for percutaneous access to avoid opening the lower urinary tract to minimize chances for neoplastic seeding.

Intraoperative complications of ureteral stent placement include hemorrhage and filling of the renal pelvis during renal parenchymal puncture, need for multiple pyelocentesis attempts, inadvertent perforation of the renal pelvis or ureter during wire passage and manipulation, need for ureterotomy or papillotomy to facilitate wire passage, stent malpositioning, urine leakage from the renal access, ureterotomy or ureteral perforation site, or cystotomy, and uroabdomen, which can occur in almost 9% of cats treated with ureteral stents [10,23,24,32,47,55–57,66]. Longer term ureteral stent complications include stent migration, encrustation and reobstruction, infection, and lower urinary tract irritation (pollakiuria, stranguria, and hematuria), with lower urinary signs being most common and occurring in 18% to 37.7% of feline cases [23,24,32,56,57]. Ureteral stent induced lower urinary tract signs are uncommon in dogs, though recurrent urinary tract infections have been documented in up to 58% of dogs and may be related to biofilm development on the stent, which is well document in human ureteral stent patients [17,20,24,25,60,61,66,67].

With the challenges and complications associated with ureteral surgery and stenting, as well as long-term stent associated discomfort, all of which are especially important in cats, an adaptation of a human ureteral bypass device was developed and patented by Drs Allyson Berent and Chick Weisse in 2010. The original subcutaneous pyelovesicular bypass graft (Detour) was developed for human urology patients with ureteral obstructions secondary to urinary tract and pelvic neoplasia, as well as postrenal transplantation ureteral strictures [68,69]. The veterinary device, called the SUB, is manufactured by Norfolk Medical and is currently in its third design iteration (SUB 3.0). The SUB 3.0 consists of a locking loop nephrostomy catheter connected directly to a straight end, multifenestrated cystostomy catheter, and a side arm catheter that is connected to a titanium subcutaneous port for urine sampling and device flushing. Most of the current literature describes the experience with the SUB 1.0 and 2.0 device as the 3.0 device only recently became commercially available. In addition, most of the literature describes its use in cats because ureteral stenting in dogs is generally easier and better tolerated.

A ventral midline laparotomy is needed for SUB placement, with wide clipping of the ventral abdomen to facilitate port placement on the ventrolateral abdominal wall adjacent to the incision. The nephrostomy tube is placed first, as this is generally the more challenging aspect of device insertion than the cystostomy tube and is important for improving patient stability for an anuric or oliguric ureteral obstruction patient so that urine drainage is re-established. If a bilateral obstruction is present, both nephrostomy tubes are placed before the cystostomy tube(s) for the same reason. After an exploratory laparotomy, the retroperitoneal fat is dissected from the kidney for nephrostomy tube insertion. The location nephrostomy tube insertion depends on the degree of renal pelvic dilation. For renal pelvic dilation greater than 5 mm, the nephrostomy tube is inserted in the caudal pole of the affected kidney for locking loop catheter positioning in the renal pelvis. For smaller renal pelvises (<4 mm), or those that are asymmetrically shaped such that coiling the locking loop of the nephrostomy catheter could be challenging, access to the renal pelvis is performed from the kidney midway between the caudal pole and greater curvature. This positioning allows the nephrostomy tube to be placed in the proximal ureter, not the renal pelvis, without locking the loop of the catheter. Once the desired renal access location is chosen, ideally in a less vascularized portion of parenchyma, an 18-g. over-the-needle catheter is passed through the parenchyma into the renal pelvis until urine is seen accumulating in the catheter hub, which is used for culture and sensitivity testing. A pyelogram is performed under constant fluoroscopic visualization with a 50:50 mixture of iodinated contrast and saline. It is important to carefully inject contrast and not to overdistend the renal pelvis and create increased pressure that can cause a subtle, partial obstruction to be missed. Once the pelvis is filled with contrast and the location of the obstruction documented on ureteropyelogram, a 0.035″ angled J-wire or 0.035″ angled hydrophilic wire is advanced in the renal pelvis or proximal ureter, respectively. The over-the-needle catheter is removed over the wire, and fluoroscopic guidance is used to ensure the wire stays appropriately positioned. The nephrostomy catheter is flushed with saline and loaded on the hollow trocar and placed over the wire. If the nephrostomy catheter is being placed in the proximal ureter, the locking suture is cut and removed before placement in the kidney to prevent inadvertent locking of the suture, which could rupture the proximal ureter on loop formation. The nephrostomy catheter/hollow trocar combination is pushed into the renal parenchyma and advanced over the wire, with simultaneous retraction of the wire and advancing the catheter/trocar to prevent wire perforation of the pelvis or ureter. In renal pelvises less than 1 cm, simultaneous catheter advancement and gentle retraction of the locking suture can help properly coil the catheter tip and position it with the renal pelvis. It is important not to overtighten the suture, which can cause the catheter to fold in half, preventing urine drainage from occlusion of the nephrostomy catheter holes. There is a black radio-opaque band on the nephrostomy catheter, distal to all of the holes in the nephrostomy catheter. The proximal edge of the black line must be in the renal pelvis to prevent subcapsular and parenchymal urine leakage. One the catheter is positioned; a repeat pyelogram is performed to ensure appropriate positioning and confirm no contrast leakage. The Dacron cuff is positioned on the renal parenchyma, followed by the clear silicone collar that prevents catheter kinking. The cuff is secured to the parenchyma with cyanoacrylate glue.

In small renal pelvises, or those that are asymmetrically shaped, the challenge of proper positioning of the nephrostomy catheter can be alleviated with a double stick technique that uses a small catheter to perform an initial pyelogram from greater curvature so that the initial nephrostomy access can be performed under visualization. This is especially important in markedly uremic patients, who may have uremia-induced thrombopathia and be at risk for hemorrhage during multiple access attempts because blood clot formation in the renal pelvis is an important consideration for reoccurrence of obstruction postoperatively. A 22-g. over-the-needle IV catheter is advanced into the renal pelvis from the greater curvature for urine sample collection and pyelogram. The 18-g. catheter is then advanced into the renal pelvis under direct fluoroscopic visualization before removal of the 22-g. catheter.

For the SUB 3.0, a single or double cytostomy catheter can be used with bilateral nephrostomy catheters as long as the appropriate Y- or X-shaped connector and kit is chosen (Fig. 4). The benefit of a single catheter is faster device placement and only one catheter in the bladder as a potential cause of lower urinary irritation. The downside of a single catheter is that should the cystostomy catheter become occluded with a blood clot, mineral debris, or a kink, both nephrostomy catheters will also become occluded. A purse string is placed in the apex of the bladder with 4 to 0 monofilament suture before a stab incision into the bladder lumen with a #11 blade. The flushed cystostomy catheter is placed on the hollow trocar, followed by placement of the catheter into the bladder to the level of the Dacron cuff, ensuring the black line is within the bladder lumen. After repeat cystogram, cyanoacrylate glue and the same monofilament suture are used to secure the cuff to the bladder.

The Y-connector is used to connect the nephrostomy and cystostomy catheters (unilateral SUB or bilateral SUBs using two unilateral systems), which are contained in the peritoneal cavity and no longer positioned across the body wall as with prior versions of the SUB. If two nephrostomy catheters and a single cystostomy catheter are used, the X-connector (bilateral SUB 3.0 kit) is used. The 3rd arm of the Y-connector/4th arm of the X-connector is attached to a small piece of catheter that is passed across the ventral body wall and connected to the titanium access port which is secured to the ventrolateral abdominal wall with 3 to 0 nonabsorbable monofilament suture. Before closure of the abdomen, an injection is performed through access port using a Huber needle and digital subtraction fluoroscopy to evaluate for appropriate filling of all catheters, the renal pelvis/pelvises, bladder, and to ensure no leaking at any of the connections or kinking of any portion of the catheter tubing. The abdomen is closed routinely, being cautious that the catheters are not damaged or incorporated during linea closure. Before recovery, lateral and ventrodorsal radiographs are taken with fluoroscopy to confirm that none of the catheters are kinked on body wall closure. Injection of Nocita into the incision during closure has greatly improved postoperative patient comfort.

Intraoperative complications associated with feline SUB placement include renal hemorrhage from renal access, perforation of the renal pelvis or ureter during wire or catheter placement, urine leakage from the kidney or bladder, or any of the catheter connections, and kinking of the catheters within the abdomen or across the body wall (SUB 1.0 & 2.0) [18,46,56,70–74]. Blood clots in the renal pelvis, bladder, or any of the catheters are an important consideration for postoperative failure of azotemia resolution or recurrence of azotemia because they generally occur in the first 1 to 4 days postoperatively. Clots are reported in up to 8% of cases, with most of them (60%) requiring surgical revision to replace the occluded catheter [56,70–72]. Long-term SUB complications include infection, mineral debris obstruction of the tubing or port, hematuria, pollakiuria, and stranguria [46,56,70–73,75].

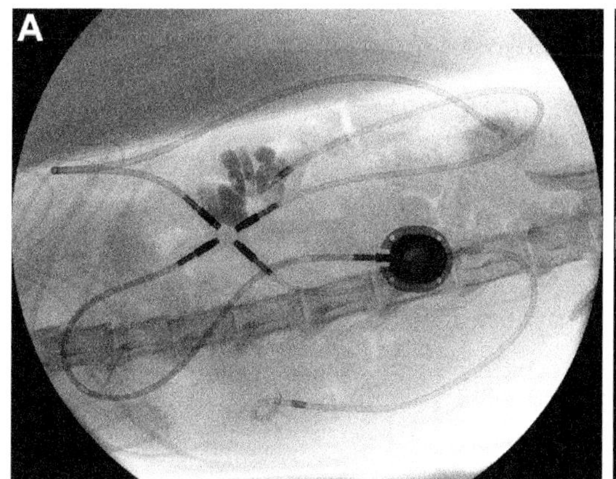

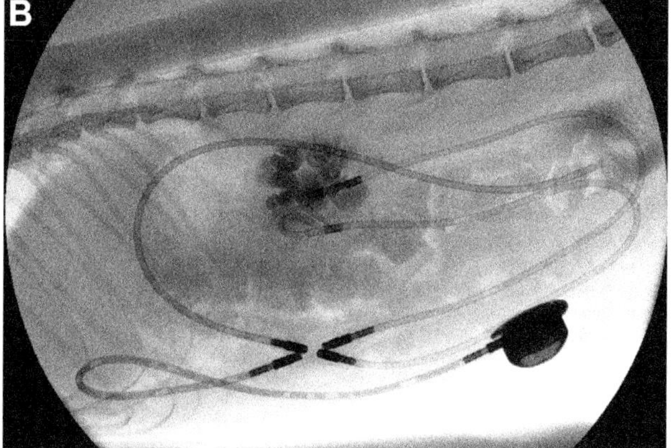

FIG. 4 (**A**) Ventrodorsal projection of an SUB 3.0 placed in a cat with 2 nephrostomy catheters, single cystostomy catheter, X-connector, and a separate catheter connecting to the port. (**B**) Lateral projection of the same cat showing the SUB 3.0 device in place.

POSTOPERATIVE MANAGEMENT

Many patients with ureteral obstructions are critically ill; therefore, anticipation and provision of intensive postoperative care is imperative for successful patient outcomes. Frequent assessment of intravascular and interstitial fluid balance, cardiovascular and respiratory stability, body weight, urine output, electrolytes, and minimum database monitoring (PCV/TS/BG) are needed for postoperative patients, especially if managing fluid overload and/or a substantial postobstructive diuresis.

Indwelling urinary catheters allow for accurate quantification of urine output, but are associated with the risk of ascending acquired infections, which is of particular concern when urinary implants (stents, SUBs) are present [46,75]. However, a recent study evaluating the incidence of urinary tract infections in cats with both SUBs and ureteral stents did not document an increased incidence of infection when indwelling urinary catheters were used postoperatively [46]. Assessment of urine production can be needed hourly when significant postobstructive diuresis is present. Use of nonabsorbent litter, plastic backed diaper pads, and catching all urine for quantification are preferred noninvasive mechanisms of objectively quantifying urine output.

Postobstructive diuresis urine production rates have been documented to range from 3 to 36.5 mL/kg/h (median = 7.75 mL/kg/h) in cats that have undergone ureteral stenting [47]. These high rates of urine output, combined with variable fluid preoperative fluid balance that can range from dehydrated to overhydrated, clearly demonstrate the need for frequent body weight assessment, quantification of urine output, blood pressure, PCV/TS, lactate and La:Ao monitoring, as fluid balance can be dynamic and require frequent adjustments in fluid therapy. Balanced isotonic replacement crystalloids are used to replace intravascular volume deficits. Both enteral and parenteral fluid therapy can be used to replace interstitial fluid deficits. Care must also be taken to avoid overhydration and volume overload, which can cause respiratory and renal compromise.

In addition to enteral water, nasoesophageal and esophageal tubes can also be used to provide nutritional support to the recovering postoperative ureteral obstruction patient. This is important as these patients may be in diminished body condition if underlying chronic renal disease is present, have had prolonged anorexia before surgery, have oral pain from uremic ulcerations, experience nausea secondary to azotemia and postoperative analgesics, and require appropriate nutrient intake for incisional healing and recovery. Postoperatively, patients are often allowed to eat any balanced diet they chose in an effort to ensure adequate nutritional intake. Renal diets, which are restricted in protein and phosphorus, may be needed for long term for residual azotemia and management of chronic renal disease.

Repeated blood sampling is often needed for electrolyte, anemia, and azotemia monitoring in the postoperative ureteral obstruction patient. Because many animals with significant azotemia have a postobstructive diuresis, but may not be ambulatory enough to void, frequent urine soaking of the hind end raises the risk of complications for venous catheters in the hind limbs. Therefore, multilumen jugular catheters are preferred for vascular sampling and ability to provide multiple simultaneous infusions, including type-specific, cross-matches packed red blood cell or whole blood transfusions, as anemia is frequently documented with ureteral obstructions in cats [21,23,24,33,47,71].

Analgesia is another essential component of managing the postoperative ureteral obstruction patient, especially those undergoing SUB placement owing to increase in ventral abdominal soft-tissue dissection compared with routine laparotomies. Local analgesia with Nocita is helpful to provide 72 hours of local incisional analgesia, decreasing requirements for systemic analgesics. In cats undergoing SUB placement, a constant rate infusion of dexmedetomidine (0.25–1 mcg/kg/h) and intermittent dosing of buprenorphine (0.01–0.02 mg/kg IV q6-8) is an effective balanced analgesic postoperative plan. Patients for whom surgical ureteral stents were placed generally require similar analgesic protocols to other laparotomy procedures. Oral analgesia is generally sufficient in patients having cystoscopic or percutaneous antegrade ureteral stenting.

There are no clear-cut guidelines for when antibiotic therapy is needed in patients with ureteral obstructions, unless infected urine from the kidney or renal pelvis is documented on culture or in cases of pyelonephritis or pyonephrosis. For cases without evidence of infection, antibiotic therapy may not be needed beyond routine perioperative use.

URETERAL INTERVENTION DECISION-MAKING

Both surgical and interventional techniques have been documented to effectively manage ureteral obstructions in veterinary patients. However, there are no standardized guidelines for when a given ureteral intervention is better than another. Considerations that must be taken into account include patient signalment, evidence of chronic renal disease, severity of illness, the nature and location of the obstruction, concurrent nephrolithiasis, other comorbidities, surgeon training, experience, and equipment availability. In addition, client considerations, including financial restrictions, ability to perform frequent follow-up, and preference also factor into decision-making for a given patient.

In general, ureteral surgical techniques and stents are preferred in dogs owing the larger ureter size, tolerance of stents, and ability to follow-up with extracorporeal shockwave lithotripsy for residual nephroureterolithiasis after the obstruction is resolved. In cats with a single ureterolith, and no evidence of nephrolithiasis, ureteral surgery remains a viable option for stone removal in the hands of surgeons comfortable with feline ureteral surgery. Ureteral stents are considered in cats with diffuse ureteral dilation, or for those in whom the ureteral stent is planned for temporary use, such as with healing after ureteral surgery owing to concerns for long-term dysuria associated with stents in cats. In cats with proximal ureteral obstructions, or in cases with strictures where passive ureteral dilation is not expected, SUBs may be best in these patients. SUBs can also be reliably quickly performed compared with surgery and stents and may therefore be preferable in unstable patients where limiting anesthesia time is crucial.

Until clear, evidence-based guidelines exist, the decision about which ureteral intervention is indicated for a given patient will likely remain controversial. In all likelihood, ureteral surgery, stents, and ureteral bypass devices will continue to remain viable options, and the decision about which procedure should be performed should be made on a case-by-case basis.

CLINICS CARE POINTS

- Diagnostic imaging, including abdominal radiographs and ultrasound, is essential for confirming a diagnosis of ureteral obstruction.
- Stabilization of hypovolemia, dehydration, electrolyte disturbances, and consequences of uremia are important before any surgical or interventional procedure for critically ill ureteral obstruction patients. In some extremely unstable patients, such as those that are anuric and/or fluid overloaded, or have refractory hyperkalemia, emergency intervention may be required.
- Ureteral surgery is generally considered in patients with a single ureterolith or midureteral to distal ureteral stricture, stone, or mass that can be resected with ureteral reimplantation or addressed with resection and anastomosis. Ureteral surgery is challenging and requires advanced training, specialized instrumentation, and magnification.
- Ureteral stents are well tolerated in dogs and can be used to address a variety of obstruction causes including ureterolithiasis, strictures, obstructive pyonephrosis, and trigonal neoplasia. Ureteral stents are also available for cats, though the size of the feline ureter makes the placement challenging. In addition, cats tend to have lower urinary tract discomfort associated with ureteral stents.
- Subcutaneous ureteral bypass (SUB) devices can be used in both dogs and cats for all forms of ureteral obstruction, though they are used most commonly in cats to avoid the downsides of ureteral stents in this species. They require long-term monitoring and flushing, because they can become obstructed or infected, and may need revision if they become infected or obstructed with blood clots, mineral debris, or the tubing kinks.

DISCLOSURE

The author has nothing to disclose.

REFERENCES

[1] Kyles AE, Stone EA, Gookin J, et al. Diagnosis and surgical management of obstructive ureteral calculi in cats: 11 cases (1993-1996). J Am Vet Med Assoc 1998;213(8): 1150–6.
[2] Kyles AE, Hardie EM, Wooden BG, et al. Clinical, clinicopathologic, radiographic, and ultrasonographic abnormalities in cats with ureteral calculi: 163 cases (1984-2002). J Am Vet Med Assoc 2005;226(6):932–6.
[3] Kyles AE, Hardie EM, Wooden BG, et al. Management and outcome of cats with ureteral calculi: 153 cases (1984-2002). J Am Vet Med Assoc 2005;226(6):937–44.
[4] Cannon AB, Westropp JL, Ruby AL, et al. Evaluation of trends in urolith composition in cats: 5,230 cases (1985–2004). J Am Vet Med Assoc 2007;231(4):570–6.
[5] Low WW, Uhl JM, Kass PH, et al. Evaluation of trends in urolith composition and characteristics of dogs with urolithiasis: 25,499 cases (1985–2006). J Am Vet Med Assoc 2010;236(2):193–200.
[6] Houston DM, Moore AEP. Canine and feline urolithiasis: examination of over 50 000 urolith submissions to the Canadian Veterinary Urolith Centre from 1998 to 2008. Can Vet J 2009;50(12):1263–8.
[7] Houston DM, Moore AEP, Favrin MG, et al. Canine urolithiasis: a look at over 16 000 urolith submissions to the

Canadian Veterinary Urolith Centre from February 1998 to April 2003. Can Vet J 2004;45(3):225–30.

[8] Lekcharoensuk C, Osborne CA, Lulich JP, et al. Trends in the frequency of calcium oxalate uroliths in the upper urinary tract of cats. J Am Anim Hosp Assoc 2005; 41(1):39–46.

[9] Westropp JL, Ruby AL, Bailiff NL, et al. Dried solidified blood calculi in the urinary tract of cats. J Vet Intern Med 2006;20(4):828–34.

[10] Zaid MS, Berent AC, Weisse C, et al. Feline ureteral strictures: 10 cases (2007–2009). J Vet Intern Med 2011; 25(2):222–9.

[11] D'Ippolito P, Nicoli S, Zatelli A. Proximal ureteral ectopia causing hydronephrosis in a kitten. J Feline Med Surg 2006;8(6):420–3.

[12] Wormser C, Clarke DL, Aronson LR. End-to-end ureteral anastomosis and double-pigtail ureteral stent placement for treatment of iatrogenic ureteral trauma in two dogs. J Am Vet Med Assoc 2015;247(1):92–7.

[13] Johnson CM, Culp WTN, Palm CA, et al. Subcutaneous ureteral bypass device for treatment of iatrogenic ureteral ligation in a kitten. J Am Vet Med Assoc 2015;247(8): 924–31.

[14] Aronson LR. Retroperitoneal fibrosis in four cats following renal transplantation. J Am Vet Med Assoc 2002;221(7):984–9.

[15] Wormser C, Phillips H, Aronson LR. Retroperitoneal fibrosis in feline renal transplant recipients: 29 cases (1998–2011). J Am Vet Med Assoc 2013;243(11): 1580–5.

[16] Cohen L, Shipov A, Ranen E, et al. Bilateral ureteral obstruction in a cat due to a ureteral transitional cell carcinoma. Can Vet J 2012;53(5):535–8.

[17] Kuntz JA, Berent AC, Weisse CW, et al. Double pigtail ureteral stenting and renal pelvic lavage for renal-sparing treatment of obstructive pyonephrosis in dogs: 13 cases (2008–2012). J Am Vet Med Assoc 2015; 246(2):216–25.

[18] Cray M, Berent AC, Weisse CW, et al. Treatment of pyonephrosis with a subcutaneous ureteral bypass device in four cats. J Am Vet Med Assoc 2018;252(6):744–53.

[19] Speakman CF, Pechman RD, D'Andrea GH. Aortic thrombosis and unilateral hydronephrosis associated with leiomyosarcoma in a cat. J Am Vet Med Assoc 1983;182(1):62–3.

[20] Berent AC. Ureteral obstructions in dogs and cats: a review of traditional and new interventional diagnostic and therapeutic options. J Vet Emerg Crit Care 2011; 21(2):86–103.

[21] Roberts SF, Aronson LR, Brown DC. Postoperative mortality in cats after ureterolithotomy. Vet Surg 2011; 40(4):438–43.

[22] Berent AC, Weisse CW, Todd KL, et al. Use of locking-loop pigtail nephrostomy catheters in dogs and cats: 20 cases (2004–2009). J Am Vet Med Assoc 2012;241(3): 348–57.

[23] Berent AC, Weisse CW, Todd K, et al. Technical and clinical outcomes of ureteral stenting in cats with benign ureteral obstruction: 69 cases (2006–2010). J Am Vet Med Assoc 2014;244(5):559–76.

[24] Wormser C, Clarke DL, Aronson LR. Outcomes of ureteral surgery and ureteral stenting in cats: 117 cases (2006–2014). J Am Vet Med Assoc 2016;248(5):518–25.

[25] Snyder D, Steffey M, Mehler S, et al. Diagnosis and surgical management of ureteral calculi in dogs: 16 cases (1990–2003). N Z Vet J 2005;53(1):19–25.

[26] Wen JG, Frøkiær J, Jørgensen TM, et al. Obstructive nephropathy: an update of the experimental research. Urol Res 1999;27(1):29–39.

[27] Coroneos E, Assouad M, Krishnan B, et al. Urinary obstruction causes irreversible renal failure by inducing chronic tubulointerstitial nephritis. Clin Nephrol 1997; 48(2):125–8.

[28] Wilson DR. Renal function during and following obstruction. Annu Rev Med 1977;28:329–39.

[29] Fink RLW, Caridis DT, Chmiel R, et al. Renal impairment and its reversibility following variable periods of complete ureteric obstruction. Aust N Z J Surg 1980;50(1): 77–83.

[30] Kerr WS. Effect of complete ureteral obstruction for one week on kidney function. J Appl Physiol 1954;6(12): 762–72.

[31] Vaughan ED, Sweet RE, Gillenwater JY. Unilateral ureteral occlusion: pattern of nephron repair and compensatory response. J Urol 1973;109(6):979–82.

[32] Nicoli S, Morello E, Martano M, et al. Double-J ureteral stenting in nine cats with ureteral obstruction. Vet J 2012;194(1):60–5.

[33] Kochin EJ, Gregory CR, Wisner E, et al. Evaluation of a method of ureteroneocystostomy in cats. J Am Vet Med Assoc 1993;202(2):257–60.

[34] Hardie EM, Kyles AE. Management of ureteral obstruction. Vet Clin North Am Small Anim Pract 2004;34(4): 989–1010.

[35] Nesser VE, Reetz JA, Clarke DL, et al. Radiographic distribution of ureteral stones in 78 cats. Vet Surg 2018;47(7): 895–901.

[36] Wormser C, Reetz JA, Drobatz KJ, et al. Diagnostic utility of ultrasonography for detection of the cause and location of ureteral obstruction in cats: 71 cases (2010–2016). J Am Vet Med Assoc 2019;254(6):710–5.

[37] D'anjou M-A, Bédard A, Dunn ME. Clinical significance of renal pelvic dilatation on ultrasound in dogs and cats. Vet Radiol Ultrasound 2011;52(1):88–94.

[38] Lamb CR, Cortellini S, Halfacree Z. Ultrasonography in the diagnosis and management of cats with ureteral obstruction. J Feline Med Surg 2018;20(1):15–22.

[39] Lemieux C, Vachon C, Beauchamp G, et al. Minimal renal pelvis dilation in cats diagnosed with benign ureteral obstruction by antegrade pyelography: a retrospective study of 82 cases (2012-2018). J Feline Med Surg 2021. https://doi.org/10.1177/1098612X20983980.

[40] Adin CA, Herrgesell EJ, Nyland TG, et al. Antegrade pyelography for suspected ureteral obstruction in cats: 11 cases (1995-2001). J Am Vet Med Assoc 2003;222(11): 1576–81.
[41] Etedali NM, Reetz JA, Foster JD. Complications and clinical utility of ultrasonographically guided pyelocentesis and antegrade pyelography in cats and dogs: 49 cases (2007–2015). J Am Vet Med Assoc 2019; 254(7):826–34.
[42] Mazzaferro EM. Complications of fluid therapy. Vet Clin North Am Small Anim Pract 2008;38(3):607–19, xii.
[43] Rishniw M, Erb HN. Evaluation of four 2-dimensional echocardiographic methods of assessing left atrial size in dogs. J Vet Intern Med 2000;14(4):429–35.
[44] Abbott JA, MacLean HN. Two-dimensional echocardiographic assessment of the feline left atrium. J Vet Intern Med 2006;20(1):111–9.
[45] Bloom CA, Labato MA. Intermittent hemodialysis for small animals. Vet Clin North Am Small Anim Pract 2011;41(1):115–33.
[46] Kopecny L, Palm CA, Drobatz KJ, et al. Risk factors for positive urine cultures in cats with subcutaneous ureteral bypass and ureteral stents (2010-2016). J Vet Intern Med 2019;33(1):178–83.
[47] Culp WTN, Palm CA, Hsueh C, et al. Outcome in cats with benign ureteral obstructions treated by means of ureteral stenting versus ureterotomy. J Am Vet Med Assoc 2016;249(11):1292–300.
[48] Adin CA, Scansen BA. Complications of upper urinary tract surgery in companion animals. Vet Clin North Am Small Anim Pract 2011;41(5):869–88.
[49] Aronson LR, Cleroux A, Wormser C. Use of a modified Boari flap for the treatment of a proximal ureteral obstruction in a cat. Vet Surg 2018;47(4):578–85.
[50] Motiwala HG, Shah SA, Patel SM. Ureteric Substitution with Boari Bladder Flap. Br J Urol 1990;66(4):369–71.
[51] Stolze KJ. Boari plastic operation and reflux. Int Urol Nephrol 1972;4(1):21–4.
[52] Vaughan ED, Gillenwater JY. Recovery Following Complete Chronic Unilateral Ureteral Occlusion: Functional, Radiographic and Pathologic Alterations. J Urol 1971; 106(1):27–35.
[53] Berent A. Interventional Management of Canine and Feline Benign Ureteral Obstructions. In: Veterinary image guided interventions. 1st edition. Somerset: John Wiley & Sons, Incorporated; 2015. p. 309–35.
[54] Adams LG. Nephroliths and ureteroliths: a new stone age. N Z Vet J 2013;61(4):212–6.
[55] Manassero M, Decambron A, Viateau V, et al. Indwelling double pigtail ureteral stent combined or not with surgery for feline ureterolithiasis: complications and outcome in 15 cases. J Feline Med Surg 2014;16(8): 623–30.
[56] Horowitz C, Berent A, Weisse C, et al. Predictors of outcome for cats with ureteral obstructions after interventional management using ureteral stents or a subcutaneous ureteral bypass device. J Feline Med Surg 2013;15(12):1052–62.
[57] Kulendra NJ, Syme H, Benigni L, et al. Feline double pigtail ureteric stents for management of ureteric obstruction: short- and long-term follow-up of 26 cats. J Feline Med Surg 2014;16(12):985–91.
[58] Berent AC, Weisse CW, Branter E, et al. Endoscopic-guided sclerotherapy for renal-sparing treatment of idiopathic renal hematuria in dogs: 6 cases (2010–2012). J Am Vet Med Assoc 2013;242(11):1556–63.
[59] Berent AC, Weisse C, Beal MW, et al. Use of indwelling, double-pigtail stents for treatment of malignant ureteral obstruction in dogs: 12 cases (2006–2009). J Am Vet Med Assoc 2011;238(8):1017–25.
[60] Lange D, Bidnur S, Hoag N, et al. Ureteral stent-associated complications–where we are and where we are going. Nat Rev Urol 2015;12(1):17–25.
[61] Saltzman B. Ureteral stents. Indications, variations, and complications. Urol Clin North Am 1988;15(3): 481–91.
[62] Runge JJ, Berent AC, Mayhew PD, et al. Transvesicular percutaneous cystolithotomy for the retrieval of cystic and urethral calculi in dogs and cats: 27 cases (2006–2008). J Am Vet Med Assoc 2011;239(3):344–9.
[63] Tong K, Weisse C, Berent AC. Rigid urethrocystoscopy via a percutaneous fluoroscopic-assisted perineal approach in male dogs: 19 cases (2005–2014). J Am Vet Med Assoc 2016;249(8):918–25.
[64] Adams LG, Senior DF. Electrohydraulic and Extracorporeal Shock-Wave Lithotripsy. Vet Clin North Am Small Anim Pract 1999;29(1):293–302.
[65] Lulich JP, Adams LG, Grant D, et al. Changing paradigms in the treatment of uroliths by lithotripsy. Vet Clin North Am Small Anim Pract 2009;39(1):143–60.
[66] Pavia PR, Berent AC, Weisse CW, et al. Outcome of ureteral stent placement for treatment of benign ureteral obstruction in dogs: 44 cases (2010–2013). J Am Vet Med Assoc 2018;252(6):721–31.
[67] Lam NK, Berent AC, Weisse CW, et al. Endoscopic placement of ureteral stents for treatment of congenital bilateral ureteral stenosis in a dog. J Am Vet Med Assoc 2012; 240(8):983–90.
[68] Desgrandchamps F, Cussenot O, Meria P, et al. Subcutaneous urinary diversions for palliative treatment of pelvic malignancies. J Urol 1995;154(2 Pt 1):367–70.
[69] Desgrandchamps F, Duboust A, Teillac P, et al. Total ureteral replacement by subcutaneous pyelovesical bypass in ureteral necrosis after renal transplantation. Transpl Int 1998;11(Suppl 1):S150–1.
[70] Livet V, Pillard P, Goy-Thollot I, et al. Placement of subcutaneous ureteral bypasses without fluoroscopic guidance in cats with ureteral obstruction: 19 cases (2014–2016). J Feline Med Surg 2017;19(10):1030–9.
[71] Berent AC, Weisse CW, Bagley DH, et al. Use of a subcutaneous ureteral bypass device for treatment of benign ureteral obstruction in cats: 174 ureters in 134 cats

(2009–2015). J Am Vet Med Assoc 2018;253(10): 1309–27.

[72] Kulendra NJ, Borgeat K, Syme H, et al. Survival and complications in cats treated with subcutaneous ureteral bypass. J Small Anim Pract 2021;62(1):4–11.

[73] Deroy C, Rossetti D, Ragetly G, et al. Comparison between double-pigtail ureteral stents and ureteral bypass devices for treatment of ureterolithiasis in cats. J Am Vet Med Assoc 2017;251(4):429–37.

[74] Palm CA, Culp WTN. Nephroureteral obstructions: the use of stents and ureteral bypass systems for renal decompression. Vet Clin North Am Small Anim Pract 2016;46(6):1183–92.

[75] Chik C, Berent AC, Weisse CW, et al. Therapeutic use of tetrasodium ethylenediaminetetraacetic acid solution for treatment of subcutaneous ureteral bypass device mineralization in cats. J Vet Intern Med 2019;33(5): 2124–32.

Immunology

Advances in Small Animal Care 2 (2021) 101–115
ADVANCES IN SMALL ANIMAL CARE

Current Knowledge on Canine Atopic Dermatitis

Pathogenesis and Treatment

Catherine A. Outerbridge, DVM, MVSc, DACVIM (SAIM), DACVD[a,*], Tyler J.M. Jordan, DVM, DACVD[b,c,1]
[a]Department of Medicine and Epidemiology School of Veterinary Medicine, University of California, Davis, Davis, CA 95691, USA; [b]Department of Clinical Sciences, College of Veterinary Medicine, North Carolina State University, 1060 William Moore Drive, Raleigh, NC 27606, USA; [c]Department of Dermatology, School of Medicine, University of North Carolina at Chapel Hill, 115 Mason Farm Road, Chapel Hill, NC 27599, USA

KEYWORDS
• Atopic dermatitis • Dog • Pathogenesis • Treatment

KEY POINTS
- Canine atopic dermatitis (CAD) is a common, genetically predisposed, chronically relapsing, progressive, pruritic, and inflammatory skin disease with characteristic clinical features and well-defined breed predispositions.
- The pathogenesis of CAD is incompletely understood but is believed to involve complex interactions between genetic and environmental factors that lead to epidermal barrier dysfunction, immune dysregulation, and dysbiosis of the cutaneous microbiome.
- CAD is a lifelong disease that requires chronic management that involves combinations of topical and systemic therapies that need to be tailored to each individual dog and dog-owner.

INTRODUCTION

Canine atopic dermatitis (CAD) is a genetically predisposed, progressive, chronically relapsing, inflammatory and pruritic skin disease with characteristic clinical features associated with immunoglobulin (Ig)E antibodies most commonly directed against environmental allergens [1]. CAD is frequently encountered in small animal clinical practice, is known to negatively impact the quality of life of affected dogs and their owners, and oftentimes requires lifelong management [2–4]. The most common and clinically significant feature of CAD is moderate to severe pruritus, which is accompanied by, and typically precedes, erythema, erythematous macular and/or papular eruptions, self-induced alopecia, excoriations, hyperpigmentation, and lichenification (Figs. 1 and 2) [5–7]. The affected skin is frequently complicated by secondary microbial infections with *Staphylococcus pseudintermedius* and *Malassezia pachydermatis*, which pose additional therapeutic challenges [6]. The distribution of skin lesions is known to vary between breeds, but generally involves the face, pinnae, ear canals, paws, axillae, ventrum, and inguinum [5–8]. Clinical signs of CAD commonly present before 3 years of age, may be either perennial or seasonal, and overlap with numerous other pruritic and inflammatory skin diseases [5]. Unfortunately,

[1] Present address: Neuroscience Research Building, Room 7135, University of North Carolina, Chapel Hill, 115 Mason Farm Road, Chapel Hill, NC 27599, USA.

*Corresponding author. Department of Medicine and Epidemiology School of Veterinary Medicine, University of California, Davis, Davis, CA 95691, USA *E-mail address:* caouterbridge@ucdavis.edu

https://doi.org/10.1016/j.yasa.2021.07.004
2666-450X/21/ © 2021 Elsevier Inc. All rights reserved.

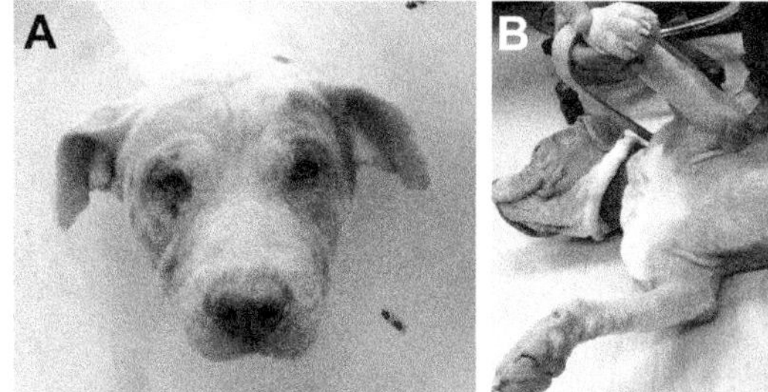

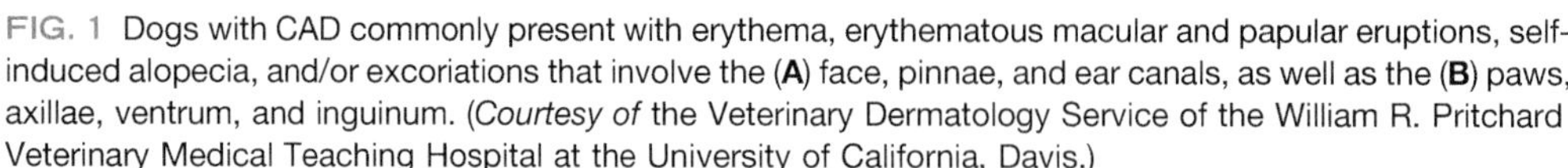

FIG. 1 Dogs with CAD commonly present with erythema, erythematous macular and papular eruptions, self-induced alopecia, and/or excoriations that involve the (**A**) face, pinnae, and ear canals, as well as the (**B**) paws, axillae, ventrum, and inguinum. (*Courtesy of* the Veterinary Dermatology Service of the William R. Pritchard Veterinary Medical Teaching Hospital at the University of California, Davis.)

there is no definitive diagnostic test or pathognomonic clinical sign that can be used to make a diagnosis of CAD. For these reasons, clinical criteria and diagnostic algorithms have been established to assist managing clinicians and clinical researchers in making a correct diagnosis [6,7]. Interestingly, striking similarities exist between CAD and atopic dermatitis (AD) in humans (ie, atopic eczema) in their clinical and immunopathological features, therapeutic approaches, and responses to treatment and CAD has been proposed as a naturally occurring, spontaneous animal model of AD in humans [9]. The objective of this review was to provide an overview of the advancements that have been made over the past decade in understanding CAD's complex pathogenesis as well as in the approaches to disease management.

PATHOGENESIS

In addition to gastrointestinal signs, urticaria, and angioedema, dogs with adverse food reactions (AFR) are also well-recognized to present with clinical signs that are indistinguishable from CAD [10–12]. Although AFR and CAD have historically been considered 2 separate and distinct clinical entities, dietary components are now recognized as flare factors of CAD in some dogs [5,6,11]. Taking this into consideration, it is critically important to perform an elimination diet trial in dogs with perennial signs of CAD to evaluate for the presence of "food-induced atopic dermatitis" [6]. For the purposes of this review, the pathophysiology of food-induced AD, and the diets used for its diagnosis and management, are not discussed.

The pathogenesis of CAD is incompletely understood, but is believed to involve complex interactions between genetic and environmental factors that lead to epidermal barrier dysfunction, immune dysregulation, and dysbiosis of the cutaneous microbiome. A significant challenge faced by researchers is determining whether epidermal barrier dysfunction, immune dysregulation, and dysbiosis of the cutaneous microbiome play critical roles in disease induction, or are secondary downstream sequela. Evidence to support a role for genetic and environmental factors, epidermal barrier dysfunction, immune dysregulation, and dysbiosis of the cutaneous microbiome are discussed herein.

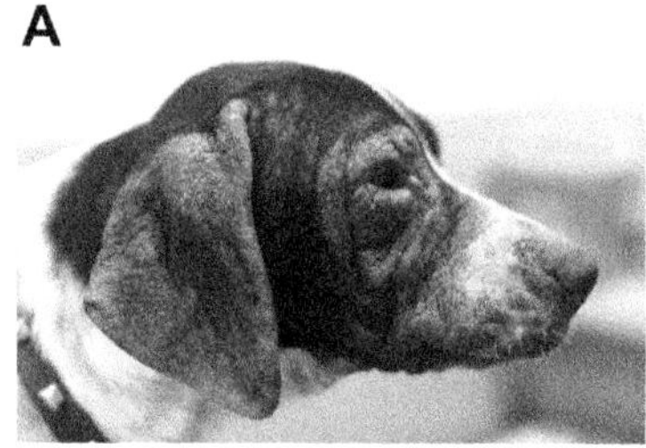

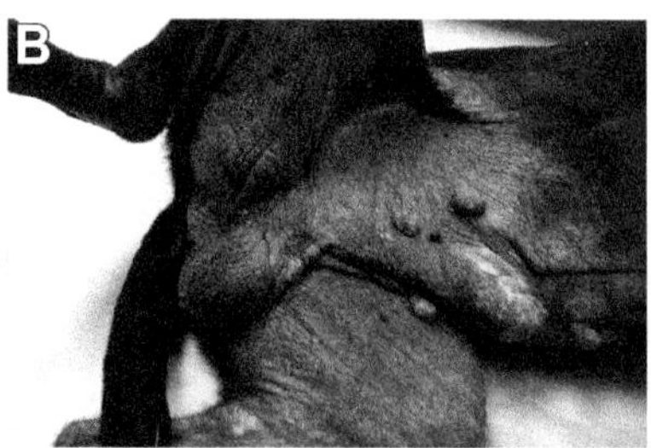

FIG. 2 With chronicity, the affect skin in CAD may develop varying degrees of (**A, B**) hyperpigmentation and lichenification. These changes are not specific to CAD and can occur in other chronic skin diseases. (*Courtesy of* the Veterinary Dermatology Service of the William R. Pritchard Veterinary Medical Teaching Hospital at the University of California, Davis.)

Genetics

Several lines of evidence have suggested a genetic basis for CAD. First, several pure breeds of dog are well-recognized to be at increased risk for developing CAD, including the golden retriever, Labrador retriever, German shepherd dog, West Highland white terrier (WHWT), and French bulldog [5,8]. Second, pedigree analyses have demonstrated the heritability of CAD [13,14]. Various approaches and methodologies have been used to investigate the genetic basis for CAD, including genome-wide linkage studies, genome-wide association studies, and candidate gene association studies [15]. Thus far, no definitive genetic markers or causative genetic variants of CAD have been identified. The candidate genes that have been implicated in CAD are summarized in Table 1.

The studies that have investigated the genetic basis of CAD to date have clearly illustrated that the disease is not a simple dominant or recessive trait. Rather, CAD appears to be a complex, polygenic disorder arising from diverse genetic mutations that vary between breeds and geographic locations. For these reasons, it is now advised that all future investigations into the genetics of CAD be performed in single breeds originating from well-defined geographic regions [15,16]. Despite the advances in our understanding of the genetic basis of CAD, much remains unknown. As such, a genetic screening and breeding program to eliminate CAD in at-risk breeds remains unfeasible and unrealistic at this time [15].

Environment

The worldwide prevalence of AD in humans has increased dramatically over the past several decades and has been attributed to changes in human lifestyles and environmental exposures [23,24]. The "hygiene hypothesis" has been proposed as a possible explanation for this phenomenon. This theory postulates that exposure to diverse microbes early in life modulate the naive immune system against the development of allergic disease by stimulating T-helper-1 (Th1) and regulatory T cell (Treg) immune responses over T-helper-2 (Th2) immune responses [23–25]. Along these lines, it is theorized that increased standards of hygiene and levels of cleanliness associated with modern lifestyles decrease the diversity of infectious agents and pathogens an individual is exposed to and promote the development of allergic inflammation. Research has been performed to better define environmental triggers of AD in humans in hopes of identifying modifiable risk factors that would prevent disease induction and exacerbation [25]. For example, urban living, exposure to air pollutants, tobacco smoke, and prenatal exposure to antibiotics have each been associated with an increased risk for developing AD in humans [25]. In contrast, larger family sizes, the presence of older siblings, exposure to farm animals, and attending childhood daycare have been suggested to protect against the disease [25].

Fewer studies have been performed to define environmental risk factors associated with CAD. Environmental factors found to be associated with CAD include living in an urban environment or in areas of increasing human density, and living primarily indoors [7,26–28]. In fact, the association between an indoor environment and CAD and has led clinical researchers to accept "living in an indoor environment" as one of several diagnostic criteria for the disease [7]. Within the household, a high level of cleanliness, permitting access to upholstered furniture, and passive exposure to high levels of tobacco smoke have been identified as risk factors associated with CAD [29,30]. Other studies have found associations between CAD and being neutered, of the male sex, being born during the autumn, and residing in regions of high average annual rainfall [26,27,29]. One study found that dogs with clinical signs of CAD, as reported by their owner, were more likely to be owned by humans with either atopic rhinitis, dermatitis, and/or asthma than healthy dogs, suggesting that CAD and allergic disease in humans are influenced by mutual environmental factors [31]. Several environmental factors appear to protect against CAD as well. For example, being born and living in a rural environment, living in outdoor facilities or a detached house, living within the household a dog was born in, and regularly walking through woodlands, fields, and/or beaches have each been found to negatively associate with CAD in various studies [28,29,31–33]. Dogs living with and having regular contact with other animals (ie, dogs, cats, farm animals) and dogs living within a family with more than 2 children have also been found less likely to have CAD [28,29,31–33].

It is well-recognized that clinical signs of CAD fluctuate seasonally in association with changing concentrations of environmental allergens in some dogs [5]. Furthermore, dogs with CAD are known to develop immunoglobulin (Ig)E antibodies against environmental allergens, and allergen-specific immunotherapy (ASIT) remains a widely prescribed therapy known to clinically benefit approximately 60% to 70% of dogs with CAD [34,35]. Taken together, there is strong evidence to support a role for environmental factors in the pathogenies of CAD. However, discrete and

TABLE 1
Candidate Genes that Have Been Implicated in the Pathogenesis of Canine Atopic Dermatitis

Gene	Breed and Location	Function of the Encoded Protein
DPP4	• Labrador retrievers residing in the United Kingdom [16].	A cell-surface glycoprotein (ie, CD26) involved in activation of T cells.
F2R	• West Highland white terriers (WHWTs) residing in the United States [17].	A g-protein coupled receptor involved in the regulation of thrombosis.
FLG	• Labrador retrievers residing in the United Kingdom [16]. • A cohort of dogs consisting of pugs, shih tzus, and poodles residing in Thailand [18].	The polypeptide, profilaggrin, which undergoes posttranslational modification to produce filaggrin peptide monomers. Filaggrin plays a vital role in forming the cornified cell envelope during terminal differentiation of keratinocytes.
INPPL1	• Shiba inus residing in Japan [16].	A protein involved in regulation of insulin function, epidermal growth factor receptor turnover, and actin remodeling.
MS4A2	• Shiba inus residing in Japan [16].	A receptor subunit of the high-affinity immunoglobulin E receptor located on a variety of immune cells (ie, mast cells, basophils, Langerhans cells).
PKP2	• German shepherd dogs residing in Sweden [19].	A component of the desmosomal plaque that plays a role in maintaining keratinocyte structure and adhesion.
PROM1	• Golden retrievers residing in the United States, United Kingdom, and Japan [20].	A transmembrane glycoprotein (ie, CD133) that binds to cholesterol in cholesterol-containing plasma membranes.
P450 26B1	• WHWTs residing in Australia [21].	A cytochrome P450 enzyme involved in retinoic acid metabolism and adipogenesis.
PTPN22	• WHWTs residing in Australia [21,22].	A lymphoid-specific tyrosine phosphatase involved in regulating intracellular signal transduction.
RAB3C	• Golden retrievers residing in the United States, United Kingdom, and Japan [20].	A GTPase involved in vesicular transport and has been shown to play a role in recycling major histocompatibility complex class 1 complexes.
RAB7A	• Labrador retrievers residing in the United Kingdom [20]. • WHWTs residing in the United Kingdom [20].	A GTPase involved in endocytosis and vesicular transport of endolysosomes and melanosomes.
SORCS2	• German shepherd dogs residing in the United Kingdom [20].	A transmembrane receptor protein is involved in neuronal function and viability.
*TSLPR**	• A cohort of dogs consisting of boxers, German shepherd dogs, Labrador and golden retrievers, shiba inus, shih tzus, pit bulls and WHWTs residing in the United States, United Kingdom, and Japan [16]. **This association was not statistically significant when each dog breed was evaluated separately.*	A subunit of the receptor complex used by "thymic stromal lymphopoietin," a keratinocyte-derived cytokine that promotes the development of Th2-polarized immune responses and induces the sensation of itch.

definitive environmental triggers of CAD, as well as their mechanisms of action, have not yet been identified. The aforementioned environmental associations do not prove causality or cause-and-effect relationships, as numerous confounding variables are likely present in each study. It is plausible that numerous environmental triggers of CAD exist that have variable effects on disease induction and exacerbation that depend on a dog's individual genetic background, as well as the environments and climates they are exposed to. Future prospective, longitudinal breed-specific and region-specific studies are needed to define precise environmental triggers of disease in genetically predisposed animals.

Epidermal Barrier Dysfunction

The skin forms a physical, immunologic, biochemical, and microbial barrier that separates the internal environment from the external environment [36]. Dysfunction of the epidermal barrier facilitates the percutaneous absorption of chemical irritants, microbes, and environmental allergens that stimulate the local immune system and induce Th2-polarized immune responses [37]. Th2-polarized immune responses are recognized to further impair epidermal barrier integrity and function by downregulating key structural proteins in the skin and by inducing pruritus, scratching, and self-trauma [24,37]. Epidermal barrier dysfunction is a consistent feature of humans with AD and mounting evidence suggests the same is true for CAD as well [23,24].

The stratum corneum (SC) is the outermost layer of the epidermis and is composed of terminally differentiated keratinocytes (ie, "corneocytes") that are embedded in intercellular lipid lamellae containing cholesterol, free fatty acids, and ceramides [36]. Ceramides comprise the largest group of intercellular lipids in the SC [36]. The deposition of intercellular lipid lamellae in the nonlesional skin of dogs with CAD has been reported to be abnormal, highly disorganized, discontinuous, and reduced in number relative to the skin of healthy dogs [38,39]. The amount of total lipids and ceramides within the lesional and nonlesional skin of dogs with CAD has also been found to be significantly decreased when compared with the skin of healthy dogs, with one study showing more pronounced decreases in the lesional skin of dogs with CAD compared with nonlesional skin [40–43]. Studies have produced conflicting results when individual ceramide subclasses have been evaluated separately, with one study demonstrating global decreases in all ceramide subclasses, and other studies have reported significant decreases only in specific ceramide subclasses [41,42,44]. In addition to decreased ceramide content, the content of fatty acids in the SC of lesional and nonlesional skin of CAD has also been found to be significantly decreased when compared with the skin of healthy dogs [43,45].

Although there is evidence to support the presence of epidermal barrier dysfunction in CAD, it has not been possible to deduce whether epidermal barrier dysfunction in CAD is a primary defect underlying disease induction, or a secondary phenomenon resulting from local skin inflammation and self-trauma [37]. Nonetheless, restoring epidermal barrier function and integrity remains an integral part of the multimodal approach to managing dogs with CAD.

Immune Dysregulation

Inflammation of the skin is a hallmark finding of both humans with AD and dogs with CAD [5,23,24]. Histologically, CAD is characterized by superficial dermal infiltration of T cells, dendritic cells, eosinophils, and mast cells [5]. Various studies have demonstrated prominent Th2-polarized immune responses in CAD with variably increased levels of interleukin (IL)-4, IL-5, and IL-13 in the serum, peripheral blood mononuclear cells, and lesional skin, as well as increased numbers of Th2 cells in the peripheral circulation of affected dogs [46–52]. Th2-polarized immune responses have been proposed to play a critical role in the development and perpetuation of CAD by promoting humoral immunity, including the production of allergen-specific IgE antibodies, and the production and recruitment of inflammatory cells associated with hypersensitivity responses (ie, eosinophils) [53]. Allergen-specific IgE binds to the surface of canine mast cells and Langerhans cells within the skin, and are believed to play a role in CAD by mediating mast cell degranulation, allergen capture, processing, and presentation [35]. In addition to their proinflammatory properties, IL-4 and IL-13 have been shown to play a direct role in inducing pruritus by activating itch-sensing neurons that innervate the skin [54]. Dysregulated Th1 and Treg immune responses have also been documented in the skin and peripheral blood of dogs with CAD, and have been proposed to play roles in the immunopathogenesis of CAD in more chronic stages of disease [48,49,53,55].

Over the past decade, IL-31 has emerged as an important mediator of pruritus in CAD. IL-31 is a cytokine that is produced by activated T cells that preferentially exhibit a Th2-polarized cytokine profile, in addition to a variety of other innate and adaptive immune cells [56]. IL-31 mediates pruritus directly by activating somatosensory neurons that innervate the skin, as well as indirectly by upregulating the release of proinflammatory mediators from keratinocytes and immune cells [56]. IL-31 has been found to be significantly increased in the serum of client-owned dogs with naturally occurring CAD and serum levels positively correlate with the severity of pruritus [57–59]. Arguably, one of the most impactful and significant advances in CAD over the past decade has been identifying IL-31 as a novel therapeutic target for drug development. Indeed, the importance and clinical relevance of IL-31 in CAD has been further established by the significant improvements reported in pruritus and dermatitis severity in dogs with CAD following administration of lokivetmab (Cytopoint, Zoetis), a commercially available and widely prescribed caninized monoclonal antibody that binds to and neutralizes IL-31 [60–64].

Dysbiosis of the Cutaneous Microbiome

Dogs with CAD have long been recognized to suffer from recurrent microbial skin infections with *S pseudintermedius* and *M pachydermatis,* which are known to exacerbate clinical disease and complicate therapeutic responses [6]. Advances in molecular techniques and bioinformatics, and the advent of next-generation sequencing have demonstrated that the skin is inhabited by complex communities of commensal bacteria, archaea, fungi, and parasites that have historically been overlooked using conventional culture-based methods [65]. These communities, their genes, and metabolic by-products are collectively referred to as the "microbiome," and are believed to play dynamic roles in modulating host immune responses and competing with pathogenic microbes [65,66]. The relationship between the microbiome and CAD has been studied by sequencing the bacterial 16S ribosomal RNA and fungal ITS gene in relatively small numbers of dogs that have variably been receiving systemic and topical therapies.

The nonlesional skin of dogs with CAD has been shown to harbor significantly lower number of observed bacterial species (ie, lower "species richness") relative to the same anatomic sites on healthy dogs [67]. Similarly, the bacterial microbiota inhabiting the skin of dogs with CAD and superficial pyoderma was found to be significantly less diverse relative to the skin of healthy dogs with increased relative abundances of *Staphylococcus* spp found across all skin sites in dogs with CAD [68]. In dogs with CAD and pyoderma, the diversity of the bacterial microbiota was found to inversely correlate with clinical disease severity scores, measures of epidermal barrier function, and relative abundances of *Staphylococcus* spp [68]. More importantly, treating pyoderma in dogs with CAD with oral and/or topical antimicrobial therapy was shown to decrease clinical disease severity scores and relative abundances of *Staphylococcus* spp, improved measures of epidermal barrier function, and increase the diversity of the bacterial microbiota across all skin sites to levels that were indistinguishable from healthy dogs [68].

Similarly, the fungal microbiota (ie, the "mycobiota") inhabiting the nonlesional skin of dogs with allergic skin disease (ie, CAD, food-induced AD, and/or flea allergy dermatitis) has also been found to be less rich in fungal species relative to the skin of healthy dogs [69]. When the composition of *Malassezia* spp was evaluated at the species level, the lipid-dependent yeasts *Malassezia globosa* and *Malassezia restricta* were found to be significantly more abundant on the skin of healthy dogs, whereas *M pachydermatis* was found to be significantly more abundant on the nonlesional skin of allergic dogs [70]. *M pachydermatis* is considered a more versatile yeast that is capable of metabolizing a broader range of lipids [70]. The shift in species composition of *Malassezia* spp in the nonlesional skin of allergic dogs was suggested to be driven by the decreased lipid content known to occur in the skin of dogs with CAD [70].

Over the past decade, there has been a dramatic rise in the frequency of methicillin-resistant and multidrug-resistant bacterial skin infections with *S pseudintermedius* in canine patients [71]. This poses a concerning and increasingly common therapeutic challenge of CAD, considering the frequency with which *Staphylococcal* pyoderma complicates management of the disease. Although dysbiosis of the cutaneous microbiome appears to be a feature of CAD, it remains unknown what specific roles the microbiota play in CAD. Additional research is needed to further define the relationship between the cutaneous microbiome and the induction and exacerbation of CAD. Future discoveries in this field may inform the development of alternative approaches to controlling staphylococcal overgrowth and pyoderma in CAD that may decrease the need for systemic antimicrobials and the promotion of antimicrobial resistance.

TREATMENT

As previously mentioned, pruritus is a hallmark clinical sign of CAD and is often the main presenting complaint when owners of dogs with CAD seek veterinary care. As such, providing immediate and sustained anti-itch relief is a primary therapeutic goal in managing CAD. It is important to recognize that the pruritus experienced by each individual dog with CAD may be complicated by various flare factors, including exposure to environmental allergens (eg, pollens, molds, house dust mites), dietary components, concurrent uncontrolled flea allergy dermatitis, and the development of microbial skin infections. For these reasons, a multimodal approach is typically required when managing CAD to ensure all contributing flare factors of disease are identified and addressed. Unfortunately, CAD cannot be cured at present and, as a chronic skin disease, requires lifelong management. When managing CAD, it is important to determine the right combination of therapies for each individual dog that will provide a safe, effective, and affordable management strategy that the respective pet owner can reliably and willingly execute. A common pitfall in the management of CAD is a failure to identify and address all disease flare factors. Consequently, whenever a dog with CAD is poorly responsive to therapy, the managing clinician should evaluate for the presence of uncontrolled flare factors that are complicating disease management. Therapeutic recommendations for CAD need to be tailored to each individual dog, including their stage and severity of disease, using a combination of topical and systemic therapies. Although significant overlap exists, there are subtle differences in the approaches to managing acute flares and the long-term maintenance of CAD. Current recommendations for the management of acute flares and long-term maintenance of CAD are summarized in Tables 2 and 3, respectively.

The Role of Topical Therapies

Topical therapies used in the management of CAD are available in a variety of different formulations, including shampoos, foaming mousses, sprays, wipes, spot-ons, creams, and ointments. There are several rationales for using topical therapy in the management of CAD. First, topical therapy directly treats the affected skin, thereby reducing, and potentially eliminating, the need for systemic medications. Depending on the active ingredients of the prescribed productions, topical therapy can also reduce surface colonization of pathogenic bacteria and yeast, improve epidermal barrier function, and deliver pharmacologic antipruritic and anti-inflammatory agents to the skin. Bathing with a medicated shampoo is frequently recommended for dogs with CAD, and the selection of shampoo should be based on the desired therapeutic goal. Regardless of the active ingredients of the prescribed shampoo, the physical act of bathing a dog with CAD can remove environmental allergens from the skin and hair coat, provide mild anti-itch relief, hydrate the skin, and remove exudate, crusting and inflammatory mediators. The efficacy of bathing with medicated shampoos is likely dependent on its frequency of administration, as well as the stage and severity of skin disease [3,72]. Bathing with a medicated shampoo twice weekly is recommended for the initial management of acute flares of CAD. Depending on the extent and severity of skin disease, additional topical products (eg, medicated sprays, foaming mousses, wipes) can be applied between medicated baths. Once a dog's skin disease is in remission and well-controlled,

TABLE 2
Therapeutic Considerations for Acute Flares of Canine Atopic Dermatitis

Therapeutic Strategy	Consider
Identification of flare factors	• Lapse in flea control or increased flea exposure • Dietary indiscretion in a dog with confirmed food-induced atopic dermatitis • Development of secondary microbial skin infections
Topical therapy	• Institute twice-weekly medicated baths with an antimicrobial shampoo • For moderate to severe clinical signs, consider daily application of antimicrobial sprays, wipes, mousses, etc., in-between medicated baths, and/or systemic antimicrobials
Reduce pruritus and cutaneous inflammation	• Brief tapering anti-inflammatory course of oral corticosteroids • And/or Tapering course of topical corticosteroids • Or oclacitinib maleate (Apoquel, Zoetis) • Or lokivetmab (Cytopoint, Zoetis)

TABLE 3
Therapeutic Considerations for the Chronic Management of Canine Atopic Dermatitis

Therapeutic Strategy	Consider
Avoidance of flare factors	• Maintain comprehensive flea control that fits with a dog's lifestyle and environment • Identification and management food-induced atopic dermatitis • Once to twice-weekly medicated baths with antimicrobial shampoos to decrease the frequency of recurrent skin infections
Interventions to restore epidermal barrier function and integrity	• Application of lipid-containing topical products (ie, shampoos, sprays, spot-ons) • Oral supplementation with essential fatty acids
Interventions to decrease pruritus and skin inflammation	• Cyclosporine (Atopica, Elanco) • Or oclacitinib maleate (Apoquel, Zoetis) • Or lokivetmab (Cytopoint, Zoetis) • And/or twice-weekly application of topical corticosteroids to localized affected body regions
Disease-modifying interventions	• Allergen-specific immunotherapy

it is recommended to continue once-weekly bathing with a nonirritating shampoo using lukewarm water for long-term maintenance [3,72].

Antimicrobial topical therapy

As previously mentioned, dogs with CAD are at increased risk for developing recurrent microbial skin infections with *S pseudintermedius* and/or *M pachydermatis*. These microbial pathogens can also colonize the external ear canals of dogs with CAD, and are frequently associated with otitis externa. For these reasons, cytologic evaluation of the skin and ear canals of dogs with CAD should be performed to identify secondary complicating skin and/or ear infections in dogs experiencing acute flares of disease as well as in dogs with chronic disease presenting for their first-time evaluation. Topical therapy containing antimicrobial agents, including combinations of chlorhexidine and azole antifungals, are an integral part of treating secondary bacterial and yeast infections in dogs with CAD. Furthermore, topical antimicrobial therapy is also recommended for the long-term maintenance of dogs with CAD to decrease surface colonization of pathogenic microbes in attempts to prevent, or at least decrease the frequency of, recurrent skin infections. However, it is important to consider that certain topical antimicrobial products may be irritating or drying to the skin and may exacerbate epidermal barrier dysfunction and adversely affect disease management. Readers are referred to recent review articles and consensus guidelines for a more comprehensive discussion on the management of staphylococcal pyoderma and *Malassezia* dermatitis [71,73,74].

Topical therapy to restore epidermal barrier integrity and function

Reparation of the abnormal epidermal barrier is considered an important therapeutic goal in the management of CAD. Essential fatty acids, cholesterol, ceramides, and phytosphingosine (ie, a ceramide precursor) have been incorporated into various topical products, including spot-ons, sprays, and shampoos, with the intent of restoring the epidermal barrier's integrity and function. In doing so, these products may decrease percutaneous absorption of irritants, allergens, and microbes, and prevent allergic sensitization and inflammation. However, limited clinical trials have been performed to evaluate the clinical efficacy of the available products.

Allerderm Spot-On (Virbac SA) is a topical product that contains ceramides, cholesterol, and free fatty acids. Allerderm has been shown to help restore the ultrastructural lipid abnormalities and significantly improve the severity of dermatitis in small numbers of dogs with CAD [39,75,76]. Similarly, significant improvements in severity of dermatitis and pruritus were reported in dogs with CAD following topical application of Dermoscent Essential 6 Spot-On (Dermoscent, LDCA, France, Bayer Animal Health, USA, Tarrytown, NJ), a topical product that contains fatty acids and essential oils [77]. More recently, a topical spot-on (Atopivet Spot-On, Bioberica S.A.U., Barcelona, Spain) containing sphingomyelin (ie, a ceramide precursor) and glycosaminoglycans (ie, hyaluronic acid) was also found to significantly improve the severity of dermatitis and pruritus in experimental laboratory model of CAD [78]. Topical emollient formulations (ie, shampoos, conditioners, and sprays) containing lipids, complex sugars, and antiseptics (Allermyl, Virbac), or phytosphingosine and raspberry oil (Douxo Calm, Ceva), have also been shown to clinically benefit dogs with CAD [79,80].

As with antimicrobial topical therapy, use of lipid-containing topical therapies are recommended for the long-term maintenance of dogs with CAD. To that goal, various antimicrobial topical therapies are now formulated with lipid complexes, thereby allowing managing clinicians and owners to treat and prevent microbial skin infections, as well as restore epidermal barrier integrity function, with one product. Many studies that have looked at topical products to address barrier dysfunction show promise but well-designed larger clinical trials are still needed to demonstrate the efficacy of the ever-increasing number of lipid-containing topical therapies marketed for CAD.

Topical antipruritic and anti-inflammatory therapies

Topical application of anti-inflammatory agents have long been a mainstay in the management of humans with mild to moderate AD [23,24]. However, frequent application of topical anti-inflammatory agents pose a unique challenge in canine patients, as dogs will often attempt to remove the products by licking, thereby increasing the risk of systemic absorption and toxicity and decreasing therapeutic efficacy. Widespread topical application of creams, gels, and ointments is challenging and impractical in dogs due to the presence of their haircoat. Nonetheless, topical therapies containing glucocorticoids and calcineurin inhibitors have been evaluated in CAD in attempts to decrease the need for systemic therapies.

There is good evidence for the use of medium potency glucocorticoid sprays, containing triamcinolone or hydrocortisone aceponate, in the short-term management of allergic pruritus [3,72,81,82]. A 0.015% triamcinolone acetonide spray (Genesis, Virbac) has been shown to be effective at treating CAD and diminishing pruritus when applied for 4 weeks following a tapering administration schedule [81]. A 0.0584% hydrocortisone aceponate spray (Cortavance; Virbac) also has demonstrated efficacy in the management of CAD [82–84]. Importantly, twice-weekly application of hydrocortisone aceponate spray has been shown to prolong the remission time in dogs with CAD between recurrences of clinical signs, demonstrating its potential role in the long-term management of CAD [85]. Both of the preceding topical glucocorticoid sprays are labeled for short-term use only and the frequency and duration of their application should be monitored closely for adverse effects of topical glucocorticoids. There are numerous topical veterinary products containing glucocorticoids, although many are untested in randomized clinical trials. Glucocorticoid-containing lotions and creams are impractical for treating large body regions, but they can be useful if the affected skin is limited to small areas, such as the paws or pinnae. The efficacy of these products and their side effects will depend on the formulation, duration of application, and potency. Chronic or habitual use of corticosteroids, particularly those of higher potency, can sometimes result in systemic side effects referable to iatrogenic hypercortisolemia from percutaneous absorption; this is of greatest concern in small-sized dogs. The most common adverse effects of prolonged application of potent, topical glucocorticoids include epidermal atrophy (ie, thinning if the skin), alopecia, superficial follicular cysts (ie, "milia"), comedones, striae, alopecia, calcinosis cutis, demodicosis, and pyoderma. Newer topical corticosteroids, like mometasone furoate and hydrocortisone aceponate, are considered "soft-steroids" as they are metabolized into inactive metabolites within the skin, thereby decreasing the risk and frequency of systemic side effects.

Tacrolimus (Protopic, Astellas Pharma, Tokyo, Japan) is a topical calcineurin inhibitor with anti-inflammatory properties that are very similar in activity to Cyclosporine A (CsA) that has been evaluated as an alternative to topical corticosteroids in the management of CAD [72]. It is available as an ointment in 2 different strengths (0.1% and 0.03%). Tacrolimus (0.1%) has been shown to be effective in the management of dogs with CAD when applied to relatively small body regions [86,87]. It is most efficacious when applied twice daily for 1 week, and then tapered as needed to control clinical signs. Tacrolimus has a slow onset of action and therefore is less useful in treating acute flares of CAD. Tacrolimus has comparatively fewer side effects relative to topical corticosteroids, but can be irritating to some patients. The clinical utility of tacrolimus in the management of CAD is somewhat limited as it is frequently cost-prohibitive for most pet owners and is challenging to apply to larger body regions.

Systemic Anti-inflammatory and Antipruritic Therapies

Systemic medications, in combination with topical therapies, are oftentimes required for the management of dogs with moderate to severe CAD. Historically, this was limited to the prescription of oral corticosteroids and oral antihistamines. Several studies have now shown that there is inconsistent evidence to support the use of antihistamines in CAD [72]. Corticosteroids have broad anti-inflammatory effects, a rapid onset of activity, and consequently can still have a useful role in the treatment of acute CAD when prescribed judiciously and appropriately. However, systemic corticosteroids should be avoided in the chronic management of CAD, whenever possible, as there are now more safe, specific, and targeted therapies available, including CsA, oclacitinib maleate (Apoquel, Zoetis), and lokivetmab (Cytopoint, Zoetis). It is important to recognize that each systemic medication is not equally efficacious in every dog with CAD and there may be different advantages or disadvantages for the selection of one medication over another, which may be dictated by their cost, associated adverse effects, or time to clinical effect. The availability of different systemic and topical therapies for CAD provides the opportunity to customize a multimodal management strategy tailored to each dog's needs and pet owner's capabilities. For the purposes of this review, the use of systemic corticosteroids in the management of CAD is not discussed.

CsA is considered an effective therapy for the chronic management of CAD and is available as a microemulsion formulated as either a capsule or liquid [3,72]. Cyclosporine inhibits intracellular calcineurin, which is an enzyme involved in the activation of T cells and the transcription of a number of proinflammatory cytokines. There have been several comprehensive reviews that have provided good evidence for the efficacy of microemulsified CsA in the management of CAD when administered at 5 mg/kg orally once daily. CsA has a delayed onset of activity and has been shown to improve dermatitis severity in dogs with CAD after 4 weeks of daily administration [88–90]. Many dogs with CAD are able to reduce the frequency of administration of CsA from once daily to every other day once their disease is in clinical remission; a minority of dogs are able to further decrease CsA administration to twice weekly [88]. Cyclosporine is metabolized by the cytochrome P450 3A4 enzyme (CYP3A4) in the liver. Drugs that inhibit CYP3A4 (ie, azole antifungals) or compete with P-glycoprotein (ie, ivermectin) can cause drug interactions with cyclosporine. For this reason, managing clinicians are advised to be cognizant of possible drug interactions whenever prescribing this medication. The most common side effects of CsA are gastrointestinal disturbances (ie, vomiting and diarrhea); however, gingival enlargement or overgrowth, opportunistic infections with fungal and/or mycobacterial pathogens, papillomatosis, and hirsutism are also known to occur [91].

Oclacitinib maleate (Apoquel, Zoetis) is a janus kinase (JAK) inhibitor approved for use in dogs and labeled for the control of pruritus associated with allergic dermatitis and the control of CAD in dogs at least 12 months of age. JAK enzymes are involved in intracellular signaling pathways once cytokines bind to their respective receptors. Oclacitinib maleate is most effective at inhibiting JAK1, which plays a key role in the mediating the intracellular signaling of IL-2, IL-4, IL-6, IL-13, and IL-31 [92]. Oclacitinib maleate is rapidly absorbed with high bioavailability and a half-life of 4 to 6 hours [93]. The labeled dose of oclacitinib is 0.4 to 0.6 mg/kg given orally every 12 hours for 14 days, then given every 24 hours for long-term maintenance. Continuing at the initial induction dose is not recommended, as the risk for adverse effects from broader immune suppression increases. Several clinical trials have demonstrated its rapid speed of onset, favorable safety profile, and clinical efficacy for both acute flares and chronic management of CAD [94–96]. Reported side effects on the package insert include vomiting and diarrhea; however, their frequency were no different from placebo. Some dogs were also reported to develop neoplasia and cutaneous growths during a 6-month continuation study; however, a recent study found no association between administration of oclacitinib maleate and the onset of new cutaneous masses [97]. Per the package insert, Oclacitinib maleate has also been associated with demodicosis and bronchopneumonia in dogs younger than 12 months of age. For this reason, oclacitinib maleate should not be used in puppies or in dogs with a history of demodicosis. Oclacitinib maleate is an effective antipruritic with some anti-inflammatory properties that can be used for both the management of acute flares and ongoing chronic management of CAD.

Lokivetmab (Cytopoint, Zoetis) is a caninized monoclonal antibody that binds IL-31, thereby preventing it from interacting with its receptor and inducing pruritus. Lokivetmab has a mean half-life of 16 days and remains in circulation for several weeks [98]. The manufacturer recommends repeated subcutaneous administration either once a month, or as needed. Lokivetmab was shown to significantly decrease pruritus within 1 to 3 days when dosed at 2 mg/kg in a dose determination study [98]. No side effects reported in the original studies cited on the package insert were found to be significantly different from the placebo control group. In several studies, lokivetmab has been demonstrated to be an effective and safe therapy for both acute flares and chronic management of CAD [60–64] (see Tables 2 and 3)

Allergen-Specific Immunotherapy

Allergen-specific immunotherapy (ASIT) is considered a first-line treatment recommendation for dogs with CAD. ASIT attempts to promote tolerance to the allergens an affected dog is sensitized to, thereby decreasing the need for systemic anti-inflammatory agents. Formulation of ASIT is based on the results of conventional allergy tests (ie, an intradermal allergy test and/or allergen-specific IgE serology). Numerous protocols exist that follow different administration schedules and routes of administration (ie, subcutaneous, sublingual, or intralymphatic) with no proven superiority of any one ASIT protocol. Published studies evaluating the efficacy of ASIT have shown that approximately 20% of dogs with CAD have an excellent response to ASIT with complete remission of clinical signs and discontinuation of all other therapies, whereas another 40% to 50% have a satisfactory response with improved clinical signs and/or a decrease in need for concurrent therapies, and the remaining 30% to 40% show insufficient response to find ASIT as a beneficial therapy [99]. In addition to managing the clinical signs of CAD, ASIT is also believed to halt, or at least slow down, the progression of disease over time. When effective, ASIT is likely associated with an increase in Treg cells, which may play a role in improving the immune dysregulation noted in CAD [100]. When ASIT is prescribed to dogs with CAD, it is recommended to be continued for at least 12 months to be able evaluate its clinical benefit. Side effects are uncommon and include localized injection site reactions and transient pruritus. Rarely, systemic side effects (ie, vomiting, diarrhea, anaphylaxis) can occur [99]. ASIT is considered a safe and effective therapy for the chronic management of CAD.

Dietary Considerations

Oral supplementation with essential fatty acids (EFAs) has long been advocated as an adjunctive therapy for CAD and has been shown to normalize lipids in the SC of dogs with CAD, similar to some topical lipid formulations [72,101]. Oral supplementation with EFAs is better suited for the chronic management of CAD as their clinical benefits, if any, may not be seen for several months [72]. Several EFA-containing commercial diets have been developed and marketed for the management of allergic skin disease. However, very few clinical trials have been performed to demonstrate their utility and efficacy in the management of CAD.

FUTURE AVENUES TO CONSIDER

AD is a heterogeneous disease in humans that is characterized by a variety of subtypes (ie, also known as "endotypes") that can be stratified by age, ethnicity, disease chronicity, and severity [24,102]. Ongoing research is being performed to define the specific molecular and cellular mechanisms that characterize each subtype [102]. For example, specific cytokine profiles and epidermal barrier defects of human AD have been shown to differ between children and adults, as well as between individuals of different ethnicities with the disease [102]. Characterizing well-defined subtypes of human AD is of particular importance and clinical relevance, as individual subtypes may respond differently to treatment [103]. Similarly, breed-specific clinical phenotypes are well-recognized to exist in CAD [8]. For example, the age of disease onset, type and distribution of skin lesions, and the predilection for skin infections with either bacteria or yeast has been shown to vary between genetically predisposed breeds [8]. Rather than representing a single disease entity, CAD may be better viewed as a clinical syndrome that is united by characteristic clinical features that originate from diverse combinations of environmental and genetic risk factors that vary depending on a dog's age, breed, and geographic location. The development of oclacitinib maleate and lokivetmab has heralded a new era in veterinary dermatology defined by the commercial availability of small molecule inhibitors and monoclonal antibodies that target specific cytokine axes. Undoubtably, the availability of targeted therapeutics for CAD will continue to grow as the pathologic mechanisms that underly the disease are better understood. Future targeted therapies in CAD may include monoclonal antibodies that bind and neutralize the receptor subunit shared by IL-4 and IL-13 (ie, IL-4Rα), or a receptor subunit used by IL-31 (ie, IL-31RA), as has been developed for humans with AD [5,23,24]. As with endotypes of human AD, it is plausible that the breed-specific clinical phenotypes of CAD may respond differently to treatment. Further characterizing the various breed-specific clinical phenotypes of CAD may therefore optimize clinical outcomes by determining what preventative and therapeutic strategies work best for each breed. In doing so, veterinarians may start to transition from a "one-size-fits-all" or "trial by error" approach to managing dogs with CAD to an approach that is defined by personalized, precision medicine.

CLINICS CARE POINTS

- Educating clients that CAD is a lifelong and progressive disease that requires chronic management will help set realistic expectations, increase owner compliance, and decrease owner frustration.

- Dogs with well-controlled CAD that flare despite no recent therapeutic changes should be evaluated for the development of secondary skin infections and/or exposure to fleas. Also consider dietary indiscretion in those dogs with a confirmed food-induced component to their allergic skin disease.
- Frequent antimicrobial topical therapy is often sufficient as a sole therapy to resolve mild to moderate superficial pyoderma in dogs with CAD and is recommended to avoid the promotion of antimicrobial resistance.
- Dogs experiencing an acute flare of CAD associated with significant inflammation of the ear canals often benefit from a short, tapering course of corticosteroids to establish clinical remission. Oclacitinib maleate and lokivetmab may not provide adequate anti-inflammatory effects for moderate to severe otitis externa.
- Corticosteroids and oclacitinib maleate may precipitate demodicosis in canine patients so deep skin scrapings and/or trichograms should be performed in previously well-controlled CAD dogs that are developing new lesions.
- Environmental allergy testing does not diagnose CAD and should only be performed in dogs that have already been determined to have CAD and if the owner is interested in ASIT. When started, ASIT should be continued for at least 1 year before evaluating its clinical efficacy. Allergen-specific IgE serology testing for food allergies is unreliable and not recommended at this time.

ACKNOWLEDGMENTS

The preparation of this manuscript was supported by US National Institutes of Health grant T320D011130 (T.J.M.J).

DISCLOSURE

The authors have nothing to disclose.

REFERENCES

[1] Halliwell R. Revised nomenclature for veterinary allergy. Vet Immunol Immunopathol 2006;114(3):207–8.
[2] Noli C, Colombo S, Cornegliani L, et al. Quality of life of dogs with skin disease and of their owners. part 2: Administration of a questionnaire in various skin diseases and correlation to efficacy of therapy. Vet Dermatol 2011;22(4):344–51.
[3] Olivry T, DeBoer DJ, Favrot C, et al. Treatment of canine atopic dermatitis: 2010 clinical practice guidelines from the international task force on canine atopic dermatitis. Vet Dermatol 2010;21:233–48.
[4] Hillier A, Griffin CE. The ACVD task force on canine atopic dermatitis (I): Incidence and prevalence. Vet Immunol Immunopathol 2001;81:147–51.
[5] Bizikova P, Santoro D, Marsella R, et al. Review: clinical and histological manifestations of canine atopic dermatitis. Vet Dermatol 2015;26:79.e24.
[6] Hensel P, Santoro D, Favrot C, et al. Canine atopic dermatitis: Detailed guidelines for diagnosis and allergen identification. BMC Vet Res 2015;11(1):196.
[7] Favrot C, Steffan J, Seewald W, et al. A prospective study on the clinical features of chronic canine atopic dermatitis and its diagnosis. Vet Dermatol 2010;21:23–31.
[8] Wilhem S, Kovalik M, Favrot C. Breed-associated phenotypes in canine atopic dermatitis. Vet Dermatol 2011;22:143–9.
[9] Marsella R, De Benedetto A. Atopic dermatitis in animals and people: An update and comparative review. Vet Sci 2017;4:37.
[10] Olivry T, Mueller RS. Critically appraised topic on adverse food reactions of companion animals (7): Signalment and cutaneous manifestations of dogs and cats with adverse food reactions. BMC Vet Res 2019;15:140.
[11] Olivry T, DeBoer DJ, Prélaud P, et al. Food for thought: pondering the relationship between canine atopic dermatitis and cutaneous adverse food reactions. Vet Dermatol 2007;18:390–1.
[12] Mueller RS, Olivry T. Critically appraised topic on adverse food reactions of companion animals (6): prevalence of noncutaneous manifestations of adverse food reactions in dogs and cats. BMC Vet Res 2018;14:341.
[13] Shaw SC, Wood JLN, Freeman J, et al. Estimation of heritability of atopic dermatitis in Labrador and golden retrievers. Am J Vet Res 2004;65:1014–20.
[14] Rostaher A, Dolf G, Fischer NM, et al. Atopic dermatitis in a cohort of West Highland white terriers in Switzerland. part II: estimates of early life factors and heritability. Vet Dermatol 2020;31:276.e6.
[15] Nuttall T. The genomics revolution: will canine atopic dermatitis be predictable and preventable? Vet Dermatol 2013;24:10.e4.
[16] Wood SH, Ollier WE, Nuttall T, et al. Despite identifying some shared gene associations with human atopic dermatitis the use of multiple dog breeds from various locations limits detection of gene associations in canine atopic dermatitis. Vet Immunol Immunopathol 2010;138:193–7.
[17] Agler CS, Friedenberg S, Olivry T, et al. Genome-wide association analysis in West Highland white terriers with atopic dermatitis. Vet Immunol Immunopathol 2019;209:1–6.
[18] Suriyaphol G, Suriyaphol P, Sarikaputi M, et al. Association of filaggrin (FLG) gene polymorphism with canine atopic dermatitis in small breed dogs. Thai J Vet Med 2011;41(4):509–17.

[19] Tengvall K, Kierczak M, Bergvall K, et al. Genome-wide analysis in german shepherd dogs reveals association of a locus on CFA 27 with atopic dermatitis. PLoS Genet 2013;9:e1003475.

[20] Wood SH, Ke X, Nuttall T, et al. Genome-wide association analysis of canine atopic dermatitis and identification of disease related SNPs. Immunogenetics 2009;61: 765–72.

[21] Roque JB, O'Leary CA, Duffy D, et al. Atopic dermatitis in west highland white terriers is associated with a 1.3-mb region on CFA 17. Immunogenetics 2012;64:209–17.

[22] Roque JB, O'leary CA, Kyaw-Tanner M, et al. PTPN22 polymorphisms may indicate a role for this gene in atopic dermatitis in West Highland white terriers. BMC Res Notes 2011;4:571.

[23] Ständer S. Atopic dermatitis. N Engl J Med 2021;384: 1136–43.

[24] Langan SM, Irvine AD, Weidinger S. Atopic dermatitis. Lancet 2020;396:345–60.

[25] Kantor R, Silverberg JI. Environmental risk factors and their role in the management of atopic dermatitis. Expert Rev Clin Immunol 2017;13:15–26.

[26] Nødtvedt A, Egenvall A, Bergval K, et al. Incidence of and risk factors for atopic dermatitis in a Swedish population of insured dogs. Vet Rec 2006;159:241–6.

[27] Nødtvedt A, Guitian J, Egenvall A, et al. The spatial distribution of atopic dermatitis cases in a population of insured Swedish dogs. Prev Vet Med 2007;78:210–22.

[28] Meury S, Molitor V, Doherr MG, et al. Role of the environment in the development of canine atopic dermatitis in Labrador and golden retrievers. Vet Dermatol 2011;22:327–34.

[29] Harvey ND, Shaw SC, Craigon PJ, et al. Environmental risk factors for canine atopic dermatitis: a retrospective large-scale study in Labrador and golden retrievers. Vet Dermatol 2019;30:396.e9.

[30] Ka D, Marignac G, Desquilbet L, et al. Association between passive smoking and atopic dermatitis in dogs. Food Chem Toxicol 2014;66:329–33.

[31] Hakanen E, Lehtimäki J, Salmela E, et al. Urban environment predisposes dogs and their owners to allergic symptoms. Sci Rep 2018;8:1585.

[32] Anturaniemi J, Uusitalo L, Hielm-Björkman A. Environmental and phenotype-related risk factors for owner-reported allergic/atopic skin symptoms and for canine atopic dermatitis verified by veterinarian in a finnish dog population. PLoS One 2017;12:e0178771.

[33] Nødtvedt A, Bergvall K, Sallander M, et al. A case-control study of risk factors for canine atopic dermatitis among boxer, bullterrier and west highland white terrier dogs in sweden. Vet Dermatol 2007;18:309–15.

[34] Deboer DJ. The future of immunotherapy for canine atopic dermatitis: a review. Vet Dermatol 2017;28:25.

[35] Pucheu-Haston CM, Bizikova P, Eisenschenk MNC, et al. Review: the role of antibodies, autoantigens and food allergens in canine atopic dermatitis. Vet Dermatol 2015;26:115.e30.

[36] Luger T, Amagai M, Dreno B, et al. Atopic dermatitis: role of the skin barrier, environment, microbiome, and therapeutic agents. J Dermatol Sci 2021;102: 142–57.

[37] Santoro D, Marsella R, Pucheu-Haston CM, et al. Review: pathogenesis of canine atopic dermatitis: skin barrier and host-micro-organism interaction. Vet Dermatol 2015;26:84.e5.

[38] Inman AO, Olivry T, Dunston SM, et al. Electron microscopic observations of stratum corneum intercellular lipids in normal and atopic dogs. Vet Pathol 2001;38: 720–3.

[39] Piekutowska A, Pin D, Rème CA, et al. Effects of a topically applied preparation of epidermal lipids on the stratum corneum barrier of atopic dogs. J Comp Pathol 2008;138:197–203.

[40] Shimada K, Yoon J, Yoshihara T, et al. Increased transepidermal water loss and decreased ceramide content in lesional and non-lesional skin of dogs with atopic dermatitis. Vet Dermatol 2009;20:541–6.

[41] Yoon J, Nishifuji K, Sasaki A, et al. Alteration of stratum corneum ceramide profiles in spontaneous canine model of atopic dermatitis. Exp Dermatol 2011;20: 732–6.

[42] Angelbeck-Schulze M, Mischke R, Rohn K, et al. Canine epidermal lipid sampling by skin scrub revealed variations between different body sites and normal and atopic dogs. BMC Vet Res 2014;10:152.

[43] Popa I, Remoue N, Hoang LT, et al. Atopic dermatitis in dogs is associated with a high heterogeneity in the distribution of protein-bound lipids within the stratum corneum. Arch Dermatol Res 2011;303:433.

[44] Reiter LV, Torres SMF, Wertz PW. Characterization and quantification of ceramides in the nonlesional skin of canine patients with atopic dermatitis compared with controls. Vet Dermatol 2009;20:260–6.

[45] Chermprapai S, Broere F, Gooris G, et al. Altered lipid properties of the stratum corneum in canine atopic dermatitis. Biochim Biophys Acta Biomembr 2018; 1860:526–33.

[46] Olivry T, Dean GA, Tompkin MB, et al. Toward a canine model of atopic dermatitis. Exp Dermatol 1999;8: 204–11.

[47] Majewska A, Gajewska M, Dembele K, et al. Lymphocytic, cytokine and transcriptomic profiles in peripheral blood of dogs with atopic dermatitis. BMC Vet Res 2016;12:174.

[48] Nuttall TJ, Knight PA, McAleese SM, et al. Expression of Th1, Th2 and immunosuppressive cytokine gene transcripts in canine atopic dermatitis. Clin Exp Allergy 2002;32:789–95.

[49] Schlotter YM, Rutten VPMG, Riemers FM, et al. Lesional skin in atopic dogs shows a mixed type-1 and type-2 immune responsiveness. Vet Immunol Immunopathol 2011;143:20–6.

[50] Hayashiya S, Tani K, Morimoto M, et al. Expression of T helper 1 and T helper 2 cytokine mRNAs in freshly

isolated peripheral blood mononuclear cells from dogs with atopic dermatitis. J Vet Med A Physiol Pathol Clin Med 2002;49:27–31.

[51] Kanwal S, Singh SK, Soman SP, et al. Expression of barrier proteins in the skin lesions and inflammatory cytokines in peripheral blood mononuclear cells of atopic dogs. Sci Rep 2021;11:11418.

[52] Früh SP, Saikia M, Eule J, et al. Elevated circulating Th2 but not group 2 innate lymphoid cell responses characterize canine atopic dermatitis. Vet Immunol Immunopathol 2020;221:110015.

[53] Pucheu-Haston CM, Bizikova P, Marsella R, et al. Review: lymphocytes, cytokines, chemokines and the T-helper 1-T-helper 2 balance in canine atopic dermatitis. Vet Dermatol 2015;26:124.e32.

[54] Oetjen LK, Mack MR, Feng J, et al. Sensory neurons co-opt classical immune signaling pathways to mediate chronic itch. Cell 2017;171:217–28.e13.

[55] Hauck V, Hügli P, Meli ML, et al. Increased numbers of FoxP3-expressing CD4+ CD25+ regulatory T cells in peripheral blood from dogs with atopic dermatitis and its correlation with disease severity. Vet Dermatol 2016;27:26.e9.

[56] Furue M, Furue M. Interleukin-31 and pruritic skin. J Clin Med 2021;10:1906.

[57] Gonzales AJ, Humphrey WR, Messamore JE, et al. Interleukin-31: Its role in canine pruritus and naturally occurring canine atopic dermatitis. Vet Dermatol 2013;24:48.e12.

[58] Messamore JE. An ultrasensitive single molecule array (simoa) for the detection of IL-31 in canine serum shows differential levels in dogs affected with atopic dermatitis compared to healthy animals. Vet Dermatol 2017;28:546.

[59] Chaudhary SK, Singh SK, Kumari P, et al. Alterations in circulating concentrations of IL-17, IL-31 and total IgE in dogs with atopic dermatitis. Vet Dermatol 2019;30:383.e4.

[60] Tamamoto-Mochizuki C, Paps JS, Olivry T. Proactive maintenance therapy of canine atopic dermatitis with the anti-IL-31 lokivetmab. can a monoclonal antibody blocking a single cytokine prevent allergy flares? Vet Dermatol 2019;30:98.e6.

[61] Michels GM, Ramsey DS, Walsh KF, et al. A blinded, randomized, placebo-controlled, dose determination trial of lokivetmab (ZTS-00103289), a caninized, anti-canine IL-31 monoclonal antibody in client owned dogs with atopic dermatitis. Vet Dermatol 2016;27:478.e9.

[62] Moyaert H, Van Brussel L, Borowski S, et al. A blinded, randomized clinical trial evaluating the efficacy and safety of lokivetmab compared to ciclosporin in client-owned dogs with atopic dermatitis. Vet Dermatol 2017;28:593.e5.

[63] Souza CP, Rosychuk RAW, Contreras ET, et al. A retrospective analysis of the use of lokivetmab in the management of allergic pruritus in a referral population of 135 dogs in the western USA. Vet Dermatol 2018;29:489.e4.

[64] Szczepanik M, Wilkołek P, Gołyński M, et al. The influence of treatment with lokivetmab on transepidermal water loss (TEWL) in dogs with spontaneously occurring atopic dermatitis. Vet Dermatol 2019;30:330.e3.

[65] Rodrigues Hoffmann A. The cutaneous ecosystem: the roles of the skin microbiome in health and its association with inflammatory skin conditions in humans and animals. Vet Dermatol 2017;28:60.e15.

[66] Bjerre RD, Bandier J, Skov L, et al. The role of the skin microbiome in atopic dermatitis: a systematic review. Br J Dermatol 2017;177:1272.

[67] Rodrigues Hoffmann A, Patterson AP, Diesel A, et al. The skin microbiome in healthy and allergic dogs. PLoS One 2014;9:e83197.

[68] Bradley CW, Morris DO, Rankin SC, et al. Longitudinal evaluation of the skin microbiome and association with microenvironment and treatment in Canine Atopic dermatitis. J Invest Dermatol 2016;136:1182–90.

[69] Meason Smith C, Diesel A, Patterson AP, et al. What is living on your dog's skin? Characterization of the canine cutaneous mycobiota and fungal dysbiosis in canine allergic dermatitis. FEMS Microbiol Ecol 2015;91:fiv139.

[70] Meason-Smith C, Olivry T, Lawhon SD, et al. Malassezia species dysbiosis in natural and allergen-induced atopic dermatitis in dogs. Med Mycol 2020;58:756–65.

[71] Morris DO, Loeffler A, Davis MF, et al. Recommendations for approaches to methicillin-resistant staphylococcal infections of small animals: diagnosis, therapeutic considerations and preventative measures. Vet Dermatol 2017;28:304.e9.

[72] Olivry T, DeBoer DJ, Favrot C, et al. Treatment of canine atopic dermatitis: 2015 updated guidelines from the international committee on allergic diseases of animals (ICADA). BMC Vet Res 2015;11:210.

[73] Bond R, Morris DO, Guillot J, et al. Biology, diagnosis and treatment of malassezia dermatitis in dogs and cats clinical consensus guidelines of the world association for veterinary dermatology. Vet Dermatol 2020;31:28–74.

[74] Hillier A, Lloyd DH, Weese JS, et al. Guidelines for the diagnosis and antimicrobial therapy of canine superficial bacterial folliculitis (antimicrobial guidelines working group of the international society for companion animal infectious diseases). Vet Dermatol 2014;25:163.e3.

[75] Marsella R, Gilmer L, Ahrens K, et al. Investigations on the effects of a topical ceramides-containing emulsion (allerderm spot on) on clinical signs and skin barrier function in dogs with topic dermatitis: a double-blinded, randomized, controlled study. Intern J Appl Res Vet Med 2013;11:110–6.

[76] Fujimura M, Nakatsuji Y, Fujiwara S, et al. Spot-on skin lipid complex as an adjunct therapy in dogs with atopic

dermatitis: an open pilot study. Vet Med Int 2011;2011: 281846.
[77] Blaskovic M, Rosenkrantz W, Neuber A, et al. The effect of a spot-on formulation containing polyunsaturated fatty acids and essential oils on dogs with atopic dermatitis. Vet J 2014;199:39–43.
[78] Marsella R, Segarra S, Ahrens K, et al. Topical treatment with sphingolipids and glycosaminoglycans for canine atopic dermatitis. BMC Vet Res 2020;16:92.
[79] Reme CA, Mondon A, Calmon JP, et al. Efficacy of combined topical therapy with antiallergic shampoo and lotion for the control of signs associated with atopic dermatitis in dogs. Vet Dermatol 2004;15:33.
[80] Bourdeau P, Bruet V, Gremillet C. Evaluation of phytosphingosine-containing shampoo and micro emulsion spray in the clinical control of allergic dermatoses in dogs: preliminary results of a multicentre study. Vet Dermatol 2007;18:177–8.
[81] DeBoer D, Schafer JH, Salsbury CS, et al. Multiple-center study of reduced-concentration triamcinolone topical solution for the treatment of dogs with known or suspected allergic pruritus. Am J Vet Res 2002;63: 408–13.
[82] Nuttall T, Mueller R, Bensignor E, et al. Efficacy of a 0.0584% hydrocortisone aceponate spray in the management of canine atopic dermatitis: a randomised, double blind, placebo-controlled trial. Vet Dermatol 2009;20:191–8.
[83] Nuttall TJ, McEwan NA, Bensignor E, et al. Comparable efficacy of a topical 0.0584% hydrocortisone aceponate spray and oral ciclosporin in treating canine atopic dermatitis. Vet Dermatol 2012;23:4.e2.
[84] Nam EH, Park SH, Jung JY, et al. Evaluation of the effect of a 0.0584 % hydrocortisone aceponate spray on clinical signs and skin barrier function in dogs with atopic dermatitis. J Vet Sci 2012;13(2):187–91.
[85] Lourenço AM, Schmidt V, São Braz B, et al. Efficacy of proactive long-term maintenance therapy of canine atopic dermatitis with 0.0584% hydrocortisone aceponate spray: a double-blind placebo controlled pilot study. Vet Dermatol 2016;27:88.e5.
[86] Bensignor E, Olivry T. Treatment of localized lesions of canine atopic dermatitis with tacrolimus ointment: a blinded, randomized, controlled trial. Vet Dermatol 2004;15:56.
[87] Marsella R, Nicklin CF, Saglio S, et al. Investigation on the clinical efficacy and safety of 0.1% tacrolimus ointment (Protopic®) in canine atopic dermatitis: A randomized, double-blinded, placebo-controlled, cross-over study. Vet Dermatol 2004;15:294–303.
[88] Steffan J, Favrot C, Mueller R. A systematic review and meta-analysis of the efficacy and safety of cyclosporin for the treatment of atopic dermatitis in dogs. Vet Dermatol 2006;17:3–16.
[89] Olivry T, Foster AP, Mueller RS, et al. Interventions for atopic dermatitis in dogs: a systematic review of randomized controlled trials. Vet Dermatol 2010;21:4–22.
[90] Olivry T, Bizikova P. A systematic review of randomized controlled trials for prevention or treatment of atopic dermatitis in dogs: 2008-2011 update. Vet Dermatol 2013;24:97.e6.
[91] Archer TM, Boothe DM, Langston VC, et al. Oral cyclosporine treatment in dogs: a review of the literature. J Vet Intern Med 2014;28:1–20.
[92] Gonzales AJ, Bowman JW, Fici GJ, et al. Oclacitinib (APOQUEL®) is a novel janus kinase inhibitor with activity against cytokines involved in allergy. J Vet Pharmcol Ther 2014;37:317–24.
[93] Collard WT, Hummel BD, Fielder AF, et al. The pharmacokinetics of oclacitinib maleate, a janus kinase inhibitor, in the dog. J Vet Pharmacol Ther 2014;37:279–85.
[94] Cosgrove SB, Wren JA, Cleaver DM, et al. A blinded, randomized, placebo-controlled trial of the efficacy and safety of the J anus kinase inhibitor oclacitinib (Apoquel®) in client-owned dogs with atopic dermatitis. Vet Dermatol 2013;24:587.
[95] Cosgrove SB, Wren JA, Cleaver DM, et al. Efficacy and safety of oclacitinib for the control of pruritus and associated skin lesions in dogs with canine allergic dermatitis. Vet Dermatol 2013;24:479.e4.
[96] Cosgrove SB, Cleaver DM, King VL, et al. Long-term compassionate use of oclacitinib in dogs with atopic and allergic skin disease: safety, efficacy and quality of life. Vet Dermatol 2015;26:171.e5.
[97] Lancellotti BA, Angus JC, Edginton HD, et al. Age- and breed-matched retrospective cohort study of malignancies and benign skin masses in 660 dogs with allergic dermatitis treated long-term with versus without oclacitinib. J Am Vet Med Assoc 2020;257:507–16.
[98] Michels GM, Ramsey DS, Walsh KF, et al. A blinded, randomized, placebo-controlled, dose determination trial of lokivetmab (ZTS-00103289), a caninized, anti-canine IL-31 monoclonal antibody in client owned dogs with atopic dermatitis. Vet Dermatol 2016;27:478.e9.
[99] Mueller R. Allergen-specific immunotherapy. In: Noli C, Foster A, Rosenkrantz W, editors. Veterinary allergy. West Sussex (UK): John Wiley and Sons; 2014. p. 85–9.
[100] Keppel KE, Campbell KL, Zuckermann FA, et al. Quantitation of canine regulatory T cell populations, serum interleukin-10 and allergen-specific IgE concentrations in healthy control dogs and canine atopic dermatitis patients receiving allergen-specific immunotherapy. Vet Immunol Immunopathol 2008;123:337–44.
[101] Popa I, Pin D, Remoué N, et al. Analysis of epidermal lipids in normal and atopic dogs, before and after administration of an oral omega-6/omega-3 fatty acid feed supplement. A pilot study. Vet Res Commun 2011;35:501.
[102] Czarnowicki T, He H, Krueger JG, et al. Atopic dermatitis endotypes and implications for targeted therapeutics. J Allergy Clin Immunol 2019;143:1–11.
[103] Cabanillas B, Brehler A, Novak N. Atopic dermatitis phenotypes and the need for personalized medicine. Curr Opin Allergy Clin Immunol 2017;17:309–15.

Urology

Advances in Small Animal Care 2 (2021) 117–129
ADVANCES IN SMALL ANIMAL CARE

Reevaluation of Prescription Strategies for Intermittent and Prolonged Renal Replacement Therapies

Cedric Dufayet, DVM[a], Larry D. Cowgill, DVM, PhD, DACVIM (SAIM)[b,*]
[a]Advanced Urinary Disease and Extracorporeal Therapies Service, University of California Veterinary Medical Center-San Diego, 10435 Sorrento Valley Road, Suite 101, San Diego, CA 92121, USA; [b]Department of Medicine and Epidemiology, University of California Veterinary Medical Center-San Diego, School of Veterinary Medicine, University of California, Davis, 2108 Tupper Hall, One Shields Avenue, Davis, CA 95616, USA

KEYWORDS
• Extracorporeal renal replacement therapy • CRRT • IHD • PIRRT

KEY POINTS

- Renal replacement therapies have become the advanced standard for the management of acute and chronic kidney failure.
- Conventional guidelines for the prescription and outcomes assessment of discontinuous therapies have become outdated, are not universally applicable across current delivery platforms and are in need of reassessment.
- Delivered urea clearance, derived from the simplified mathematical relationship between fractional patient urea clearance, and urea reduction ratio, is proposed as a unifying link to the prescription and outcome assessment of discontinuous renal replacement therapy across currently available delivery platforms and modalities.

INTRODUCTION

Extracorporeal renal replacement therapy is now acknowledged as the advanced standard of care for animals with acute and chronic kidney failure and has become increasingly available worldwide. During the past 25 years, these therapies transitioned from the exclusive purview of nephrologist and now are provided equally by nephrologists and criticalists. Dialysis equipment has expanded in veterinary therapeutics to include both intermittent and continuous platforms, and each has been exploited beyond their conventional designs to provide a broad spectrum of dialytic modalities therapeutically adapted to the requirements of animal patients [1]. Despite the evolution of these modalities of therapy, delivered on fundamentally diverse extracorporeal platforms, there has been no recent attempt to reevaluate current prescription criteria or to provide a unifying approach to prescription across these differing platforms.

Standard, catheter-based, venous dialytic techniques include intermittent hemodialysis (IHD) and intermittent hemodiafiltration and continuous renal replacement therapy (CRRT), including continuous hemodialysis, continuous hemofiltration, and continuous hemodiafiltration [1–10].

More recently, modifications of these standard IHD and CRRT therapies have emerged to better accommodate patient needs and practical constraints of veterinary therapeutics. These discontinuous therapies provided over variable ranges of time have been

No conflicts of interest.

*Corresponding author, *E-mail address:* ldcowgill@ucdavis.edu

https://doi.org/10.1016/j.yasa.2021.07.001
2666-450X/21/ © 2021 Elsevier Inc. All rights reserved.

described variously in the veterinary literature as slow low-efficiency dialysis or prolonged intermittent renal replacement therapy (PIRRT, includes H, HD, and hemodiafiltration [HDF] modalities). Other variant modalities have emerged, including dialysate-based IHD treatments in which dialysate flow (below the operational parameters of the machine) controls treatment intensity, and IHD bypass treatments in which dialysis intensity is controlled by discontinuous pulses of "no dialysis" and "dialysis" by placing the IHD machine alternatively "in" and "out" of bypass, respectively, while maintaining a variable blood flow [1–3,6,7]. Each of these various terminologies embrace an alteration of the configuration or prescription of dialysis with regard to the modality of therapy, intensity of treatment, and duration of the treatment session. Collectively, variations from traditional IHD or CRRT therapies are designated simply as "hybrid therapies" with attendant descriptors to identify the modification(s).

The necessity for veterinary IHD hybrid treatments emerged at a time when CRRT platforms were not available widely, and the existing IHD platforms had to be adapted to mimic features of CRRT by providing less intensive and more prolonged treatments. Similarly, the evolution of hybrid modalities delivered on continuous platforms arose from the constraints to provide expert staffing for continuous sessions and the requirements for a single CRRT machine to span a broader spectrum of dialytic indications [1]. Compared with standard IHD treatments, hybrid treatments are configured to provide considerably decreased intensity for urea clearances (K• t) on the order of 0.3 to 0.8 L/kg delivered over extended treatment sessions of 6 to 12 hours. Similarly, compared with standard CRRT treatments delivered continuously spanning multiple days, a hybrid treatment on a CRRT platform is delivered discontinuously over a 6- to 12-hour treatment shift on sequential days.

A veterinary renal replacement center may embrace both IHD and CRRT delivery platforms and prescribe a variety of treatment modalities on any given day. Alternatively, a center may be established with a singular platform required to provide a spectrum of therapies. Current guidelines for veterinary IHD prescriptions were derived empirically more than 30 years ago and have remained relatively unchanged [1–8]. CRRT prescription, although more contemporary, is founded on recommendations exclusive of hybrid therapies, which are more typical in veterinary therapeutics [9,10]. An updated unifying approach to the prescription and delivery of these varied modalities of therapy would facilitate the establishment of comparable treatment guidelines and benchmarks for outcomes assessments across all platforms.

Renal replacement prescription must be tailored to the unique requirements of individual patients and adapted to changing requirements on sequential dialysis sessions. The delivery platform must accommodate the size diversity of veterinary patients (from <1 to >100 kg) and simultaneously accommodate the requirements for different phases of kidney failure and differing degrees of azotemia, fluid balance, and electrolyte and acid–base dysregulation.

The foundation of blood purification by dialytic modalities is based on the capacity to transfer dysregulated or toxic solutes from the patient into the dialysate or effluent across the membrane of the extracorporeal filter. Uremia is characterized by a broad classification of retained solutes, but dialysis intensity and efficacy generally are characterized by the transfer of small solutes and prescribed in terms of the clearance of urea. In human medicine, prescription standards and guidelines for human patients are based on the fractional clearance of urea from the patient (Kt/V_{urea}) derived from formal urea kinetic modeling [11–14] and for CRRT are based on the intensity of urea clearance, defined as the normalized effluent volume (in milliliters per kilogram per hour) [14].

Both of these standards have been described for veterinary dialysis, but guidelines based on formal kinetic modeling may be less applicable or valid for veterinary patients, where acute kidney injury is the most frequent indication [14,15]. For acute kidney injury, the assumptions of the steady-state nitrogen balance, constant urea generation, and a uniform distribution volume for urea (V_{urea}) required for kinetic modeling are not likely present; nor is the analytical rigor to define these outcomes in veterinary therapeutics readily applied. Consequently, treatment intensity and efficacy outcomes have been relegated to a more indirect standard, the urea reduction ratio (URR; see Equation 1a). Although the URR is mechanistically linked to urea clearance (Box 1, Formula 1b), it oversimplifies solute transfer and ignores many of the complexities inherent with solute clearance. Despite these deficiencies and the simplicity of URR as a basis for prescribing and quantifying dialysis delivery, it is highly ingrained in veterinary therapies and likely will not be replaced by more rigorous clearance-based standards. It is the authors' intent to broaden the understanding of the inherent relationship between URR and fractional clearance (Kt/V_{urea}) across renal replacement platforms and modalities of therapy. From this understanding, we

BOX 1
Equations

$$URR = (BUN_{pre} - BUN_{post}) / BUN_{pre}; \mathrm{URR}(\%) = [(BUN_{pre} - BUN_{post}) / BUN_{pre}] \times 100 \qquad \textbf{1-a}$$

$$\frac{Kt}{Vurea} = -\ln(1 - target\ URR) \qquad \textbf{1-b}$$

$$Kd_{urea} = Q_b(BUN_{in} - BUN_{out}) / BUN_{in} \qquad \textbf{1-c}$$

propose a reprised approach to the prescription of discontinuous therapies with applicability across all currently used delivery platforms and modalities of therapy. The unifying link to prescription across these diverse modalities of therapy is the urea clearance delivered to the patient. In this article, we hope to expose the limitations of current prescription patterns and explore the practicality and rational to standardize prescriptions based on delivered clearance. To this goal, we have established a clinical strategy and prescription calculator to facilitate a uniform and cross-platform approach to the delivery of extracorporeal renal replacement therapy.

CURRENT INTERMITTENT HEMODIALYSIS AND INTERMITTENT HEMODIALYSIS HYBRID PRESCRIPTION AND DELIVERY ASSESSMENTS

The prescription intensity for IHD-based dialysis treatments for dogs and cats with acute or chronic kidney failure has been founded on URR predictions from the "total blood processed" through the hemodialyzer during a treatment session (*Qb•t*), where *Qb* is the average blood flow rate (in milliliters per minute) during the treatment, and *t* is dialysis time (in minutes) (Fig. 1). This empiric basis for prescribing IHD was founded on the direct relationship between *Qb* and urea clearance of the hemodialyzer (*Kd*) (see Box 1 Equation 1c) and the observational correlation between "total blood processed" and the intensity of the treatment as predicted by URR for specific hemodialyzers [1,3,6,8]. "Total blood processed" became the de facto operational parameter to guide dialysis prescription and delivery for a desired URR treatment outcome. The usefulness of this simple relationship was adopted widely owing to the flow dependency of clearance at low blood flow rates and the time dependency of total clearance at faster blood flow rates. At a low *Qb* used during the initial dialysis treatments for acute kidney injury, urea extraction across the dialyzer approaches 100%, and urea clearance (*Kd*) is approximately equal to Q_b and independent of hemodialyzer selection. Under these conditions, *Qb•t* becomes a reasonable surrogate for patient clearance, *Kd•t*. At the faster blood flow rates used for maintenance treatments, the relationship between *Qb* and clearance flattens, because *Kd* is influenced to a greater extent by membrane characteristics dependent on hemodialyzer selection and to a lesser extent from increasing *Qb*. Under these conditions, the relationship between *Qb•t* and the URR also flattens reflecting contributions to patient clearance owing to an increased *t* (see Fig. 1). Published URR prediction charts based on "blood processed" became widely used despite their applicability to only specific hemodialyzers and species [1,3,6,8]. As a result, practice patterns for prescribing and quantitating IHD dosing promoted little recognition or understanding of clearance beyond URR.

For hybrid therapies including IHD bypass and low-intensity IHD dialysate-based techniques, treatment prescriptions also have been based on the same total blood processed–URR outcome predictions used for more intensive treatments. For these low-intensity treatments, the blood processed projections reflect the volume of blood to be dialyzed during the "out of bypass" intervals for IHD bypass modalities or the volume of dialysate required for low-intensity dialysate-based IHD modalities, respectively. For these low-intensity treatments, the predicted blood processed is essentially equivalent to the total dialyzer clearance (*Kd•t*) and patient urea clearance during the treatment session. For IHD bypass modalities, the prescribed volume is distributed over small intervals of the treatment time (*t*) when the machine is out of bypass. It is important to distinguish this effective volume of processed blood from the total blood volume passed through the hemodialyzer during both bypass and out of bypass

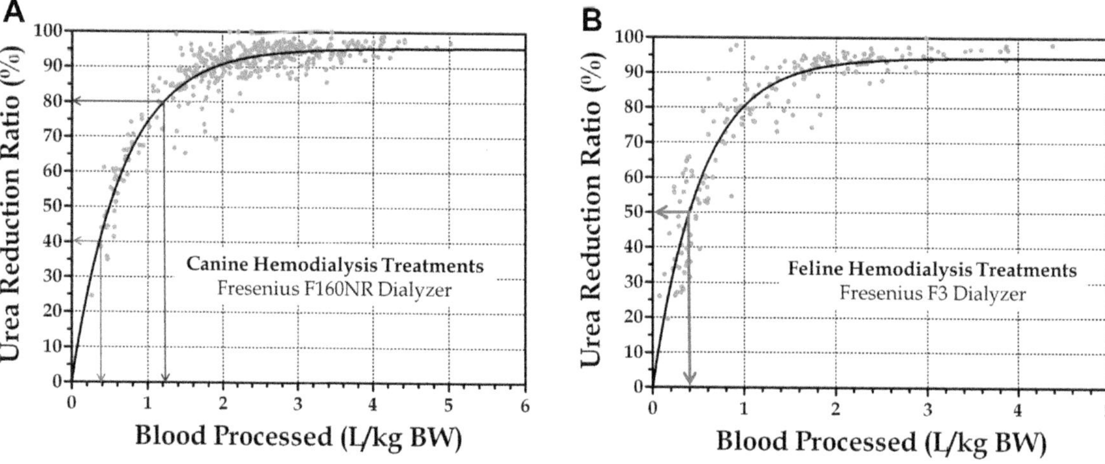

FIG. 1 IHD treatment nomograms to predict the required volume of blood to process in liters per kilogram of body weight (L/kg BW) through a Fresenius F160 NR hemodialyzer for dogs (**A**) and cats treated using a Fresenius F3 hemodialyzer (**B**) to achieve a prescribed URR outcome for a treatment session. The *arrows* illustrate the estimated volume of blood to be dialyzed ($Qb \bullet t$) to achieve specific URR outcomes of 40%, 50%, and 80%.

intervals. For low-intensity dialysate-based IHD modalities, this effective volume of blood to process (see Fig. 1), divided by the appropriate treatment time, predicts the required *Qd* for the URR outcome. Again, the actual volume of blood passing through the hemodialyzer will be many times greater than this URR predicted volume. The slow *Qd* also will be equivalent to *Kd* if it is saturated completely during transit through the hemodialyzer. As can be seen from these examples, the common prescription and outcome link through the varied modalities delivered on a IHD platform is patient clearance.

Patient urea clearance also functions as the delivery link for the prescription of hybrid therapies delivered on a CRRT platform. For a low-intensity $PIRRT_{HD}$ treatment, *Qd*, not *Qb*, controls the delivery of the desired URR for the treatment. Currently, that parameter commonly is predicted from blood processed URR nomograms derived for IHD treatments or empirically derived effluent versus URR nomograms rather than more universal predictions from the URR–clearance relationships.

A REASSESSED PARADIGM FOR DIALYSIS PRESCRIPTION AND DELIVERY

A shift from the historical paradigm of prescribing the delivery of dialysis based on the processed blood volume to a strategy based on patient clearance, would establish a more uniform and rational strategy for prescribing renal replacement treatment applicable to either IHD or CRRT platforms. For a unifying strategy, the URR likely would remain the outcome measure of treatment efficacy, given its conceptional simplicity and deep roots in veterinary dialysis. However, the fractional clearance of urea (Kt/V_{urea}) over the session would define the delivery of therapy necessary to achieve the prescribed URR outcome.

For example, consider a hybrid prescription for a cat with an historical weight of 4.6 kg presented for dialysis with a blood urea nitrogen of 285 mg/dL (102 mmol/L) and current weight of 4.9 kg. For the first hybrid treatment, a URR treatment outcome of 50% over an 8-hour treatment session is elected with a plan to remove approximately 7 mL/kg/h of fluid to resolve the fluid burden. From the relationship between URR and Kt/V_{urea} (see Box 1, Equation 1b; Fig. 2), it is necessary to clear 70% of the urea burden from the cat ($Kt/V_{urea} = 0.7$) to achieve the 50% URR outcome for the treatment. Predicting the urea distribution volume, *V*, is approximately 65% of the cat's body weight owing to the 300 g weight gain; the urea volume of the cat is 3185 mL (4.9 kg × 0.65 × 1000 mL/kg), and the treatment requires approximately 2208 mL (3185 mL × 0.7) of total clearance ($Kd \bullet t$) or 276 mL of clearance per hour of treatment. Because ultrafiltration for the fluid removal contributes 35 mL/h (7 mL/kg/h) of clearance to the treatment goal, an additional 240 mL/h of diffusive and/or convective clearance is required to achieve the outcome URR. This component of the treatment

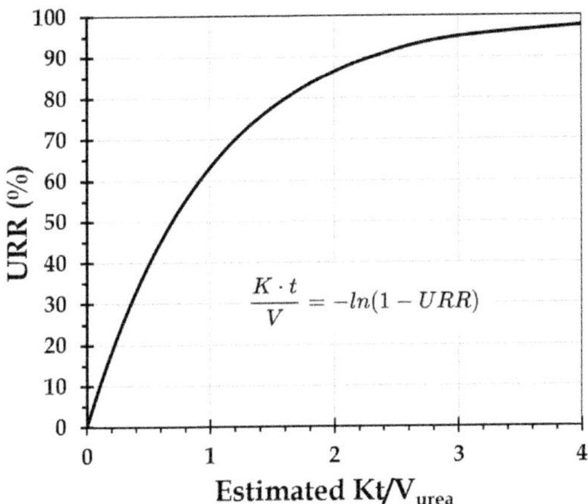

FIG. 2 Graphical nomogram relating the URR and fractional clearance of urea (Kt/V_{urea}) estimated from the simplified single pool kinetic modeling of urea removal (Equation 1b, insert) in the absence of urea generation, G, and changes in the urea distribution volume, V.

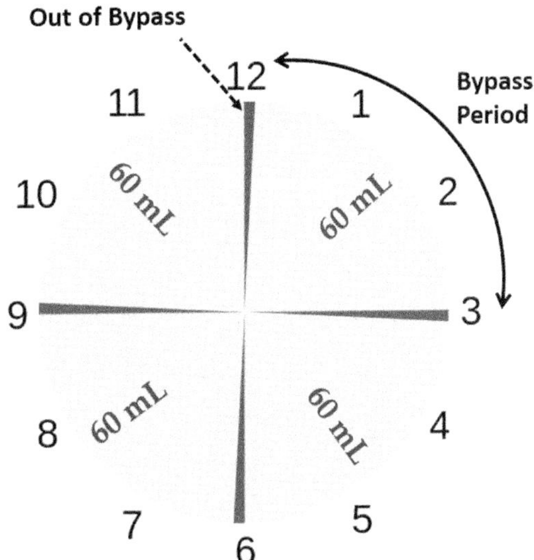

FIG. 3 Schematic representation of the IHD bypass modality to deliver low-intensity treatments on an IHD hemodialysis platform. The illustration depicts an hour of treatment performed with a Fresenius F3 hemodialyzer. At the beginning of the hour, the delivery system briefly is "taken out of bypass" mode (*red area*) to establish 30 to 40 seconds of dialysate flow sufficient to refresh the dialysate compartment of the hemodialyzer with the blood pump temporarily stopped. When the delivery system is placed into bypass mode (*yellow area*), the refreshed dialysate is entrapped in the dialyzer as the blood flow is reestablished. For the Fresenius F3 hemodialyzer, the dialysate compartment contains 60 mL of dialysate, which becomes progressively saturated with urea during 10 to 15 minutes of bypass, establishing 60 mL of blood clearance. When this process is repeated at 15-minute intervals the process delivers 240 mL/h of diffusive clearance. If a greater hourly clearance is required, brief periods (2–5 minutes) of dialysis at a reduced *Qb* can be delivered between the bypass intervals.

could be delivered by any hybrid method over the 8-hour session (t = 480 minutes) by providing 4 mL/min (1928 mL/480 min) or 240 mL/h of clearance as an appropriate treatment intensity for this degree of azotemia. This predicted clearance is essentially the same as the 4.2 mL/min (249 mL/h) *Qb* predicted from Fig. 1B for the Fresenius F3 hemodialyzer, but was derived independent of empirical nomograms as a direct clearance projection applicable universally on any delivery platform.

Procedurally, the treatment could be delivered using an IHD bypass modality with a Fresenius F3 hemodialyzer and a *Qb* of greater than 30 mL/min (Fig. 3) simply by stopping the blood pump and taking the machine out of bypass for 30 to 60 seconds to refresh the dialysate compartment, and then placing the machine back in bypass and restarting the blood pump. The F3 hemodialyzer provides approximately 60 mL of clearance as the dialysate compartment containing approximately 60 mL of new dialysate at the start of the interval reequilibrates with plasma water during the bypass period. When the procedure is repeated every 15 minutes, it provides the 240 mL of hourly clearance, and the prescribed 1920 mL of diffusive clearance would be delivered in an 8-hour session. The convective component of the treatment for the fluid removal would be prescribed independently at 35 mL/h. The urea profile for a treatment of this intensity is illustrated by the graph depicted in Fig. 4 (see Prescribing Tool, elsewhere in this article).

For a low-intensity $PIRRT_{HD}$ treatment on either an IHD platform (using an external dialysate controller) or on a CRRT platform, the treatment is achieved simply by setting *Qd* to 4 mL/min (240 mL/h) for the duration of the 8-hour treatment and prescribing ultrafiltration at 35 mL/h. On a CRRT platform, the treatment alternatively could be delivered by a purely convective prescription of 240 mL/h of postfilter replacement fluid, or any desired combination of convection and diffusion providing 240 mL/h of saturated effluent flow in addition to the 35 mL/h of ultrafiltration for a total effluent flow of 275 mL/h.

For treatments on a CRRT platform or low-intensity IHD dialysate-based treatments, it generally is accepted

PIRRT Calculator

Patient	72-29-35 Prince
Date	
BW (kg)	4.9
Estimated V (%)	65
V (ml)	3185
Starting BUN (mg/dL)	285
PCV (%)	33

Treatment URR target (%):	50%	Time (hours)	8
KT/V_{urea}	0.69	*Kt* (mL)	2208
		K (mL/h)	276

	Hour 1	Hour 2	Hour 3	Hour 4	Hour 5	Hour 6	Hour 7	Hour 8	
Prescription									
Qb (mL/min)	65	65	65	65	65	65	65	65	
Qd (mL/hr)	240	240	240	240	240	240	240	240	
Qd (mL/min)	4.0	4.0	4.0	4.0	4.0	4.0	4.0	4.0	
Qrep pre (mL/h)	0	0	0	0	0	0	0	0	
Qrep pre (mL/min)	0.0	0.0	0.0	0.0	0.0	0.0	0.0	0.0	
Qrep post (mL/h)	0	0	0	0	0	0	0	0	
Qrep post (mL/min)	0.0	0.0	0.0	0.0	0.0	0.0	0.0	0.0	
Qpfr (mL/h)	35	35	35	35	35	35	35	35	
Qpfr(mL/min)	0.6	0.6	0.6	0.6	0.6	0.6	0.6	0.6	
Qeff (mL/h)	275	275	275	275	275	275	275	275	
Saturation ratio (%)	100%	100%	100%	100%	100%	100%	100%	100%	
Caculated values									
Filtration fraction	1%	1%	1%	1%	1%	1%	1%	1%	
Qb/Qd	16.3	16.3	16.3	16.3	16.3	16.3	16.3	16.3	
PFR Rate (mL/kg/h)	7.1	7.1	7.1	7.1	7.1	7.1	7.1	7.1	
Volume of distribution	3150	3115	3080	3045	3010	2975	2940	2905	
Calc.clearance (mL/h)	275	275	275	275	275	275	275	275	
Calc. Clearance (mL/min)	4.6	4.6	4.6	4.6	4.6	4.6	4.6	4.6	
							Total Effluent	2200.0	
Treatment Time (min)	0	60	120	180	240	300	360	420	480
Predicted BUN	285	261	240	219	201	183	167	153	139
%hourly URR	8%	8%	8%	9%	9%	9%	9%	9%	9%
Overall URR	0%	8%	16%	23%	30%	36%	41%	46%	51%

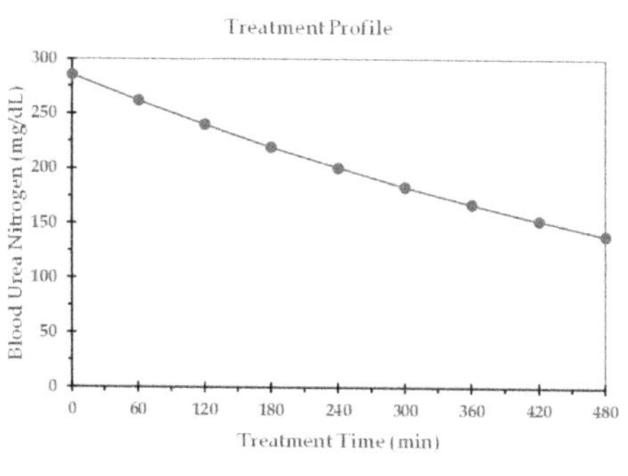

FIG. 4 Illustration of a prescription tool developed to generate clearance delivery targets (Kt/V, Kt, and K) from prescription inputs to achieve a defined URR outcome goal. The example demonstrates prediction of the hourly clearance required for a 50% URR outcome in a 4.9 kg patient requiring 300 mL of ultrafiltration over an 8-hour $PIRRT_{HD}$ session (see text). The prescription could be delivered on a CRRT platform or as a low-intensity IHD dialysate–based treatment. The calculator also plots the expected treatment profile. Box 2 provides the formulas for the treatment projections.

that 1 mL of effluent or dialysate is equivalent to 1 mL of clearance. This concept is true if the effluent (or dialysate) is fully saturated, meaning the urea concentration of the dialysate or effluent are the same as the inlet blood water concentration. This assumption may not hold when delivering more intensive treatments over shorter treatment times and higher *Qd* prescriptions (Fig. 5). Effluent (and dialysate) typically is considered saturated if *Qb* is at least 3 times faster than *Qd*, but this generalization does not consider dialyzer size or membrane performance and may not be valid universally.

As illustrated in Fig. 5, at a *Qb* of 100 mL/min using a Prismaflex HF20 blood set, the effluent will become undersaturated when the *Qd* exceeds 1.5 L/h, even at a Qb/Qd ratio of greater than 3. To ensure greater accuracy in the delivery of PIRRT treatments, it is important to consider the concept of saturation ratio, the ratio between effluent (or dialysate) and inlet urea concentrations. When the saturation ratio is less than 100%, the effluent flow will not equal the *Kd*, but the effective *Kd* can be estimated as the product of effluent flow and saturation ratio.

Prescribing standard or hybrid treatments based on delivered clearance permits the formulation of treatment parameters independent of patient size, degree of azotemia, available platform, and duration of the treatment session. It fosters a consistent understanding of treatment prescription and delivery across distinctly different delivery platforms, which otherwise can be confusing.

THERAPEUTIC AND PRESCRIPTION PRESUMPTIONS

The URR is likely to remain the prescription and outcome standard for veterinary dialysis for the foreseeable future, based on current treatment indications and the inherent difficulties to validate more rigorous outcome standards in animal patients. Prescribing and delivering treatment based on fractional clearance using simplified assumptions for the estimation of Kt/V_{urea} (see Fig. 2; Equation 1b) may differ from its more rigorous estimation by formal urea kinetic modeling. Formally modeled Kt/V_{urea} more accurately predicts the required and delivered fractional clearance by consideration of nutritional intake and catabolic status of the patient, urea distribution, compartmentation, and sequestration, fluid removal, filter kinetics, residual kidney function, and access flow [16–21]. Failure to consider the influence of these variables in the

BOX 2
PIRRT Calculator Formulas

$$V(mL) = BW(kg) * \%Vd * 1000$$

$$\frac{Kt}{Vurea} = -\ln(1 - target\ URR)$$

$$\mathrm{Kt} = \frac{Kt}{V} * \mathrm{V}$$

$$\mathrm{Qeff} = \mathrm{Qd+Qreppre+Qreppost+Qpfr}$$

$$\mathrm{FF} = \frac{(Qd+Qreppre+Qreppost+Qpfr)}{Qreppre+Qb\left(\frac{1-PCV}{100}\right)}$$

$$\text{PFR rate} = \frac{Qpfr}{BW}$$

$$\text{Calculated clearance } K = SR * \frac{Qeff}{1+\frac{Qreppre}{Qb}}$$

$$\mathrm{URR} = 1 - e^{-\frac{Kt}{V}}$$

formulation of the treatment can result in substantial deviations from expected outcomes [17–21]. Exaggerated urea appearance from excessive dietary intake or a high nitrogen turnover in catabolic patients causes an apparent undertreatment and a higher than expected URR outcome. The urea distribution volume (V) is not quantitated readily by clinical assessment, and inaccurate estimates of hydration, lean body mass, or fat mass can cause the underestimation or overestimation of the V and corresponding undertreatment and overtreatment prediction by URR. Similarly, overestimates of Kd owing to inaccurate Qb measurements, clotting of the filter, access recirculation, or incomplete dialysate or effluent saturation can overpredict actual

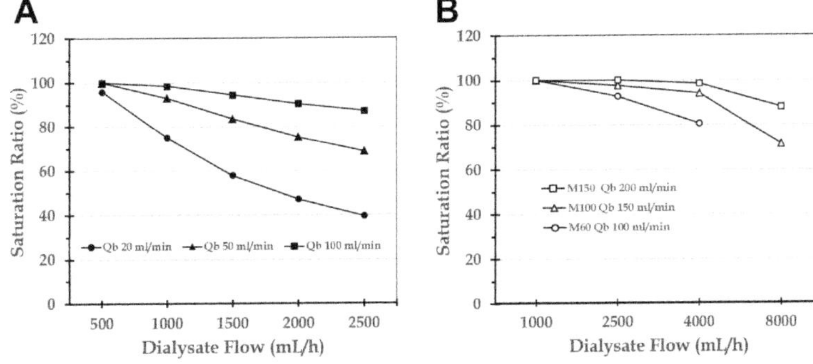

FIG. 5 Influence of dialysate and blood flow rates on effluent saturation ratio. Saturation ratios are calculated from manufacturer's clearance estimations for the Baxter HF20Set (**A**) during continuous hemodialysis treatments at blood flow rates (Qb) of 20, 50, and 100 mL/min and (**B**) the Baxter M150, M100, and M60 Sets at blood flow rates of 200 mL/min, 150 mL/min, and 100 mL/min, respectively. Note that significant effluent undersaturation is possible with small hemofilters and Qb/Qd ratios of less than 3.

delivery of the treatment. Any influences affecting the true treatment delivery can be expected to alter actual outcome from projected outcome.

The application of the *URR* versus Kt/V_{urea} relationship to establish clearance delivery targets ignores many important assumptions incorporated into Kt/V_{urea} quantitation by formal urea kinetic modeling. However, the relationship is sufficiently robust to direct the prescription of therapies that are inherently subject to clinical and treatment variables that positively or negatively bias treatment outcomes. Clearance targets stand on more theoretic validity across all delivery platforms than conventional prescriptions formulated from the URR normograms derived for specific treatment platforms and specific hemodialyzers with their own inherent variance (see Fig. 1).

The precise estimation of the Kt/V_{urea} requires documentation of residual renal clearance (*Kr*); ultrafiltration volume; dialysis time (*t*); measurement of pretreatment, post-treatment, and the subsequent pretreatment urea concentrations; average clearance of the filter (*Kd*); *Qb*; *Qd*; and iterative estimation of urea appearance (*G*) and urea distribution volume (*V*) for a treatment session [7,12,17–20]. For practical and economic considerations, this degree of precision is not likely to direct veterinary dialysis. The precision of URR outcomes from the delivery prescriptions based on Kt_{urea} will be dictated by the same clinical uncertainties that influence all dialysis outcome analyses. Parameters determined with reasonable certainty include only *Qd* and *t*. All other determinants of treatment outcome are subject to variable errors of clinical assessment or cannot be assessed directly.

Residual urea clearance, *Kr*, rarely is assessed in animal patients undergoing acute or maintenance dialysis and typically is considered negligible over the treatment session. However, even low rates of *Kr* can contribute to total session clearance and promote a lower than predicted post-treatment urea concentration and increased URR [12,13].

Similar to *Kr*, filter clearance, *Kd*, rarely is measured. Most commonly, *Kd* is overestimated owing to filter clotting, inaccurate *Qb* measurements, access recirculation, periods of dialysate bypass, or excessive periods of pump stoppage owing to poor access performance. The overestimation of *Kd* results in less treatment than prescribed and a lower URR outcome than predicted [18,20]. During IHD bypass treatments, total patient clearance may be underestimated significantly if the clearance produced by dialysate equilibration during bypass intervals is ignored. Patient clearance will be increased from the prescribed clearance, and URR will be greater than prescribed for the session. Ionic dialysance can help to predict real-time *Kd* and unexpected decreases owing to clotting, access recirculation, or blood flow inaccuracies [22–25].

Dialysis time, *t*, can be overestimated if the session time or clock time is used to deliver the treatment rather than actual treatment time. Discrepancies between session time and treatment time occur if the session is burdened with excessive alarm conditions during which treatment does not occur, or during prolonged or continuous treatments if the patient is disconnected temporarily for procedural necessities. These situations promote underdialysis from decreased delivered clearance and lower URR outcomes.

URR outcomes can deviate from prescribed projections owing to errors in post-treatment blood sampling. A delay in post-treatment sampling by even several minutes causes an increase in the urea concentration from rebound compared with samples taken immediately after treatment [20]. A 5% to 25% increase in the urea concentration owing to delayed sampling would cause a corresponding decrease in the session URR and a seemingly inadequate treatment. In contrast, dilution of the post-treatment sample by access recirculation would decrease the measured urea concentration and artificially increase the measured URR for the session [20].

Urea distribution volume, *V*, and urea appearance, *G*, directly influence urea kinetics and patient clearance for all modalities of renal replacement, but cannot be measured directly or predicted accurately by clinical assessment. Estimates of *V* and *G* are derived by iterative calculation using urea kinetic modeling to compute Kt/V_{urea} [12,18,20,25]. Simplified algorithms to estimate the Kt/V_{urea} incorporating adjustment of the *V* owing to ultrafiltration during the treatment, and estimates of *G* have been derived for human patients but have not been explored or validated in animals [17,26,27]. Until these compensations have been defined, and in the absence of formal urea kinetic modeling, Equation 1b provides a reasonable surrogate for the prescribed intensity (*Kt*) and efficacy (Kt/V_{urea}) of the delivered therapy to meet URR goals for individual treatments.

When formulating a clearance-based prescription, consideration should be given to the variable influences of the *G* and *V* and the caveats for the other influences, as described elsewhere in this article, to better match the clearance requirements to the patient's clinical state.

For normally hydrated animal patients, the *V* generally is estimated as 60% (53%–66%) of body weight; however, V changes according to hydration status and directly influences both the required and delivered patient clearance [28]. In an overhydrated patient, the V is predictably more than 60% of the body weight. The prescription should be adjusted for a greater estimate of V to provide greater patient clearance, Kt, than predicted for normal hydration and body condition. Because the fluid burden is corrected with ultrafiltration, fractional clearance may increase, leading to a higher than predicted URR outcome. Obese patients have a relatively lower V as a percentage of body weight, and may have greater URR outcomes when the V is estimated for a normal body composition.

Urea appearance rate (G) from hepatic urea generation generally is ignored in both the prescription and outcomes assessment of renal replacement therapies in animals.

The extremes of urea generation and nitrogen balance significantly influence URR outcomes, and should be considered when formulating the prescription. Infectious or inflammatory causes or comorbidities associated with kidney injury generally cause a catabolic state and increased urea appearance rate that increase the requirement for delivered clearance and URR outcome. Urea appearance also increases as patients are provided enteral or parenteral nutrition. Increases in the blood urea nitrogen by more than 25 mg/dL/d between renal replacement sessions suggest a hypercatabolic state that may require the prescription of increased patient clearance.

REPRISED UREA REDUCTION RATIO APPROACH AND PROLONGED INTERMITTENT RENAL REPLACEMENT THERAPY CALCULATOR TO DELIVER RENAL REPLACEMENT BY FRACTIONAL UREA CLEARANCE

With the increased application of renal replacement therapy in veterinary medicine over the past 25 years, it is timely to reassess prescription strategies to provide a unifying approach applicable across all conventional platforms and modalities of delivery. The vast majority of renal replacement treatments are provided discontinuously rather than as continuous modalities, so we have limited this discussion to discontinuous therapies. Despite its inherent shortcomings, we also have reprised URR as the operative outcome parameter, owing to its simplicity and engrained foothold in veterinary medicine. However, conventional URR prescriptions based on "processed blood volume" nomograms are not universal to all dialysis modalities and should be respectfully retired [3,6–8]. In its place the fractional urea clearance (Kt/V_{urea}) is proposed as a prescription delivery target, as it is universally applicable to all renal replacement platforms and modalities of therapy. It has been validated as the standard of therapy for human patients and has a practical mathematical relationship to URR (see Fig. 2). [11–14,18,21]. This kinetic relationship provides an opportunity to maintain the current URR heritage while embracing patient clearance as a more appropriate operational parameter to prescribe and deliver renal replacement therapies.

We propose an approach and calculating tool to facilitate a transition for the operational delivery of renal replacement therapies (see Fig. 4). The calculating tool provides opportunity to perform "what if" manipulations of URR, URR/h, t, Qb, Qd, UF, effluent saturation, filtration fraction, prefilter versus postfilter replacement, and Qb/Qd ratio to establish treatment parameters appropriate across platforms and modalities. Therapy delivered on the basis of clearance is logical and imposes less confusion when confronting differing platforms and modalities of therapy. Without the calculating tool, the prescription requirements can be configured from a simple strategic approach.

Step 1: From the patient weight and clinical estimate of hydration status, V is estimated as a percentage of the patient weight subject to the caveats and uncertainties as discussed elsewhere in this article. A value of 60% of body weight can be used for euhydrated patients, and proportionate adjustments used for dehydrated (50%–59% of body weight) or overhydrated (61% to $\geq$70% of body weight) patients as predicted from historical weight or clinical judgment.

Step 2: The desired URR outcome and appropriate treatment time (t) are determined to define the treatment goals for the patient during the session.

Step 3: The operational Kt/V_{urea} for the selected URR outcome for the treatment (Step 2) is determined from Equation 1b (see Fig. 2), or the calculating tool. From the operational Kt/V_{urea}, the required patient clearance (Kt) is determined by multiplying the unitless Kt/V_{urea} value by the estimated V determined in Step 1.

Step 4: Dividing the total patient clearance (Kt) by time (t) provides the hourly clearance required to establish the treatment goals by hemodialysis, hemofiltration, or hemodiafiltration independent of the treatment platform (IHD, $PIRRT_{HD}$, IHD-bypass, or low-intensity IHD dialysate-based modalities on an IHD platform; or $PIRRT_{H}$, $PIRRT_{HD}$, or $PIRRT_{HDF}$ using hemofiltration, hemodialysis, or hemodiafiltration on a CRRT platform, respectively).

For treatment modalities delivered on an IHD platform, the hourly treatment goals are delivered as follows.

Standard or $PIRRT_{HD}$

The hourly and session urea clearance goals are delivered by the selection of the hemodialyzer and the prescribed *Qb*. Establishing the appropriate *Qb* requires some understanding of the performance characteristics of the selected hemodialyzer. Its instantaneous urea clearance, *Kd* (mL/min), at typical dialysate flow rates of more than 300 mL/min, is predicted by *Qb* times the extraction ratio at the selected *Qb*. For nearly all hemodialyzers, at a *Qb* less than 50 mL/min, the extraction ratio approaches 100% and the *Kd* is approximately equal to the *Qb*. The prescribed hourly clearance equals the *Qb* (mL/min) times 60 minutes. At faster blood flow rates, the *Kd* increases exponentially, and the instantaneous *Kd* and hourly clearance must be predicted from its mass transfer area coefficient (KoA), historical or real-time measurements of *Kd* or ionic dialysance at the selected Qb, or manufacturer's references. If the initially prescribed hourly clearance cannot be delivered owing to limitations of access flow or performance of the hemodialyzer, the clearance goals for the session can only be achieved by extension of the treatment time, such that the product of *Kd* and session time (*t*) matches the prescribed patient clearance goal (*Kt*).

IHD bypass modality

The IHD bypass technique was conceived to enable the delivery of a very slow, low-efficiency treatment, especially in small patients on an IHD platform ill-designed to deliver such therapies. The strategy is to provide small discontinuous intervals of diffusive clearance within the platform's capabilities of *Qb* and *Qd* followed by prolonged intervals of no clearance while maintaining the *Qb* as fast as possible to prevent clotting in the extracorporeal circuit. Cumulatively, over the session, these intervals of clearance sum to achieve the prescribed patient clearance goal (*Kt*). The diffusive clearance is interrupted by placing the IHD platform in bypass to stop delivery of dialysate to the hemodialyzer. To deliver the treatment, the desired hourly URR is divided into the URR goal to determine the required session time in hours. For example, a 50% URR treatment goal providing 6% URR per hour would require an 8-hour treatment. The hourly clearance is determined next by dividing the calculated session clearance goal (*Kt*)by the treatment time (see Fig. 4). Because the *Kd* will be very low for these treatments, one component of the hourly clearance is determined by the product of *Qb* (mL/min) and the number of minutes the system is out of bypass. However, during bypass, there is additional clearance equivalent to the volume of the refreshed dialysate contained in the hemodialyzer during the bypass interval, as this fluid equilibrates with flowing blood. This component of clearance must be configured into the total hourly clearance to prevent overtreatment of the patient. Fig. 3 illustrates the IHD bypass method providing 240 mL of hourly diffusive clearance (4 mL/min) delivered during bypass alone. Equilibration of the refreshed dialysate during bypass contributes 1900 mL of cumulative clearance as a component of the total 2208 mL of clearance required for a 4.9 kg patient over an 8-hour session (see example in Fig. 4). In this example, the equilibrating static dialysate provides the entire diffusive clearance while the system is in bypass. There is no requirement to provide additional clearance out of bypass. Ultrafiltration for fluid removal provides the small additional component to the total clearance. This prescription will deliver the 0.7 Kt/V_{urea} required to achieve the 50% URR outcome for the treatment. As discussed elsewhere in this article, the prescription can be delivered simply by equilibrating the 60 mL of dialysate retained in the hemodialyzer (Fresenius F3) during the bypass intervals to achieve 60 mL of clearance. Repeating this procedure every 15 minutes for the 8-hour session provides both the required hourly and cumulative session clearances, respectively, while maintaining the *Qb* within machine capabilities sufficient to prevent clotting in the circuit. If a greater hourly clearance is required, brief periods (2–5 minutes) of dialysis at a decreased *Qb* can be delivered between the intervals bypass.

Low-intensity IHD dialysate–based modalities

This hybrid technique also was conceived to enable the delivery of a very slow, low-efficiency diffusive treatment to small patients on an IHD platform. Much like on a CRRT platform, dialysis intensity is controlled by delivering a very slow *Qd* rather than a slow *Qb*. At *Qb*/*Qd* ratios of greater than 3, the dialysate approaches 100% saturation, and the *Kd* will be equivalent to the *Qd*. The treatment is delivered simply by providing a dialysate flow equal to the prescribed hourly clearance at a *Qb* at least 3 times this flow. IHD platforms are not designed to deliver dialysate at such slow flows, so an external pump can be configured to divert a small portion of the bulk dialysate flow to the hemodialyzer at the desired rate (Fig. 6).

The configuration and delivery of hybrid treatments based on clearance are more intuitive on CRRT platforms, because the components of the effluent volume are more predictably equivalent to clearance.

Prolonged Intermittent Renal Replacement Therapy with Hemofiltration

For purely convective modalities, the total clearance required for a given URR outcome is determined by setting the effluent rate (*Qeff*) to the required hourly clearance (postfilter replacement) or to the adjusted effluent rate to accommodate dilution from prefilter replacement and/or net ultrafiltration. The delivery of these effluent rates must be prescribed with consideration of the obtainable *Qb* and appropriate filtration fraction.

Prolonged Intermittent Renal Replacement Therapy with Hemodialysis

A purely diffusive treatment on a CRRT platform is analogous to a low intensity IHD-dialysate-based modality, as described elsewhere in this article. Typically, the *Qd* will be sufficiently slow to promote a *Qb/Qd* ratio of greater than 3 to provide saturation of the effluent. Under these conditions, the *Qd* will approximate the prescribed hourly clearance. The *Qd* should be decreased by the rate of ultrafiltration for net fluid removal to prevent an increased treatment intensity and excessive URR outcome.

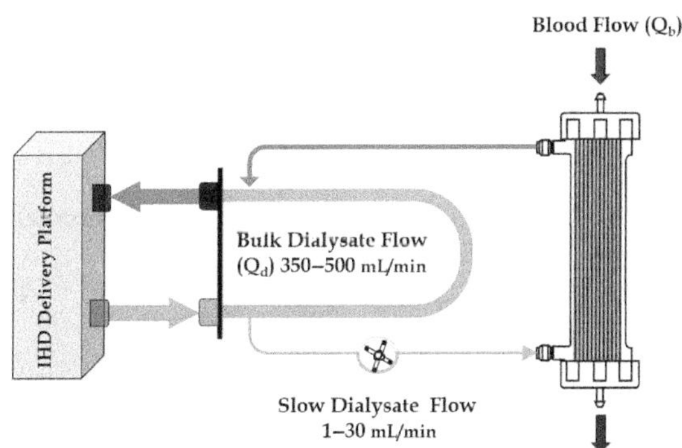

FIG. 6 Schematic illustration of a low-intensity IHD dialysate–based circuit designed for use on a conventional IHD platform. The bulk dialysate flow from the IHD platform circulates in a loop, and a variable slow flow is diverted by an external pump and delivered to the hemodialyzer. The equilibrated dialysate (including any ultrafiltration) is returned to the bulk dialysate stream. The slow dialysate flow controls the intensity of the treatment and generally is equivalent to Kd_{urea}. This configuration does not require modification to the IHD platform and does not interfere with any of the monitoring alarm or systems functions of the platform. (*Courtesy of* Dr. LD Cowgill.)

Prolonged Intermittent Renal Replacement Therapy with Hemodiafiltration

For this modality, clearance is provided by both diffusion and convection, and the required patient clearance can be achieved by variable distribution of among these modalities. Once the total (*Kt*) and hourly clearances are determined the different combinations of filtration, diffusion, and ultrafiltration, can be configured to determine the best combination to maximize effluent saturation, Qb/Qd ratio, filtration fraction, prefilter versus postfilter replacement, and fluid removal. Commonly, the distribution is arbitrarily set to 50% diffusion and 50% convection, in which the *Qd* and *Qrep* would each contribute one-half of the hourly clearance, presuming conditions permitting complete effluent saturation prevail (see Fig. 5).

SUMMARY

As veterinary renal replacement therapy completes its first 50 years of inception, establishment, and evolution, it is opportune to reflect on its impact to advanced veterinary therapeutics. It is also opportune to look to our past and current guidelines for the delivery of these therapies to assess their future applicability and relevance. We have exploited the mechanistic relationship between the URR and the fractional urea clearance of the patient (Kt/V_{urea}) in an attempt to provide greater uniformity of understanding dialysis across the diversity of platforms for its delivery. From this understanding we propose reevaluating the approach to the prescription of standard and hybrid extracorporeal therapies with applicability across the current modalities of therapy.

CLINICS CARE POINTS

- Prescribing dialysis intensity and outcomes based on "blood processed" nomograms provides a highly generalized and indirect estimate of the required clearance for a delivered URR outcome, but such nomograms are specific to a targeted filter, blood flow rates, species, IHD modality, and solutes and should not be generalized to therapeutic conditions beyond their defined characteristics.

- Blood processed nomograms to predict URR outcomes predict clearance only at relatively slow blood flow rates and low URR goals when the extraction ratio for urea approximates 100%. At progressively faster blood flow rates and progressively higher URR outcome goals, the predicted blood volume to process is more significantly influenced by treatment time as blood flow rate (*Qb*) becomes limiting.
- The *Kt/V* versus URR relationship (see Box 1, Equation 1b) proposed to prescribe dialysis treatment intensity and delivered URR outcome also generalizes this complex relationship and oversimplifies the influences of urea distribution volume, generation rate, compartmentation, and treatment schedule, among other clinical factors.
- The *Kt/V* versus URR relationship (see Box 1, Equation 1b) proposed to prescribe dialysis treatment intensity and delivered URR outcome promotes a reasonably simplified yet generalizable approach for dose prescription and outcomes monitoring of discontinuous renal replacement therapies within the inherent clinical and technical variabilities of these therapies.
- The treatment session clearance estimated from the Kt/V versus URR relationship (see Box 1, Equation 1b) can be delivered by variable combinations of diffusive or convective modalities independent of the delivery platform.
- Clinical estimates of urea distribution volume based on hydration status and body composition and predictions of the catabolic status of the patient should be incorporated into dose prescription for discontinuous renal replacement treatments.
- For bypass-based hybrid treatments, the clearance provided during the bypass intervals must be included in the prescription of the total clearance provided to the patient during the treatment session.

REFERENCES

[1] Cowgill LD, Guillaumin JJ. Extracorporeal renal replacement therapy and blood purification in critical care. J Vet Emerg Crit Care 2013;23:194–204.

[2] Cowgill LD, Langston CE. History of hemodialysis in dog and other companion animals. In: Ing TS, Rahman MA, Kjellstrand CM, editors. Dialysis: history, development and promise. Singapore: World Scientific Publishing Co. Pte. Ltd; 2012. p. 901–13.

[3] Cowgill LD, Francey T. Hemodialysis and extracorporeal blood purification. In: DiBartola SP, editor. Fluid, electrolyte, and acid-base disorders in small animal practice. 4th edition. St. Louis: Elsevier (Saunders); 2012. p. 680–712.

[4] Cowgill LD, Langston CE. Role of hemodialysis in the management of dogs and cats with renal failure. Vet Clin North Am Small Anim Pract 1996;26:1347–78.

[5] Langston CE, Cowgill LD, Spano JA. Intermittent hemodialysis for small animals. J Vet Intern Med 1997;11: 348–55.

[6] Cowgill LD, Francey T. Hemodialysis. In: DiBartola SP, editor. Fluid, electrolyte, and acid-base disorders in small animal practice. Philadelphia: Saunders/Elsevier; 2006. p. 650–77.

[7] Cowgill LD. Urea kinetics and intermittent dialysis prescription in small animals. Vet Clin North Am Small Anim Pract 2011;41:193–225.

[8] Langston C. Hemodialysis. In: Bartges J, Polzin DJ, editors. Nephrology and urology of small animals. Oxford: Wiley-Blackwell; 2011. p. 255–85.

[9] Acierno MJ. Extracorporeal renal replacement therapy and blood purification in critical care. Vet Clin North Am Small Anim Pract 2011;41:135–46.

[10] Acierno MJ. Continuous renal replacement therapy. In: Bartges J, Polzin DJ, editors. Nephrology and urology of small animals. Oxford: Wiley-Blackwell; 2011. p. 286–92.

[11] Lowrie EG, Laird NM, Parker TF, et al. Effect of the hemodialysis prescription of patient morbidity: report from the National Cooperative Dialysis Study. N Engl J Med 1981;305(20):1176–81.

[12] Gotch FA, Sargent JA. A mechanistic analysis of the National Cooperative Dialysis Study (NCDS). Kidney Int 1985;28:526–34.

[13] National Kidney Foundation. KDOQI clinical practice guideline for hemodialysis adequacy: 2015 update. Am J Kidney Dis 2015;66(5):884–930.

[14] Kidney Disease Improving Global Outcomes (KDIGO). Acute kidney injury work group. KDIGO clinical practice guideline for acute kidney injury. Kidney Int Suppl 2012; 2:1–138.

[15] Liang KV, Zhang JH, Palevsky PM. Urea reduction ratio may be a simpler approach for measurement of adequacy of intermittent hemodialysis in acute kidney injury. BMC Nephrol 2019;20(1):82.

[16] Lowrie EG, Sargent JA. Clinical example of pharmacokinetic and metabolic modeling: quantitative and individualized prescription of dialysis therapy. National Cooperative Dialysis Study. Kidney Int Suppl 1980;10: S11–6.

[17] Daugirdas JT. Simplified equations for monitoring Kt/V, PCRn, eKt/V, andePCRn. Adv Ren Replace Ther 1995;2: 295–304.

[18] Depner TA. Prescribing hemodialysis: a guide to urea modeling. Boston: Kluwer Academic Publishers; 1991.

[19] Coyne DW, Delmez J, Spence G, et al. Impaired delivery of hemodialysis prescriptions: an analysis of causes and an approach to evaluation. J Am Soc Nephrol 1997;8: 1315–8.

[20] Yeun JY, Depner TA. Complications related to inadequate delivered dose: recognition and management in

acute and chronic dialysis. In: Lameire N, Mehta RL, editors. Complications of dialysis. New York: Marcel Dekker, Inc; 2000. p. 89–115.

[21] Ding L, Johnston J, Pinsk MN. Monitoring dialysis adequacy: history and current practice. Pediatr Nephrol 2021. https://doi.org/10.1007/s00467-020-04816-9.

[22] Aslam S, Subodh J, Moro S, et al. Online measurement of hemodialysis adequacy using effective ionic dialysance of sodium-a review of its principles, applications, benefits, and risks. Hemodial Int 2018;22(4):425–34.

[23] Petitclerc T, Ridel C. Routine online assessment of dialysis dose: ionic dialysance or UV-absorbance monitoring? Semin Dial 2021;34(2):116–22.

[24] Mercadal L, Ridel C, Petitclerc T. Ionic dialysance: principle and review of its clinical relevance for quantification of hemodialysis efficiency. Hemodial Int 2005;9(2):111–9.

[25] Daugirdas JT, Depner TA, Greene T, et al. Solute-solver: a web-based tool for modeling urea kinetics for a broad range of hemodialysis schedules in multiple patients. Am J Kidney Dis 2009;54(5):798–809.

[26] Daugirdas JT, Leypoldt JK, Akonur A, et al. Improved equation for estimating single-pool Kt/V at higher dialysis frequencies. Nephrol Dial Transpl 2013;28(8):2156–60.

[27] Sternby J, Daugirdas JT. Theoretical basis for and improvement of Daugirdas' second generation formula for single-pool Kt/V. Int J Artif Organs 2015;38(12):632–7.

[28] Wellman ML, DiBartola SP, Kohn CW. Applied physiology of body fluids in dogs and cats. In: DiBartola SP, editor. Fluid, electrolyte, and acid-base disorders in small animals. St. Louis: Elsevier-Saunders; 2011. p. 2–25.

Advances in Small Animal Care 2 (2021) 131–142
ADVANCES IN SMALL ANIMAL CARE

Activated Carbon Hemoperfusion and Plasma Adsorption

Rediscovery and Veterinary Applications of These Abandoned Therapies

Jeff Barnes[a,*], Larry D. Cowgill, DVM, PhD, DACVIM (SAIM)[b,c], Jose Diaz Auñon, PhD[d]

[a]AimaLojic Animal Health, 3620 Homestead Street, Rapid City, SD 57703, USA; [b]University of California Veterinary Medical Center-San Diego; [c]Department of Medicine and Epidemiology, School of Veterinary Medicine, University of California-Davis, 2108 Tupper Hall, One Shields Avenue, Davis, CA 95616, USA; [d]ImmutriX Therapeutics, Inc., 3620 Homestead Street, Rapid City, SD 57703, USA

KEYWORDS

- Hemoperfusion • Hemoadsorption • Plasma adsorption • Blood purification • Intoxication • Poisoning • Cytokines • Extracorporeal

KEY POINTS

- Hemoperfusion witnessed a rise in adoption in the 1970s and 1980s and then a decline in the 1990s as modern dialytic devices dramatically improved. With new improvements in adsorbent technology, there is promise of a comeback for this extracorporeal therapy.
- Modern hemoadsorbents are extremely effective at removing drugs and other toxins from blood and is poised to play a significant role in other disease conditions moving forward.
- The availability of equipment to deliver stand-alone hemoperfusion has never been commercially available. New dedicated equipment will open up the therapy to be delivered in any clinical setting.

INTRODUCTION

Hemoperfusion (HP), or what may be better described as hemoadsorption, is an extracorporeal blood purification therapy delivered in a method similar to hemodialysis (HD). Blood is continuously withdrawn from a vein and pumped through a tubing circuit and a filtering device and then returned to the patient via a standard dual lumen dialysis catheter. The filtering device (HP column) contains adsorbent media which can remove a large quantity of specific or spectrum of molecules that are associated with drug overdose, poisoning, or other disregulated molecules associated with disease conditions. This must be done without extracting or affecting normal blood components.

BACKGROUND

HP was first introduced in the 1940s, refined in the 1950s and 1960s, introduced as a therapeutic procedure in the 1970s, and used frequently throughout the 1970s and 1980s. Biomass-derived activated charcoal has been the primary adsorbent used because of its large surface area and excellent filtering capability. High-quality charcoal can be produced by using a biomass such as coconut shells or bamboo and heating it to a very high temperature in the absence of oxygen. The result is an extremely porous carbon that is then activated using superheated CO2, steam, or chemicals to further increase the surface area and to create microscopic transport channels to connect the individual voids or pores.

*Corresponding author, *E-mail address:* jbarnes@immutrix.com

https://doi.org/10.1016/j.yasa.2021.07.010
2666-450X/21/ © 2021 Elsevier Inc. All rights reserved.

The historical challenges with activated charcoal as it pertains to purifying blood were numerous. Charcoal particles derived from plants are irregularly shaped with sharp edges that caused activation of platelets and blood complements and may damage or destroy cellular components such as red blood cells (Fig. 1). Hemolysis and thrombocytopenia were commonly observed in legacy HP procedures [1]. Other complications occur due to the soft and crumbly nature of activated charcoal forming microparticles that can leach out of the device and cause emboli. Lastly, the pore structure of plant-derived charcoal is designed by nature to transport water, and the micropores are somewhat random and vary in size, shape, and consistency. Charcoal is a powerful adsorbent that will remove a wide range of molecules, but the specific molecules and kinetics are somewhat uncontrollable. Hemodynamic instability, hypocalcemia, hypokalemia, hypoglycemia, and inflammatory responses were also commonly observed with early activated charcoal HP devices.

The bioincompatibility issue of charcoal sorbents was first addressed in 1969 (T M S. Chang) by applying a thin coating of cellulose nitrate and albumin to the charcoal particles [2]. The coating improved hemocompatibility and biocompatibility to an acceptably safe level but at the same time reduced the adsorptive performance and capacity, diminishing the effectiveness of the therapy. Subsequent coating attempts were made by others using acrylic hydrogel, cellulose, collodion, cross-linked gelatin, and modified hydrogel with varying yet similar results.

Animal studies [3] demonstrated the effectiveness of charcoal HP in the treatment of acute intoxication of glutethimide, pentobarbital, and salicylate leading to the first clinical trials for adult patients with suicidal or accidental drug poisoning. The success of the first human clinical trial [4], led to routine clinical use in patients around the world.

Throughout the 1970s, HP was used for removal of uremic metabolites because the devices were much more effective for the clearance of creatinine, uric acid, and middle molecules than the dialyzers available at that time. Clinical investigators also studied HP in series with HD [5] for patients with dialysis-resistant uremic toxins. Results showed improvement in "well-being" and decreased treatment times when compared with HD alone. Since then, modern HD membranes have significantly improved clearance for middle molecules; however, even the most modern dialyzers are not as effective for middle molecule clearance as legacy HP devices. The introduction of new and more efficient dialytic devices created a steady decline in the use of HP to the point where it has become essentially forgotten in modern medicine (Fig. 2).

Extracorporeal therapies (ECTs) in veterinary medicine, including HP and HD, are performed infrequently; however, HP has been an accepted extracorporeal modality since the inception of ECTs in animal patients, and its interest and application is growing among the Internal Medicine and Emergency and Critical Care specialties. Reasons for historical low adoption of these therapies are the cost of the treatments and equipment, lack of an established network of dialysis units, lack of training programs, and lack of veterinary-specific devices and delivery systems.

The growing number of veterinary dialysis programs relies on devices designed for adult human patients, and special considerations and procedures need to be used to treat smaller companion animals. Access to a blood bank may be required for very small animals as extracorporeal circuit volume can exceed safe extracorporeal limits or even the total blood volume of the animal. HP in veterinary medicine makes up only a small percentage of the totality of ECTs. Existing HP columns need to be connected to HD or other continuous renal replacement treatment (CRRT) machines to deliver the

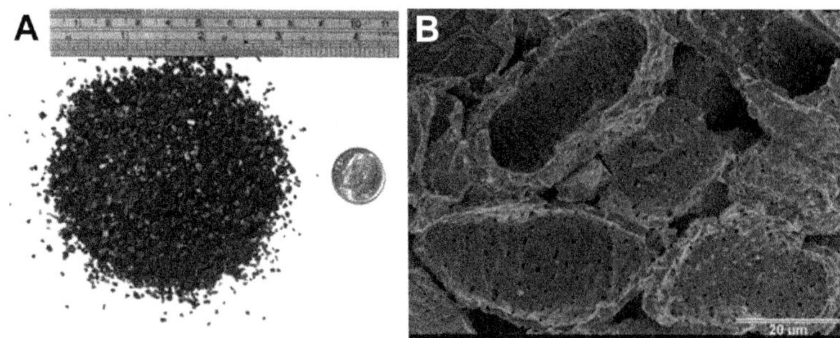

FIG. 1 **(A)** Activated charcoal. **(B)** Scanning electron micrograph (SEM) of naturally derived activated charcoal showing irregular shaped surface and rough edges. (*Courtesy of* John Dinsley, Crawford, NE.)

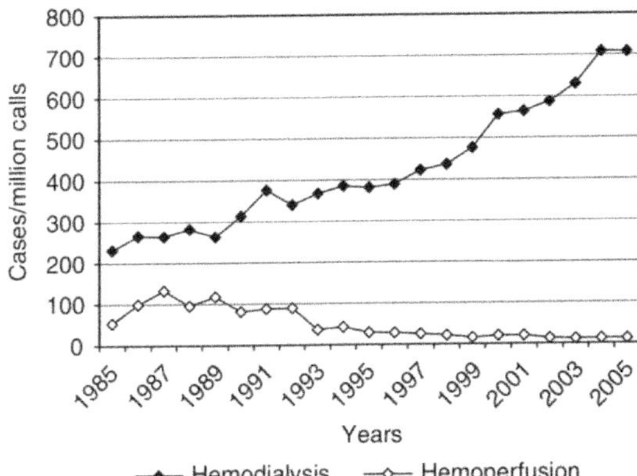

FIG. 2 Human cases reported to U.S. poison centers that required extracorporeal toxin removal. The number of hemodialysis procedures has grown while hemoperfusion is all but forgotten. (*From* Holubek WJ, Hoffman RS, Goldfarb DS, Nelson LS. Use of hemodialysis and hemoperfusion in poisoned patients. Kidney Int. 2008 Nov;74(10):1327-34.)

therapy, which requires the prescriber to have a high degree of skill as these machines were not designed to deliver HP, and no commercially available HP-specific delivery systems have been available until recently.

HEMOPERFUSION DEVICES

There are several HD and CRRT machines available and capable of running either a direct HP treatment or a combination therapy in line with dialysis. Conventional systems are designed for human patients and are not intuitively adaptable for routine use in smaller veterinary patients. These systems also were not specifically designed for HP, so a user must seek training to learn the nuances of each platform to use them for HP.

There are advantages to a combination of the HD–HP extracorporeal circuit including the control of body temperature, balancing electrolytes, and adding convective and diffusive clearance capability; however, in routine use, a combination circuit may not be necessary and adds cost and complexity to the procedure. For some acute toxicities, adsorptive clearance of the toxin may be all that is needed.

A new dedicated delivery system for direct HP is now available for use in veterinary patients. It consists of an extracorporeal tubing circuit, blood pump, disposable adsorption column, and integrated monitoring system to ensure the safety of the procedure (Fig. 3). The system perfuses blood through the extracorporeal circuit and provides anticoagulation delivery and pressure monitoring. Pressures are measured on the inlet line, precolumn, and postcolumn to allow detection and location of catheter restrictions and circuit clotting.

ADSORPTION FUNDAMENTALS

The mechanism at work in HP is adsorption, not to be confused with absorption. Absorption is the process of a fluid going within an absorbent like a sponge. Adsorption is the adhesion of atoms, ions, or molecules to the surface of an adsorbent. Confusing the matter is the fact that activated carbon (AC) has adsorptive surface distributed throughout the material, so in reality, solutes are going within the carbon structure where they are being attached to the carbon surface via adsorption.

Adsorption is the result of four forces: van der Waals force, hydrogen bonds, ionic bonds, and covalent bonds. van der Waals force is a weak bond comprising London dispersion forces and stronger dipole–dipole interactions. Hydrogen bonds are 10 times stronger than van der Waals force although weaker than ionic bonds. Covalent bonds or chemical adsorption also can occur and are the strongest bond. van der Waals force is the primary force participating in adsorption. These are weak electrical forces that attract molecules to one another.

Another fundamental property of adsorption is size exclusion. Modern sorbents can be designed with very precise pore sizes, with nanometer precision. Large structures, like RBCs, can be excluded completely while molecules that fit into the pore structure may be bound to the inner pore surface of the adsorbent. Molecules with physical dimensions smaller than the pore size are typically adsorbed if they are susceptible to adsorption forces (electrical charge and van der Waals force). Pore size can be precisely controlled and adjusted to target a specific range of molecules associated with intoxication or other disease conditions. Pore size is characterized as microporous, mesoporous, and macroporous based on pore diameter (Table 1).

Typically, molecules targeted for drug overdose and poisoning are between 150 Da and 1,500 Da, which also includes drug metabolites. These molecules can be effectively cleared by microporous adsorbents if pharmacokinetic parameters are met (see "*Use of Hemoperfusion In Drug Overdose and Poisoning*"). Pathologic molecules associated with other disease conditions can exceed 50 kDa or even 100 kDa, and mesoporous or macroporous structured adsorbent is needed. Legacy activated charcoal is almost purely microporous in structure. Modern ACs in contrast can be manufactured in virtually any pore size, either broadly or narrowly distributed, depending on the needs of the application.

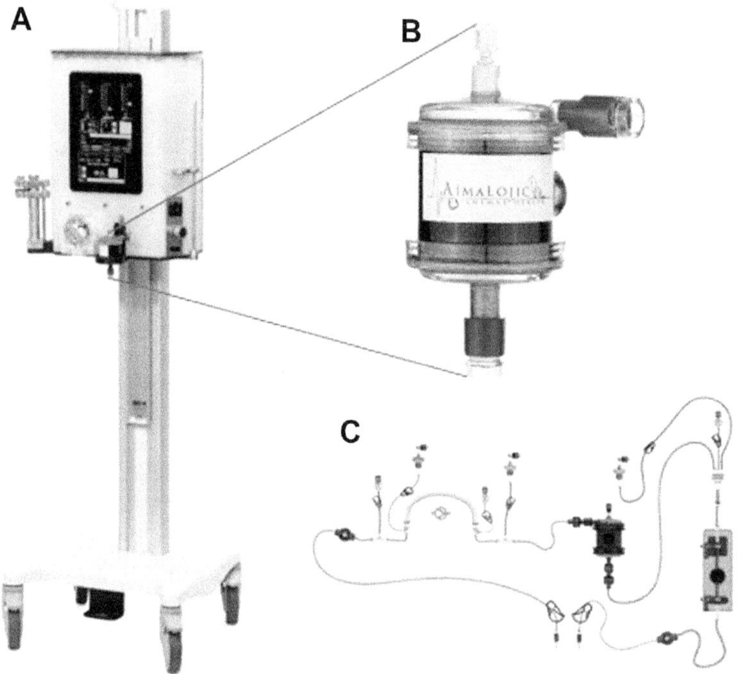

FIG. 3 (**A**) AimaLogic direct hemoperfusion system. (**B**) Hemoperfusion column. (**C**) Diagram of extracorporeal circuit.

Surface area is one of the principal determinants of how much and how fast a solute will be adsorbed. Surface area is created in modern synthetic sorbents by forming a series of voids in a cured polymer resin with alcohols or other agents that can be removed easily via solvent dissolution or burning it off at high temperature. The precursor polymer resin subsequently is transformed into a porous pure carbon adsorbent through the process of pyrolysis (heating the resin to high temperatures in the absence of oxygen), and in this process, anything that is not carbon is burned off. Porous carbon at this stage can have surface area in excess of 600 m2/g; however, the created voids (pores) in the original polymer are not yet interconnected.

TABLE 1
Characteristic of Pore Size

Microporous	**<2 nm**
Mesoporous	2nm – 50 nm
Macroporous	>50 nm

The final step is activation, a thermal–chemical reaction, where fractures and channels are created within the porous carbon to open the internal structure of the carbon and thus create a massive internal surface area of interconnecting pores. These fractures and channels are known as transport pores and are responsible for making the internal surface area available for adsorption. Transport pores are critical for a rapid rate of adsorption. After activation, modern carbon sorbents can have a surface area greater than 2,000 m^2/g, and a single modern therapeutic HP column can have a surface area greater than 30 football fields.

Thermal activation is measured in "burn-off" or the mass reduction percentage attained during the process. Surface area increases as burn-off increases to a critical point, and then, surface area declines (with decreasing carbon mass) as burn-off surpasses this point. One hundred percent (100%) burn-off would mean there is no solid product left, and everything has been converted to gas, primarily CO2. Adsorbents with larger surface areas will have faster adsorption kinetics and a larger adsorptive capacity.

A final characteristic controlling which adsorbates will bond to an adsorbent is determined by the surface chemistry of the adsorbent. Point of zero charge (PZC) is the pH value required for the net surface charge of AC to be zero. A low PZC-AC has a positively charged surface, and a high PZC will have a negative surface charge. Normally, it is easier to adsorb a cation onto a negatively charged surface and an anion onto a positively charged surface. Other interactions may be stronger than electrostatic forces which can make the surface charge less important. PZC of AC can be made to be very high, very low, or neutral. One can think of PZC as the characteristic that gives the adsorbent a greater affinity for one molecule over another.

LEGACY AND MODERN SORBENTS

In 1973, research began in Ukraine (V. Nikolaev and colleagues) (Vladimir Nikolaev, personal communication, 2018) at the then Soviet Union National Institute of Science to develop an AC specifically intended for HP from synthetic resins (Note the distinction of activated charcoal vs AC. The author will use "carbon" to distinguish synthetically derived "carbon" vs "charcoal" which is carbon derived from natural materials.). These new synthetic hemoadsorbents were the first of their kind possessing a uniform spherical shape, larger surface area (1,200 m2/g – 1,600 m2/g), and a smooth external surface that were hemocompatible without additional polymeric coatings. Somewhat later this team developed specialized ACs for targeting highly protein-bound molecules, which were named "deliganding" or HemoSorbent Granulated Deliganding AC with an even larger surface area of 2,000 m2/g to 3,000 m2/g. These sorbents form the basis for the highly specialized ACs for HP that are manufactured today (Fig. 4).

Considerable research and clinical experience was gained in the Soviet Union over two decades on the applications of AC in HP in a wide variety of disease conditions including acute radiation sickness, chronic glomerulonephritis, biliary and portal cirrhosis, severe forms of leptospirosis, skin psoriasis, psoriatic arthritis, idiopathic dilated cardiomyopathy, chronic kidney failure, and gonadotoxic side effects of intense cancer chemotherapy.

Other modern sorbents have been formulated for therapeutic HP from polymer beads (Cytosorbents, Inc, Exthera Medical, Alteco Medical). These manufactured sorbents also are highly porous and work in a similar fashion as AC. Synthetic sorbents also can be functionalized with a drug or other substance to provide selective adsorption capabilities. An example is the heparin functionalization of Seraph 100 (ExThera Medical Corporation, Martinez, CA), for adsorption of broad-spectrum pathogenic toxins, and Polymixin B functionalization of LPS Adsorber (Alteco Medical AB, Lund, Sweden) to promote adsorption of endotoxin.

Activation of carbon (as discussed earlier) is the step that opens the internal structure and connects the pores of a carbon-based adsorbent. In contrast, polymer-based beads are not activated, limiting the inner pore accessibility of these sorbent materials which consequently limits their functional surface area. Nitrogen porosimetry and mercury porosimetry are analytical techniques used to quantify surface area, pore size, pore structure, and density of porous materials (Table 2). Examining polymer beads by these methods demonstrates the relatively low functional surface area of this category of sorbents. While polymer sorbents can have unique capabilities, the sorbent columns need to be larger and necessitate longer treatments to compensate for the relatively low surface area compared with AC counterparts. They often can suffer earlier saturation that carbon-based devices undergo.

Saturation of HP sorbents can be difficult to predict in a living model and is an ongoing challenge during therapy. Sorbents can be measured for saturation points for different solutes ex vivo in a solution such as water, polyelectrolyte solution, or blood. As the carrier solution becomes more complex with a large number of constituents as is the case with plasma or blood, the predictability of saturation becomes more complicated. Interactions between molecules in the carrier solution and adsorption affinities and competition between solutes become more involved with more constituents. Add in a multicompartment living subject where solute distribution and generation rates might be occurring in real time, and the system and predictability becomes more complex still. Testing blood *in vitro* can provide some prediction for saturation at various toxicity concentrations but only in the most simplistic cases does it equate directly to *in vivo* treatment conditions.

Until there are better patient-side diagnostics and available clinical experience, the rule of thumb for HP is to use the largest, highest capacity device that is safe for the size of the patient. HP should be provided until clinical signs improve (for acute toxicity) with the anticipated possible need to replace the HP column based on any available manufacturer recommendations if provided. Saturation is concentration dependent, and it is rarely known what the actual toxin or solute concentration is before treatment. Mild to moderate toxicities based on estimated exposure or clinical signs may be treatable with a single device, while more severe toxicities may require exchange of a second or third column.

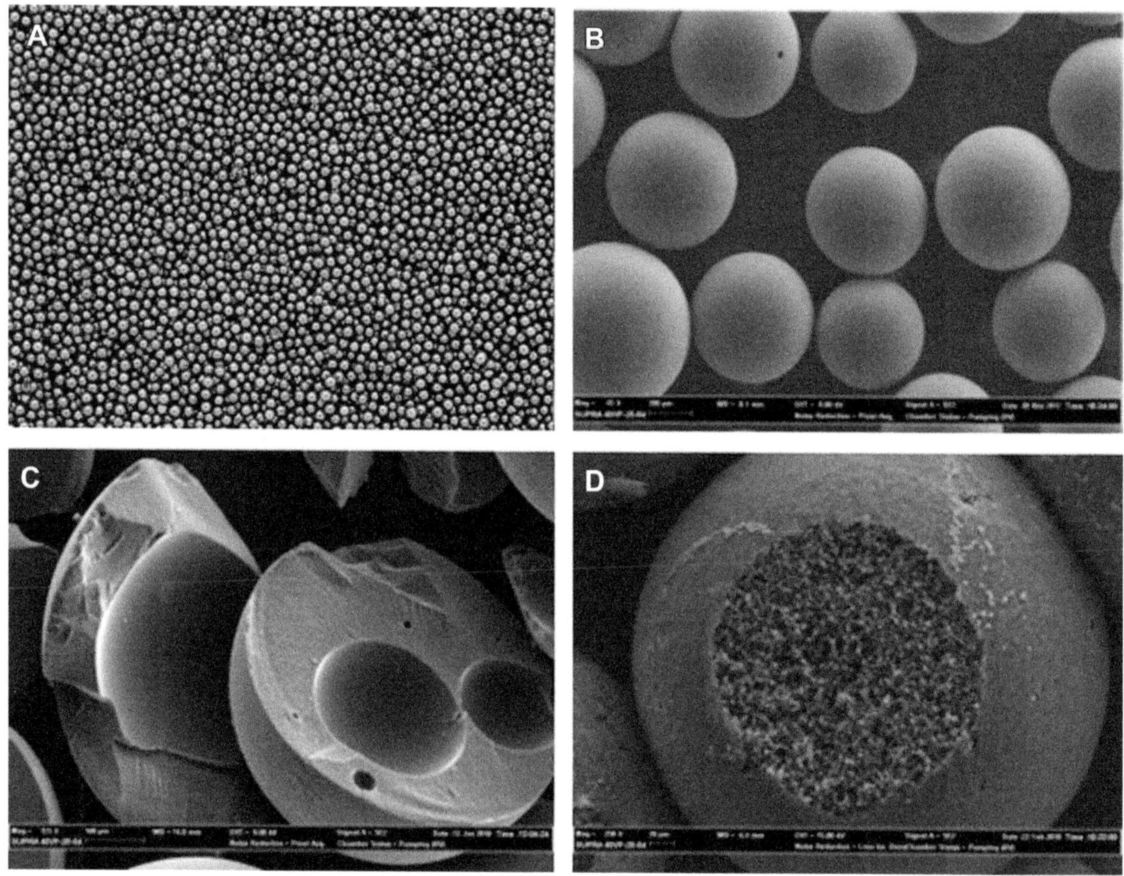

FIG. 4 (**A**) Photograph of synthetically derived activated carbon beads. (**B**) SEM illustrates the smooth surface and uniformity of beads. (**C**) SEM of crushed activated carbon illustrates the inner structure of 20 nm pore size. The craters are air bubbles that were trapped inside the resin as it cured. (**D**) Activated carbon bead with surface stripped off revealing 3,000 nm pore size inner structure. (*Courtesy of* ImmutriX Therapeutics, Inc.)

TABLE 2
Characteristics of Contemporary Adsorbents

Name	Pore Size (nm)	Surface Area (m2/g)	PZC
AimaLojic #1	24	1956	10.4
AimaLojic #2	78.7	2162	10.72
AimaLojic #3	82	1902	10.4
Activated charcoal	4	1390	7.1
Pitch-based AC	3.85	1776	10.9
Polymer Sorbent	45	473.29	3.04

The requirement to exchange HP devices becomes more likely for devices with lower adsorptive surface areas.

USE OF HEMOPERFUSION IN DRUG OVERDOSE AND POISONING

Volume of Distribution and Water Solubility

Toxins that are most susceptible to rapid clearance via HP have a low volume of distribution (Vd), may be protein bound or nonprotein bound, and have a molecular weight between 150 Da and 50,000 Da. Toxins with a larger Vd or high water solubility may not be susceptible to clearance with HP.

Toxins with low Vd (<0.2 L/kg) are distributed primarily in the vascular compartment and subject to faster removal by HP. Toxins with a higher Vd are distributed beyond the vascular compartment, and only the amount of toxin within the blood can be effectively removed. Redistribution (compartment equalization) of the toxin into the blood is required to clear these broader compartments by HP and detoxify the patient. Little is known about the distribution volume and redistribution rate of specific drugs or intoxicants at different intoxicating dosages, and it may be required to treat a longer time or to repeat a treatment to allow for vascular redistribution of the drug or toxin to facilitate therapeutic clearance or reappearance of clinical signs.

Pharmacokinetic data for drugs are based on therapeutic dose ranges, and in severe intoxications, Vd and the elimination half-life of a drug might be significantly different than published information for a drug or toxin. An example would be ibuprofen which has a small Vd at a therapeutic dose but appears to have a much larger Vd and half-life with massive overdose. Patients undergoing HP treatments for intoxication with a drug with a large Vd can experience symptomatic rebound of the intoxication after treatment is discontinued, and additional treatments may be required for total body clearance.

Solutes with very high water solubility such as salts and alcohols may not be suitable for clearance with HP owing to their high affinity to water and the difficulty for the adsorbent to separate the target solute from water. For these intoxicants, diffusive and convective dialytic treatments may be more effective as clearance across the dialyzer membrane is more efficient at clearance of small molecular weight water-soluble solutes.

Historically, the indications for use of HP in intoxication put it in a category between HD and therapeutic plasma exchange (TPE). For small molecular weight water-soluble solutes like ethylene glycol, HP is not effective, and HD is preferred. For highly protein-bound solutes like ibuprofen, HD is minimally effective, and HP is indicated. On the other hand, for exceptionally tightly protein-bound molecules, TPE has been suggested. With modern adsorptive technologies, the role of HP may be expanded to include indications historically indicated by HD or TPE (Fig. 5).

Currently, there is not a comprehensive list of candidate toxins that can be removed via modern HP adsorbents and devices. With expanding expertise in veterinary ECT, there is a growing understanding of known toxins susceptible to clearance by ECTs; however, until adoption of these therapies becomes more widespread, this list will be slow to develop with toxin-specific clearance data. The Extracorporeal Treatments in Poisoning Workgroup (EXTRIP, www.extrip-workgroup.org), a group of participants from nephrology, medical toxicology, pediatrics, emergency medicine, and critical care and clinical pharmacologists, has issued guidance on indications for the extracorporeal treatment of specific toxins. EXTRIP's guidance is largely focused on HD, as it is the primary modality used in human medicine, but these guidelines might help to predict candidate indications for HP, if a listed intoxicant is ineffectively cleared by hemodialysis.

Limited literature exists for HP role in intoxications including snake envenomation [6] and marijuana toxicity [7] which shows promise, but too little experience exists currently to know if HP is a preferred therapy for these indications. If and when HP becomes more readily available and prescribed, data will accumulate more rapidly, and standards of care may embrace these new techniques.

HEMOPERFUSION IN OTHER DISEASE CONDITIONS

There was considerable interest and research in HP indications and efficacy for use in numerous disease conditions during the 1970s and 1980s. Endotoxemia and sepsis were evaluated extensively [8], as well as its role in the clearance of bilirubin, phenols, and middle molecular weight substances in patients with acute liver failure [9]. Outcomes of these efforts showed remarkable promise; however, development in this area stalled abruptly possibly due to a lack of significant improvements in adsorbent technologies and the dramatic improvements in dialytic devices and pharmaceuticals since that time.

Typically, the uncontrolled release of cytokines is triggered by endotoxins (ETs). ETs are lipopolysaccharides (LPSs) molecular weight ranging between 4 kDa and 20 kDa; however, these molecules tend to form micelles of the size between 300 kDa and 1000 kDa. Though the release of some cytokines could be initiated by uremic or other toxins, targeting cytokines and the solutes creating the release of cytokines may be a visionary strategy to control, modify, or manage cytokine-mediated diseases. Modern carbon sorbents are very effective at removing LPSs.

Adsorption of cytokines by HP devices has been the subject of dozens of studies over the last several decades as the uncontrolled release of cytokines (cytokine storm) is associated with high mortality in many diseases such as sepsis [10]. Cytokines are a group of relatively small proteins (5 kDa-20 kDa) produced by blood and tissue cells. They often exist in blood as dimers or trimers, making them difficult to remove with

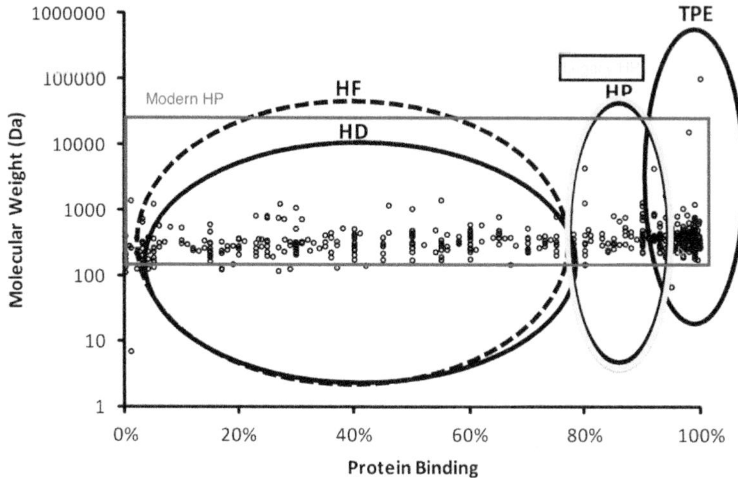

FIG. 5 Traditionally, hemoperfusion has been indicated for use only in those cases not well served by hemodialysis or therapeutic plasma exchange (*yellow circle*). Modern HP devices are capable of and may be another treatment option for many indications (*red rectangle*) historically addressed by HD or TPE. (*From* Ghannoum M, Roberts DM, Hoffman RS, Ouellet G, Roy L, Decker BS, Bouchard J. A stepwise approach for the management of poisoning with extracorporeal treatments. Semin Dial. 2014 Jul-Aug;27(4):362-70.)

dialytic techniques owing to their large size. While legacy microporous sorbents have shown some effectiveness in extraction of cytokines, studies show mesoporous and macroporous sorbents are decisively more effective [11].

Sepsis is associated with a rapid increase in inflammatory cytokines IL-6, IL-8, IL-23, and TNFa. Broad-spectrum antibiotic therapy is the current standard of care to reduce cytokine concentrations, but to date, the results of conventional medical therapies are inconclusive, and severe sepsis remains a deadly condition with few good treatment options. Owing to the extensive surface area and cytokine binding capacity of modern sorbents, HP holds promise as an extracorporeal option for the management of sepsis and other cytokine-mediated inflammatory diseases.

Sepsis is a very complex condition resulting from a wide variety of causes and is a very challenging model to study. Like sepsis, heat stroke also is associated with cytokine storm, systemic inflammatory response syndrome, shock, multiple organ failure, and death. In many ways, heat stroke may serve as a better model for evaluating proof of concept effectiveness of HP to treat cytokine storm than sepsis. A study has been initiated in canines (AimaLojic Animal Health, Rapid City, SD USA/Hebrew University, Jerusalem, IL) to assess the effectiveness of modern sorbent HP on the morbidity and mortality in patients with heat stroke compared with conventional treatment.

Other disease conditions that beg to be studied in veterinary medicine are leptospirosis, immune-mediated hemolytic anemia, pneumonia, pancreatitis, and acute kidney injury/acute lung injury to name a few. In most illness, there is some pathologic contribution of a blood component, interaction, or response associated with the expression of the disease. Modulating blood components with new extracorporeal devices portends a novel redirection to the conventional therapeutic approaches and extension of the role of ECT as an adjunct or alternative to current approaches.

Other modern carbon technologies exist in recent years and are being used in many ways in modern pharmacy and medicine. Carbon nanotubes have been successfully applied for drug delivery, tissue regeneration, and biosensor diagnosis owing to their small size, high surface area, and other traits. Studies of cytokine elimination by ultramodern carbon nanoforms (Y.Gogotsi, 2018) [12] demonstrated that graphene platelets outperformed all other carbon materials studied, both in adsorption kinetics and capacity. Nevertheless, none of the adsorbent strategies evaluated in these studies are cost effective. They either lack the adsorption rate and capacity, blood, and biological compatibility or currently are too expensive for mass production methods. As a plausible alternative, synthetic porous carbons can be widely modified, manufactured inexpensively, and are essentially inert, biocompatible, and infinitely scalable.

Synthetic carbon adsorbents derived by pyrolysis of various polymers have controllable porosity, and numerous studies have evaluated the effects of pore size on the kinetic and thermodynamic parameters of adsorption of ETs and cytokines. *Ex vivo* studies of synthetic carbons with three different pore sizes have been performed (ImmutriX Therapeutics, Inc., Rapid City, SD) to evaluate cytokine removal from solutions of human serum albumin (HSA) (Fig. 6). These studies documented that pore size influences cytokine clearance, but other parameters including pore volume and surface area also contribute to the carbon's ability to bind these molecules.

There remains a considerable lack of understanding about cytokine structure and adsorbent interactions. Some cytokines form dimers, trimers, and even multimers in certain pathologic conditions. This affects the structure and size of targeted cytokines and consequently influences the efficacy of carbon sorbents to clear cytokines under varying conditions. The binding capacity of the carbon decreases with size and complexity of the cytokine (Fig. 7).

Collectively, these data demonstrate that AC can be formulated to bind 90% to 100% of cytokines between 14 kDa and 50 kDa and approximately 50% for cytokines greater than 50 kDa in solution of HSA. Despite an overall efficacy of ACs to bind a spectrum of cytokines, it is apparent that formulation of the adsorptive properties of the carbon can be tailored to improve the efficacy of targeted cytokines as exemplified by formulation AC4 in Table 3. Evidence indicating modern AC can remove proinflammatory cytokines *ex vivo* suggests their potential to modulate disease states associated with their dysregulated production in cytokine-mediated inflammatory disease. Clearly, extensive study is still required to translate these exciting observations to clinical application and therapeutic benefit *in vivo*.

HEMOPERFUSION; THERAPY DELIVERY

HP as an extracorporeal procedure can be delivered with adaptation of conventional CRRT or Intermittent hemodialysis delivery platforms; however, these extracorporeal platforms were not designed specifically for HP. Their use is appropriate if HP is purposefully combined with a dialytic modality but somewhat inconvenient if HP is intended or indicated as a stand-alone treatment.

Vascular access is a required component of any ECT, and establishing and maintaining vascular access sufficient to deliver the required blood flow is critical to successful treatments. Typically, a large bore, dual lumen dialysis catheter, appropriate to the size of the patient and requisite blood flow is necessary to deliver HP. Proper training in the placement and management of the vascular access is paramount. In contrast to hemodialysis, vascular access for HP is generally limited to one or 2 days but should be approached with the same rigor and attention to asepsis as required for more prolonged ECTs.

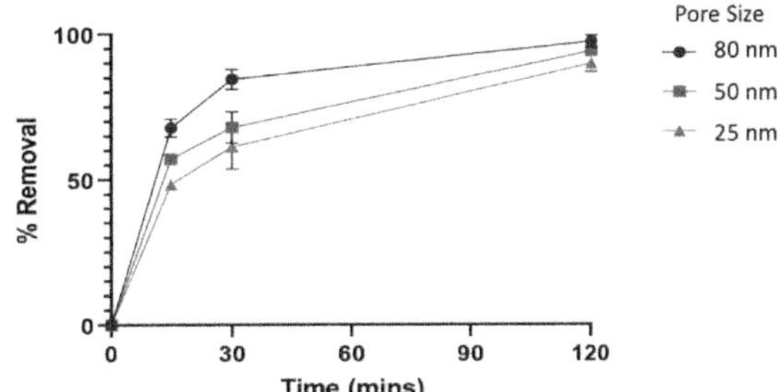

FIG. 6 Removal of cytokine IL-6 from HSA using three different formulations of activated carbon with different pore sizes.

Blood flow during HP is regulated by a peristaltic roller pump located on the IHD, CRRT, or HP delivery platform. Pressure transducers are used to measure circuit pressures to ensure the integrity of the extracorporeal blood flow rate, blood flow path, and to alert for clotting in the circuit. HP typically requires blood flow rates between 50 and 200 mL/min and consequently requires appropriate vascular access to achieve these flow rates.

HEMOPERFUSION; COMPLICATIONS

There are risks and complications that are common to all ECTs, and there are some that may be more pronounced with HP.

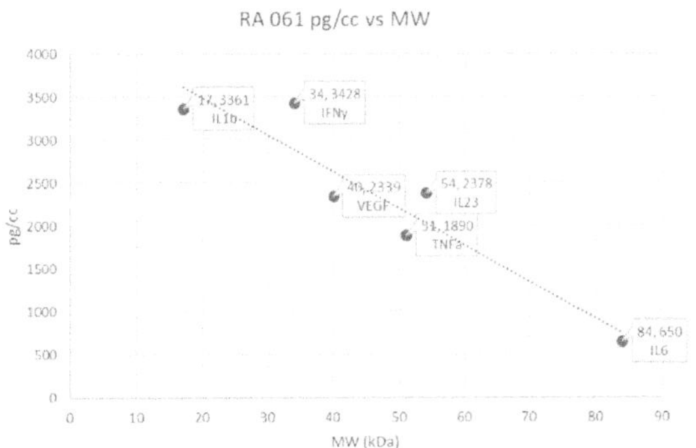

FIG. 7 Removal of cytokines per cc of activated carbon. This illustrates that the larger and more complex a molecule is, the less it will be adsorbed. IL-6 in this experiment was a trimer explaining its high MW.

TABLE 3
Removal of Cytokines by Differing Formulations of Synthetic Carbon Adsorbents from Albumin Solutions

Cytokine	MW (kDa)	AC4% Removal 30 min	AC4% Removal 120 min	AC3% Removal 30 min	AC3% Removal 120 min	AC5% Removal 30 min	AC5% Removal 120 min
GM-CSF (monomer)	14	68%	98%	48%	78%	52%	87%
IL-7 (monomer)	17	66%	90%	45%	75%	45%	76%
IL-1 Beta (monomer)	17	71%	93%	49%	62%	58%	84%
IL-6 (monomer)	21	88%	99%	58%	93%	67%	94.7%
IFN-Gamma	17 (34)	93%	100%	85%	92%	72%	85%
VEG-F (dimer)	21 (40)	91%	95%	79%	91%	76%	92%
TNF-alpha (trimer)	17 (51)	76%	97%	49%	74%	58%	82%
IL-23 (heterodimer)	27 (54)	32%	53%	21%	32%	11%	16%
IL-12 (heterodimer)	70	51%	77%	24%	50%	29%	50%

- Vascular access issues include bleeding, clotting, vessel damage, infection, and air embolism.
- Systemic anticoagulation with heparin may predispose to bleeding if provided in excess or in patients predisposed to bleeding due the underlying intoxication or disease condition. Oppositely, a patient may be predisposed to clotting of the extracorporeal circuit or thromboembolic complications if the systemic anticoagulation is inadequate or the patient is hypercoagulable.
- Thrombocytopenia is common in ECTs to a degree but may be pronounced with HP.
- Clotting of extracorporeal circuit may cause disruption or discontinuance of treatment and potential blood loss if circuit needs to be discarded without returning blood to patient.
- Inflammatory or allergic response to circuit components is uncommon as modern extracorporeal devices and HP sorbents have mitigated most of these concerns. Clinical signs of allergic or inflammatory incompatibility should be monitored throughout and after treatment.
- Changes in electrolyte and serum chemistries, while greatly mitigated with combined HD and HP and modern sorbents, can occur and should be monitored. Serum glucose concentrations are particularly susceptible to priming techniques which can promote profound hypoglycemia or hyperglycemia.
- Particle embolization has been an historical concern with sorbent materials and HP. With modern materials and HP devices, these concerns have become extremely unlikely.
- Hypothermia remains a concern on extracorporeal platforms like HP that may not incorporate blood warming capabilities for the extracorporeal circuit. This is not a significant factor in HP when a blood warmer is used on the return blood circuit, but hypothermia can be profound especially in small patients. External warming with blankets and warming devices is recommended.

The most common unintended effect of HP is thrombocytopenia, which is a consistent and well-known phenomenon across all HP devices. On initiation of HP, platelet count (and usually white blood cell count) is likely to drop by 30% to 50% within 15 to 40 minutes but generally recovers to about 60% to 80% of baseline over the course of treatment. For treatments terminated within 2 hours of initiating HP, the platelet count may not recover from the initial nadir. Adverse clinical effects of this transient thrombocytopenia are not expected but may predispose to increased bleeding risk. HP should be initiated very cautiously in patients with an initial platelet count less than 75,000/uL.

Attempts to understand and reduce the effect of synthetic carbon HP on platelets have been made, and enlargement of the size of the spherical carbon bead used in the HP column appears to minimize the platelet drop during treatment. For currently available synthetic carbon HP devices, there has not been a direct attempt to modify bead size as this is known to decrease adsorption kinetics. Because resolution of the attending acute toxicity is the primary concern, maximizing adsorption kinetics is deemed a higher priority to transient thrombocytopenia which fully recovers within days following treatment.

SUMMARY

Modulating or purifying blood composition via ECT to ameliorate disease has been practiced for over 70 years. If you subscribe to the notion that bloodletting was once a therapy to remove toxins from the body, one could argue the idea has been around for many millennia. Medical technologies have evolved in an amazing and ever-increasing fashion of complexity. Modern science gives us the opportunity to look back at ideas that were ahead of the technical capabilities available at their time with far better tools. With modern material science, chemistry, and improved diagnostic and disease understanding, perhaps, powerful therapies like HP will make a resurgence.

CLINICS CARE POINTS

- Require complete asepsis for catheter placement
- Appropriate size catheter for the size of the patient and required blood flow rate
- Avoid triple lumen catheters
- If the catheter is maintained after the treatment, the heparin lock concentration should be proportional to the size of the patient and the interval between reuse. In cats, it is usually 200 U/ml; for medium-sized dogs, it is 500 to 1000 U/ml; for large dogs, it is 1500 to 3000 U/mL.
- *Do not allow any other use of the catheter except hemoperfusion or extracorporeal therapies.*
- Enclose securely in a neck bandage

FUNDING

This research has been privately funded by the stock holders in ImmutriX Therapeutics, Inc.

DISCLOSURE

J.Barnes is an employee of AimaLojic Animal Health, a division of ImmutriX Therapeutics, Inc., Rapid City, SD, USA, and a manufacturer of an activated carbon hemoperfusion system.

REFERENCES

[1] Chang TMS. Hemoperfusion: clearance, blood compatibility and safety. Int J Artif Organs 1979;2(6):276–7.
[2] Chang TMS. Clinical experience with ACAC coated charcoal hemoperfusion in acute intoxication. Clin Toxicol 1980;17(4):529–42.
[3] Chang TMS. Artificial cells, monograph, 212 pp. Springfield (IL): Charles C Thomas; 1972. Available at: http://www.medicine.mcgill.ca/artcell/1972book-Covercr.pdf.
[4] Chang TMS, Coffey JF, Barré P, et al. Microcapsule artificial kidney: treatment of patients with acute drug intoxication. Can Med Assoc J 1973;108:429–33.
[5] Winchester JF, Apiliga MT, Mackay JM, et al. Combined hemodialysis-charcoal hemoperfusion in the dialysis patient. Kidney Int 1976;10(Suppl 7):S315–9.
[6] Oliveira ME, Campanholi J, Cavalcante RL, et al. Experimental model for removal of snake venom via hemoperfusion in rats. J Vet Emerg Crit Care 2020;30:286–94.
[7] Culler CA, Vigani A. Successful treatment of a severe cannabinoid toxicity using extracorporeal therapy in a dog. J Vet Emerg Crit Care (San Antonio) 2019;29(6):674–9.
[8] Nolan JP. The Role of Endotoxin in Liver Injury. Gastroenterology 1975;69(6):1346–56.
[9] Hughes R, Williams R. Clinical Experience with Charcoal and Resin Hemoperfusion. Semin Liver Dis 1986;6(2).
[10] Kellum JA, Kong L, Fink MP, et al. Understanding the Inflammatory cytokine response in pneumonia and sepsis: results of the genetic and inflammatory markers of sepsis (GenIMS) Study. Arch Intern Med 2007;167:1655–63.
[11] Mikhalovsky SV. Emerging technologies in extracorporeal treatment: focus on adsorption. Perfusion 2003;18(1_suppl):47–54.
[12] Yachamaneni S, Yushin G, Yeon SH, et al. Mesoporous carbide-derived carbon for cytokine removal from blood plasma. Biomaterials 2010;31(18):4789.

Advances in Small Animal Care 2 (2021) 143–155
ADVANCES IN SMALL ANIMAL CARE

Vaccine-Enhanced Adoptive T-Cell Therapy to Treat Canine Cancers

Noe Reyes, DVM*, Gary W. Wood, PhD
ELIAS Animal Health, 10900 S Clay Blair Boulevard, Suite 700, Olathe, KS 66061, USA

KEYWORDS
• Immunotherapy • Immuno-oncology • Canine cancer • Adoptive T-cell therapy • Osteosarcoma • Autologous vaccine • Apheresis

KEY POINTS

- Adoptive T-cell immunotherapies can be used to treat various canine cancers.
- Autologous cancer cell vaccines can be used to familiarize immune cells to cancer-specific neoantigens.
- Apheresis is used to harvest vaccine-primed lymphocytes which are *ex vivo* activated and expanded.
- In a pilot study, fully responsive canine patients did not require additional therapy for their cancer after treatment.
- Treatment protocol has shown efficacy in canine osteosarcoma and also against human cancer types.

INTRODUCTION

The advent of immunotherapies has changed the manner in which cancers are treated. The potential to stimulate a patient's own immune system to ameliorate or eradicate cancer introduces promising new treatment modalities for clinicians. Various cancer immunotherapies used either as monotherapy or in combination with other therapies are being actively researched and developed, with some already achieving regulatory approval as human therapeutics (eg, ipilimumab, rituximab, and tisagenlecleucel). Examples of these various immunotherapeutics include autologous cancer vaccinations, antibodies, checkpoint inhibitors (drugs that "unmask" the cancer cells to the immune system), and adoptive T-cell transfer therapies such as chimeric antigen receptor (CAR-T) and tumor infiltrative lymphocyte (TIL) technologies. Adoptive T-cell therapies (ACTs) use the patient's own immune cells to recognize distinct highly tumor-specific antigens referred to as "cancer neoantigens" and eliminate cancer cells. It is precisely these cancer neoantigens that have allowed development of highly targeted therapeutics such as ACTs [1–3].

Some ACT protocols use genetic manipulation of a patient's T cells to have them recognize a known specific target(s) on cancer cells (CAR-T), while others use T cells harvested from excised tumor tissue which have become primed with the tumor cell antigens (TIL). In both ACT examples, the sourced T cells are activated and expanded *ex vivo*. The process of T-cell activation and expansion increases the number of (neo)antigen-specific effector T cells delivered to the patient, where they enter cancer tissue and generate a cascade of cytokine-mediated immunologic events that result in

Both authors are employed at ELIAS Animal Health, a company developing canine cancer therapies including the subject adoptive T-cell therapy. N. Reyes is the Chief Medical Officer at ELIAS Animal Health and G.W. Wood is the Chief Scientific Officer at ELIAS Animal Health. G.W. Wood is also employed as Chief Scientific Officer at TVAX Biomedical, a company developing the human version of the subject adoptive T cell therapy.

*Corresponding author, *E-mail address:* nreyes@eliasah.com

https://doi.org/10.1016/j.yasa.2021.07.007
2666-450X/21/ © 2021 Elsevier Inc. All rights reserved.

cancer cell killing and, in best responders, rejection of the growing cancer [2–4].

Some of the immunotherapeutics causing excitement in human medicine recently have become available to veterinary clinicians. Here we discuss an ACT for the treatment of canine osteosarcoma (OSA), as well as potentially other cancer types. This therapy, referred to as vaccine-enhanced adoptive cell therapy (VACT), uses autologous cancer cell vaccines, manufactured from the patient's excised tumor tissue, to condition T cells to the cancer neoantigens *in vivo*. After a series of three vaccinations, the primed T cells are harvested via leukocytapheresis ("apheresis") to be *ex vivo* expanded and activated before their reinfusion back into the patient. After infusion, a short course of low-dose interleukin-2 (IL-2) is administered to stimulate continued T-cell multiplication.

GENERAL OVERVIEW, BACKGROUND, AND STUDY RATIONALE FOR VACCINE-ENHANCED ADOPTIVE CELL THERAPY

Proof-of-concept studies for the general form of immunotherapy discussed later have been performed using rodent cancer models [5,6]. Studies in mice have demonstrated immunity to cancer is mediated by T cells [7,8], which has led most studies of immunotherapy to focus on T cells. Those studies demonstrated cancer immunity could be adoptively transferred from one inbred mouse to another with T cells but not with antibodies. Early mouse studies also demonstrated that, while primed T cells removed from immune animals are unable to kill cancer cells, T cells could be removed from immune animals and restimulated with an antigen *in vitro* to generate cytotoxic effector T cells that killed cancer cells in an major histocompatibility complex-restricted cancer neoantigen–specific manner [9,10]. Subsequent studies aided by the availability of recombinant human IL-2 demonstrated polyclonal populations of cancer neoantigen–specific effector T cells could be generated by stimulating cancer neoantigen–primed T cells with the antigen and rhIL-2 [11,12]. Those studies demonstrated adoptive transfer of the *ex vivo* activated effector T cells into cancer-bearing animals resulted in those animals being cured in a cancer neoantigen–specific manner [11,13]. These studies were repeatedly and independently reproduced with histopathologically distinct cancers growing in virtually any body location where cancers could be implanted or to which the cancers spontaneously metastasized [11,14].

Preclinical studies used inbred strains of rodents and cancers that either arose naturally or were carcinogen induced and then transplanted between genetically identical individuals. These are generally referred to as syngeneic rodent models and are designed to mimic cancer antigen–specific immunotherapy of naturally occurring cancers arising in any mammalian species. In a syngeneic rodent model, the immune system of the individual in whom the cancer arose is used to generate immunotherapeutic effects that are focused on genetic differences between the cancer and its host. Because all members of inbred strains of animals are genetically identical, immunotherapy in a syngeneic model is comparable with performing autologous immunotherapy in a single dog with a naturally occurring cancer.

Several fundamental observations relating to mammalian immune systems and their interaction with patients' cancers suggest findings obtained in rodent models are relevant to the use of cancer antigen–specific immunotherapy to treat canine OSA.

- Although there are some species differences, all mammalian immune systems are organized in the same fundamental way.
- The adaptive immune system protects all mammals from attack by infectious agents such as viruses in the same fundamental way. The same basic mechanisms also are involved in the adaptive immune system's response to cancer cells and viruses. When the immune system is exposed to a cancer cell vaccine or to a viral vaccine, the ensuing protective immune response is T cell mediated.
- All cancers that have been systematically tested, which includes both rodent and human cancers, have been shown to be immunogenic. Immunogenicity is independent of the cancer's histopathology. One would predict from those observations that canine OSAs are similarly immunogenic.
- All cancers that have been systematically tested, which includes both rodent and human cancers, have been shown to be susceptible to killing by T cells. Therefore, one would predict from those observations that canine OSAs are similarly susceptible to killing by T cells. The ability to be killed by T cells is independent of the type of cancer being targeted and the species in which the cancer occurred.

Experimental rodent cancers were first demonstrated to be immunogenic in the 1950s [1]. Immunity to cancer antigens is mediated by T cells, and the immune response is exquisitely specific for the cancer used for immunization [2,3]. Vaccination with live attenuated cancer cells and a powerful immunologic adjuvant induces a T cell–mediated immune response against even the least immunogenic cancers [15]. Generally, the approach used in rodent studies was to immunize normal syngeneic animals and then to test the vaccinated animals for the development of protective immunity by injecting them with live cancer cells. Positive protection assays demonstrate T cells (1) kill cancer cells *in vivo* and (2) kill all cancer cells in a cancer. The main immunologic adjuvants used for cancer vaccine studies have been bacterial and cytokine. The primary bacterial adjuvants have been Bacillus Calmette-Guerin (BCG), which is an attenuated form of *Mycobacterium tuberculosis,* and killed *Propionobacterium acnes* [*P. acnes* (formerly *Corynebacterium parvum*)]. The primary cytokine adjuvant used is granulocyte macrophage colony-stimulating factor (GM-CSF). These bacterial and cytokine adjuvants have approximately equivalent immunologic adjuvant capabilities. *P. acnes* has been used in most rodent studies, and BCG and GM-CSF, which are Food and Drug Administration–approved drugs, were used in most human studies.

T cells removed from immune animals and stimulated with antigen and the T-cell growth factor, IL-2, acquire the ability to kill cancer cells in an antigen-specific manner *in vitro* [9,11,16]. These cells are called cytotoxic T cells (CTLs). Subsequent studies demonstrated a similar *ex vivo* T-cell activation strategy could produce bulk populations of polyclonal cancer antigen–specific effector T cells. These polyclonal populations contain CTLs as well as other types of cancer antigen–specific effector T cells that mediate their effects by activating bystander cells (macrophages and natural killer cells) to kill cancer cells. These T cells may be either CD4+ T cells (Th1) or CD8+ T cells (Tc1) and mediate their effects mainly through the production of interferon gamma.

Adoptively transferred cancer antigen–specific effector T cells initially were shown to reject growing cancers and cure cancer-bearing animals during the 1980s and 1990s [11,17,18]. Although pretreatment with certain chemotherapeutic agents could augment the clinical effects [17], the anticancer effects of adoptively transferred cancer antigen–specific effector T cells could be produced in the absence of any other form of treatment [11,18]. That is, animals that had not been treated with surgery, radiotherapy, or any form of chemotherapy before or after receiving immunotherapy could be treated effectively. Cancer antigen–specific effector T cells are responsible for the therapeutic effects.

This general treatment strategy that exploits the effects of cancer antigen–specific effector T cells has been shown to be effective against a wide range of rodent cancers, including the brain [18], mammary [19–21], colon [22], fibrosarcoma [9], kidney [23], lung [22],leukemia [17,24], lymphoma [25], melanoma [26,27], and prostate [28,29]. Additional studies have demonstrated cancers growing in the bone marrow [30], brain [16], liver [31], lung [6], and skin [32] and in unknown sites to which the cancer spontaneously metastasized [26,27] could be treated effectively. These observations are directly relevant to the treatment of individuals, including dogs, with stage 4 (metastatic) cancers of all kinds, including metastatic OSA. In all rodent studies, therapeutic efficacy was improved by treating animals with a course of systemic IL-2 after adoptive transfer of the cancer antigen–specific effector T cells.

Extensive human studies also have demonstrated adoptive transfer of cancer antigen–specific effector T cells combined with a course of systemic IL-2 produces dramatic anticancer effects in patients with a variety of advanced cancers [33–39]. Genetically engineered effector T cells have proven effective against B-cell lymphomas and leukemias [40,41]. Cancer antigen–specific effector T cells produce significant durable objective clinical responses in all of the studies. Studies also have demonstrated outcomes in both rodents and humans could be improved by pretreatment with cyclophosphamide [14,17,36–39,42–44].

The following summarizes the general relevance of these rodent model studies to canine cancer treatment:

- Cancer immunotherapy using adoptive transfer of cancer antigen–specific effector T cells is effective against rodent and human malignancies, suggesting that it would be similarly effective against canine malignancies, including OSA.
- Cancers are rejected wherever they are growing in the body. The experimental testing conditions were not identical to treating a naturally progressing canine cancer, but the various conditions provided as close an approximation to the canine condition as one could generate in rodent models.
- Invariably, in all models and in all experiments, there was a direct relationship between response rate and survival. In all models studied, even those that used a very weakly immunogenic, highly metastatic mammary cancer, growing cancers were rejected and the cancer-bearing animals were permanently cured when the effector T cells were used to treat minimal disease. This observation suggests that ECI could potentially be highly effective against the minimal residual disease that exists in dogs after cytoreductive chemotherapy.
- A variety of T-cell stimuli have been used to generate cancer antigen–specific effector T cells in vitro. Most commonly, the T-cell activating agent was a specific antigen, antiCD3, or superantigen. Also, most commonly, the T-cell growth factor that was used

for stimulating T-cell proliferation both *in vitro* and *in vivo* was IL-2, but other T cell–stimulating cytokines, including IL-7, IL-15, and IL-21, have proven effective.

There are two caveats that should be applied to the rodent studies. The first is, in most studies, the immune cells used to generate cancer antigen–specific effector T cells were obtained by immunizing normal healthy animals. Normal healthy rodents may not be comparable with patients who have advanced cancers and definitely are not comparable with patients who have received treatments that have the side effect of damaging the patient's immune system. The closest that one could get to the rodent conditions during a natural treatment scenario would be to use immunotherapy to treat patients immediately after diagnosis or to treat patients who only have been treated at diagnosis with surgery. The latter is necessary when an autologous cancer cell vaccine is used as part of the treatment. These individuals would have relatively healthy immune systems, and human studies have demonstrated that these individuals mount vigorous immune responses to their own cancers [20,45,46]. However, with some cancers, it may be necessary to use some other agent, such as chemotherapy, to cytoreduce the cancer to provide sufficient time for the immunotherapy to be delivered and to generate its anticancer effects.

The other caveat is that application of this general strategy to a dog with cancer would require all steps be performed in the same individual. That is, the dog is vaccinated, immune cells are collected from that dog, and then, after those immune cells are converted into effector T cells *ex vivo*, those activated T cells are returned to the same dog.

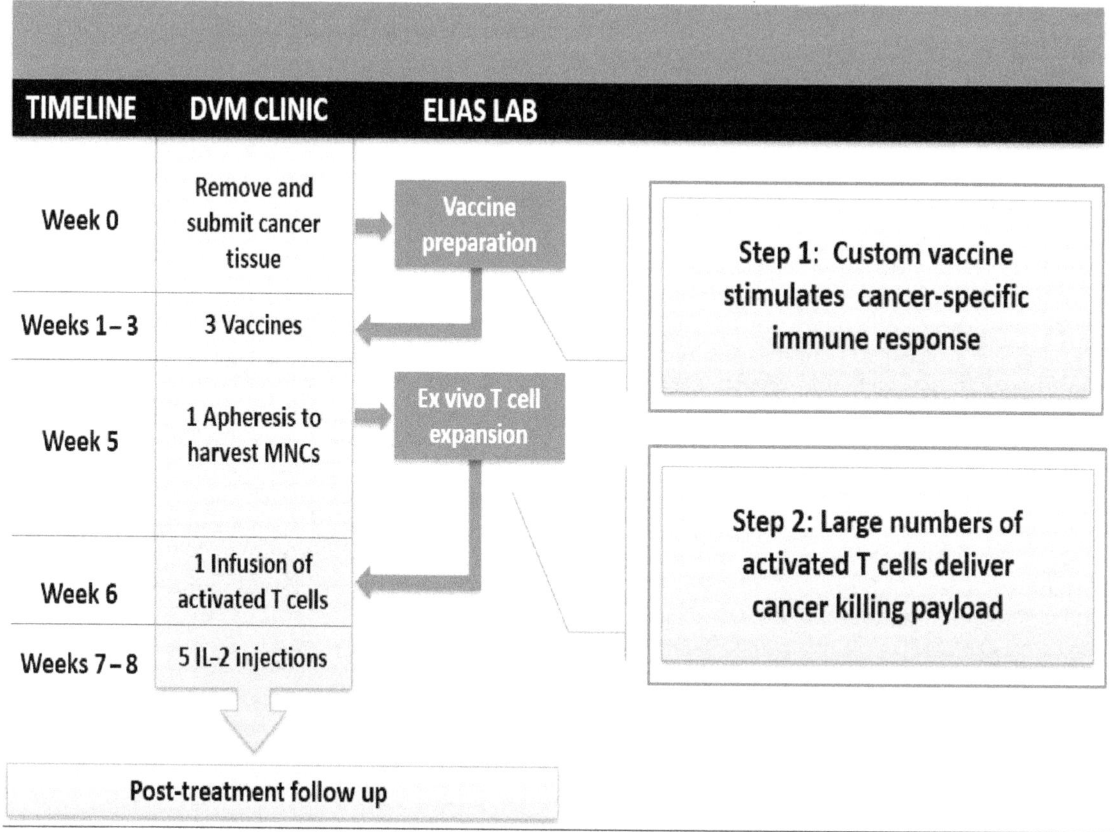

FIG. 1 Overview of the canine VACT protocol shows each step in the 7- to 8-week protocol. Schedule can be divided into two general processes: tumor collection and vaccine manufacture and apheresis, activation of T cells and IV reinfusion. (*From* Sonderegger FL, Fitzpatrick J, and Wood G., Phase I Clinical Trial to Evaluate the Safety of ELIAS Cancer Immunotherapy, Research Poster presented at 2016 ACVIM conference.)

At the time those various rodent studies were performed, there was a full awareness of the fact that nonspecific immune stimuli have the ability to stimulate immune responses, including stimulating immune responses in cancer bearing animals. Thus, consider the individual components of vaccine-enhanced adoptive T-cell therapy. The individual components included (1) an attenuated autologous cancer cell/immunologic adjuvant vaccine, (2) adoptively transferred cancer neoantigen–specific T cells, and (3) IL-2.

VACCINE-ENHANCED ADOPTIVE CELL THERAPY IN DOGS: PROTOCOL AND COMPONENTS

VACT requires two broad steps: (1) the tissue harvest and vaccination phase and (2) leukocytapheresis, T-cell infusion, and IL-2 phase [47,48]. Fig. 1 gives an overview of the protocol steps and its two general phases. As noted earlier, VACT currently is undergoing evaluation in human clinical trials for the treatment of malignant glioma and renal cell carcinoma with impressive and lasting results in responding patients [34,35]. The VACT protocol was adapted for use in canines to evaluate its safety and efficacy in OSA.

OSA was selected as the initial cancer indication to evaluate the canine VACT protocol as OSA comprises 5% to 10% of canine cancers, and up to 75% of canine bone cancers are OSAs [49,50]. Curative intent treatment options include surgery and some form of adjuvant systemic chemotherapy to eliminate the cancer cells that remain after surgery. Chemotherapy designed to suppress metastatic disease often can be ineffective unless combined with surgery to remove the primary bone cancer. Chemotherapy is not curative; only a portion of the cancer cells remaining after surgery are killed by cytotoxic chemical agents.

OSA is an excellent potential target for immunotherapy because removal of the primary cancer by amputation generally creates minimal residual disease. Studies in rodent models have demonstrated VACT has the ability to cause long-term remission against minimal disease and produce only transient inflammatory-type side effects. Surgery combined with VACT has the potential to dramatically prolong the survival of treated and responsive dogs without significantly compromising their quality of life.

Individual Vaccine-Enhanced Adoptive Cell Therapy Components and Sequence

Surgical harvest of the cancer cells for vaccine-enhanced adoptive cell therapy vaccine

Surgical removal of the primary bone cancer by amputation is the recommended first-line treatment for canine bone cancer [51]. As a palliative treatment, surgery reduces or eliminates bone pain and eliminates the risk of fracture. Surgery is also required to obtain cancer tissue to manufacture the attenuated autologous cancer cell vaccine, an essential component of VACT. Surgical removal of the cancer also reduces the total amount of cancer tissue present in a patient's body, thereby minimizing the residual disease to be eliminated potentially by VACT.

Irradiated harvested cancer cells. The primary objective of vaccination is to induce an immune response that ultimately leads to cancer antigen–specific destruction of cancer cells. Harvested cancer cells obtained from the surgical amputation are irradiated for using in the VACT vaccine to ensure the same

TABLE 1
Mean Values of Leukapheresis and Activated T-Cell Products of Normal, Healthy Laboratory Dogs

	Total Cells (Billions)[a]	Viability (%)[a]	Lymphocyte (%)[a]	Lymphoblast (%)[a]	Monocytes (%)[a]	Total T Cells (%)[b]	CD4 (%)[b]	CD8 (%)[b]	CD25 (%)[b]
Leukapheresis	5.4	89	52	<1	31	54	43	11	<5
Activated T cell	22	80	39	56	5	87	57	31	>95

All percentages are based on % of total cells in population. Note the increase in proportion of CD4+ and CD8+ cells with the majority carrying the CD25+ activation marker.

[a] Cell analyses before freezing sample: based on morphologic characterization (cytosph and Wright stain).

[b] Cells analyses after thawing frozen samples: gated on total live/nondoublet cells.

From Flesner BK, Wood GW, Gayheart-Walsten P, Sonderegger FL, Henry CJ, Tate DJ, Bechtel SM, Donnelly LL, Johnson GC, Kim DY, Wahaus TA, Bryan JN, Reyes N. Autologous cancer cell vaccination, adoptive T-cell transfer, and interleukin-2 administration results in long-term survival for companion dogs with osteosarcoma. J Vet Intern Med. 2020 Sep;34(5):2056-2067; with permission.

unique antigens are used to generate immune responses as would be the specific targets for the immune-mediated, cancer antigen–specific destructive process yet attenuated and incapable of further growth. Preclinical studies demonstrated live cancer cells attenuated by irradiation invariably produce the most potent anticancer immune responses when compared with other sources of cancer antigens. Human studies demonstrated further, when combined with an immunologic adjuvant (bacterial or cytokine), live cancer cells that are attenuated by irradiation induce detectable immune responses in vaccinated patients in the presence of growing cancers [52–57].

Immunologic adjuvant and vaccination. Killed *P acnes* (Neogen Corporation) are the immunologic adjuvant used in this study. *P acnes* polarize immune responses into the Th1 (T cell–mediated immunity) arm of the immune system, which is essential because cancer cell killing is exclusively mediated by T cells. *P acnes* augment immune responses by inducing an inflammatory response at the vaccination site, which results in activation and recruitment of antigen-presenting cells (dendritic cells) at vaccination sites.

Nearly all preclinical rodent studies of cancer antigen–specific immunotherapy that used intradermal vaccination with an irradiated cancer cell vaccine used killed *P. acnes* as the immunologic adjuvant. No toxicity was observed in those rodent studies. Killed *P. acnes* also have been tested in large, randomized studies as a systemic cancer treatment in humans. Minimal toxicity was observed when high doses (2 mg/M2) of *P. acnes* were repeatedly administered subcutaneously at 1- to 2-week intervals [58–61]. Most treated individuals developed mild fevers, and a portion of treated individuals developed injection site reactions that subsided within a few days. Killed *P. acnes* have been tested and shown to produce minimal toxicity in dogs [62] and are commercially available as a United States Department of Agriculture-approved immune stimulant for companion dogs and horses (Neogen).

Using an immunologic adjuvant strategy and intradermal vaccination protocol that maximizes immune responses is essential because cancer antigens are relatively weak immunogens. The stronger the immune response, the higher the number of cancer antigen–specific effector T cells that are generated. The higher the number of cancer antigen–specific effector T cells generated, the greater the potential for producing significant anticancer effects.

Leukocytapheresis. Mononuclear cells are collected from the vaccinated dog by leukocytapheresis to generate cancer antigen–specific effector T cells. The required immune cell precursors are contained within the mononuclear white blood cell compartment. Leukocytapheresis is used because it is an established method for obtaining high numbers of mononuclear white blood cells from a donor without significantly compromising the donor's health. Leukocytapheresis generates high numbers of mononuclear white blood cells because the procedure can selectively target these cells, and other essential blood components are returned to the donor as mononuclear white blood cells

TABLE 2
Schedule of Events for Vaccine-Enhanced Adoptive Cell Therapy

Study Visit		**V1**	**V2**	**V3**	**V4**	**V5**	**V9**	**V10–14**	**V15**
Study visit days	Screen	0	7	14	21	35	42	43–51	57[a]
Diagnosis	X								
Thoracic rads	X								X
Surgery		X							
Vaccination			X	X	X				
Apheresis performed						X			
Activated T-cell infusion							X		
IL-2 injections								X	
Follow-up assessment									X

Includes posttreatment assessment visits (from ELIAS Animal Health protocol).
[a] Thoracic radiographs repeated q3mos after day 57.

are removed, which allows essential blood functions to be maintained. The mononuclear white blood cells that are removed are rapidly replaced by the body. The harvested T cells are *ex vivo* activated and expanded. Table 1 shows a typical example of the high degree of T-cell activation achieved during the *ex vivo* activation process indicated by the increase in the percentage of CD25+ T cells. CD25 is an indicator of T-cell activation being, as it is, one of several cell surface molecules that are upregulated after T-cell activation [63].

Intravenous infusion of ex vivo activated effector T cells. Approximately 1 week after cell collection, the activated T cells are delivered intravenously to the patient on arrival to the clinical site. Dogs receive a pretreatment of diphenhydramine (2 mg/kg, IM) and maropitant (1 mg/kg, SC) approximately 1 hour before infusion to mitigate potential adverse events. After infusion, the administered activated T cells can then travel to and attack cancer cells where they are located. During and after the infusion, the clinician will need to be vigilant for signs of cytokine release syndrome (CRS). CRS is caused by a large, rapid release of cytokines into the blood from immune cells affected by the immunotherapy [64]. Many patients receiving adoptive T cells experience mild to moderate CRS-like effects after their infusions, and in some cases, CRS signs can worsen and quickly become life-threatening. Dogs exhibiting worsening CRS signs (eg, hypotension, fever spike, dyspnea) could be treated with glucocorticoids (dexamethasone 0.25 mg/kg, i.v., qd) to control infusion-related adverse events. All dogs received a pretreatment of diphenhydramine (2 mg kg, IM) and maropitant (1 mg/kg, SC) approximately 1 hour before infusion to assist in mitigating these adverse events.

Injections of interleukin-2. IL-2 (20,000 IU/kg) is injected subcutaneously beginning approximately 24 hours after infusion of activated T cells to continue stimulating T-cell multiplication *in vivo*. Four subsequent doses of IL-2 are delivered at 48-h intervals (5

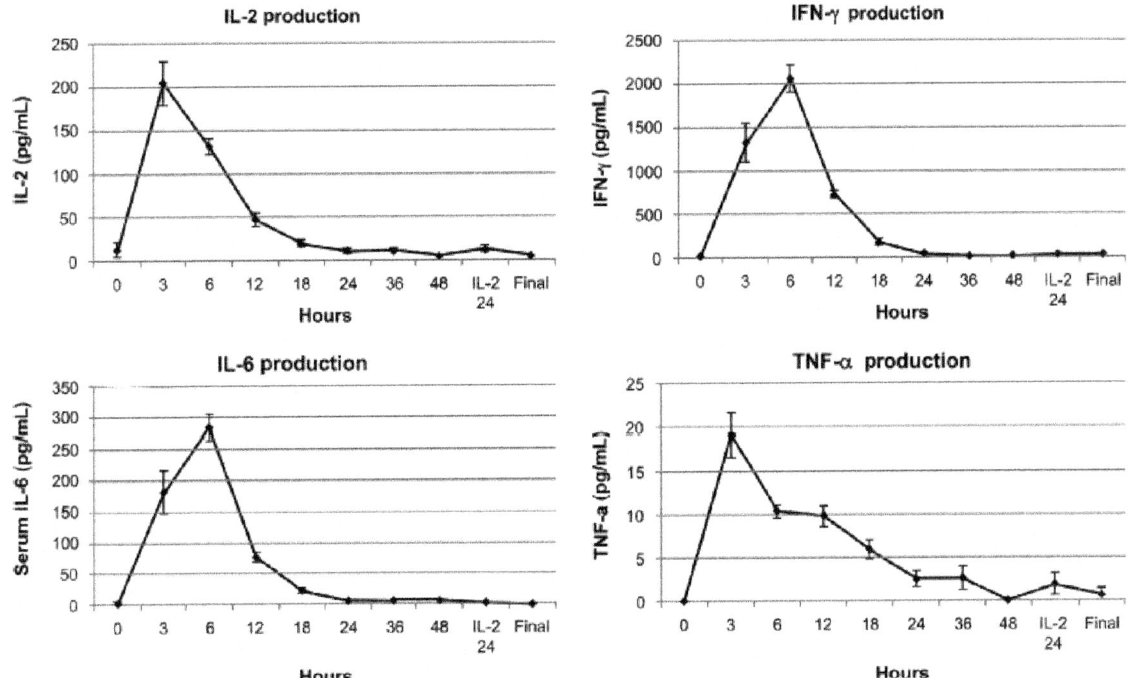

FIG. 2 Cytokine levels in the serum of 4 non–cancer-bearing dogs after activated cellular therapy (ACT). IL-2, IL-6, TNF-α, and IFN-γ were elevated above baseline for 12 hours after the infusion of the activated T cells. Presented are cytokine levels by time point ±SEM. Minimum limits of detection are less than approximately 10 pg/mL. TNF-α lower limit of detection is approximately 6 pg/mL. SEM, standard error of the mean. (*From* Sonderegger FL, Fitzpatrick J, and Wood G., Phase I Clinical Trial to Evaluate the Safety of ELIAS Cancer Immunotherapy, Research Poster presented at 2016 ACVIM conference.)

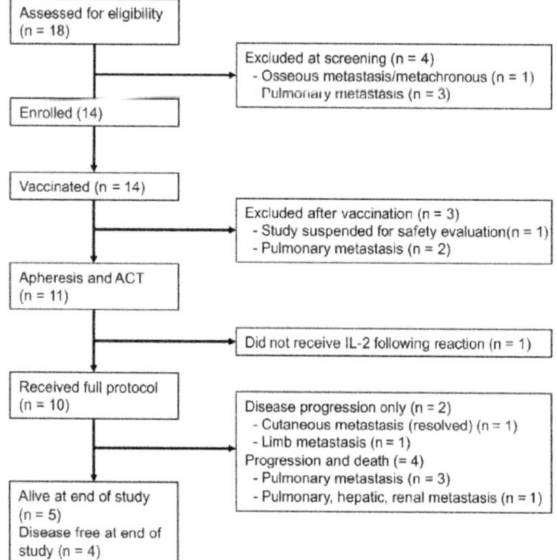

FIG. 3 CONSORT diagram illustrating the outcomes of evaluated and enrolled dogs. (*From* Flesner BK, Wood GW, Gayheart-Walsten P, Sonderegger FL, Henry CJ, Tate DJ, Bechtel SM, Donnelly LL, Johnson GC, Kim DY, Wahaus TA, Bryan JN, Reyes N. Autologous cancer cell vaccination, adoptive T-cell transfer, and interleukin-2 administration results in long-term survival for companion dogs with osteosarcoma. J Vet Intern Med. 2020 Sep;34(5):2056-2067; with permission.)

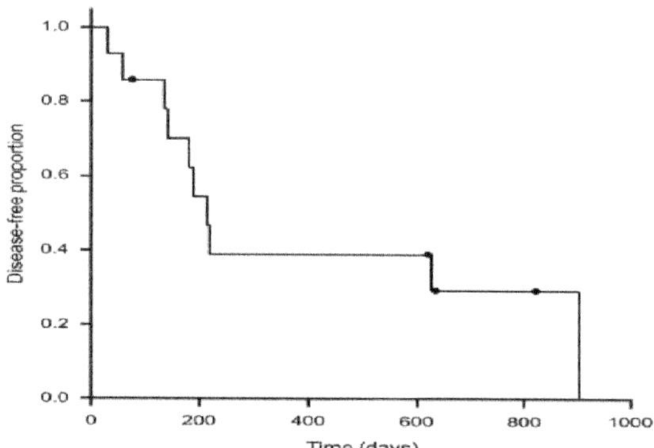

FIG. 4 Disease-free interval (DFI) for all dogs on an intent-to-treat (ITT) basis. The median DFI for all dogs (n = 14) was 213 days. Dogs that were alive at the end of the study (n = 5) were censored (*dots*) as well as 1 dog which was euthanized at the primary veterinarian without disease progression having continued to be monitored for metastasis at the trial site. (*From* Flesner BK, Wood GW, Gayheart-Walsten P, Sonderegger FL, Henry CJ, Tate DJ, Bechtel SM, Donnelly LL, Johnson GC, Kim DY, Wahaus TA, Bryan JN, Reyes N. Autologous cancer cell vaccination, adoptive T-cell transfer, and interleukin-2 administration results in long-term survival for companion dogs with osteosarcoma. J Vet Intern Med. 2020 Sep;34(5):2056-2067; with permission.)

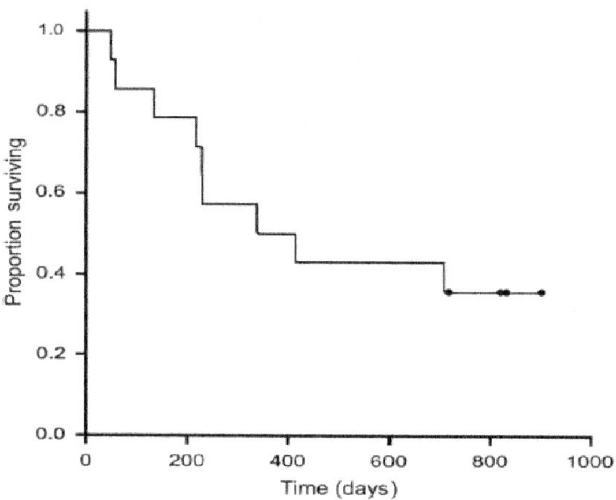

FIG. 5 Overall survival time (OST) for all dogs on an intent-to-treat (ITT) basis. The median OST for all dogs (n = 14) was 415 days. Dogs that were alive at the end of the study (n = 5) were censored (*dots*). The median survival of these 5 dogs at the time of analysis was 822 days. (*From* Flesner BK, Wood GW, Gayheart-Walsten P, Sonderegger FL, Henry CJ, Tate DJ, Bechtel SM, Donnelly LL, Johnson GC, Kim DY, Wahaus TA, Bryan JN, Reyes N. Autologous cancer cell vaccination, adoptive T-cell transfer, and interleukin-2 administration results in long-term survival for companion dogs with osteosarcoma. J Vet Intern Med. 2020 Sep;34(5):2056-2067; with permission.)

doses total). The dosing regimen is designed to continue exposure of infused effector T cells to IL-2 for a prolonged period of time after the administered T cells would have entered cancer tissue, thereby potentially augmenting the anticancer effect generated by those T cells. The dosing regimen used generally is described as low-dose IL-2, to distinguish it from high-dose IL-2, which is used therapeutically as a treatment for metastatic renal cell carcinoma and melanoma in humans [65].

The protocol schedule for VACT immunotherapy is summarized in Table 2.

Vaccine-Enhanced Adoptive Cell Therapy Use in Canine Osteosarcoma

Safety evaluation of vaccine-enhanced adoptive cell therapy procedures in non–cancer-bearing dogs

VACT immunotherapy has been evaluated in canines in two studies examining the safety and efficacy in cancer-bearing and non–cancer-bearing dogs (safety only) [47,48]. In the initial safety study, four healthy dogs followed the VACT protocol from the leukocytapheresis step onward. T-cell activation data and postinfusion

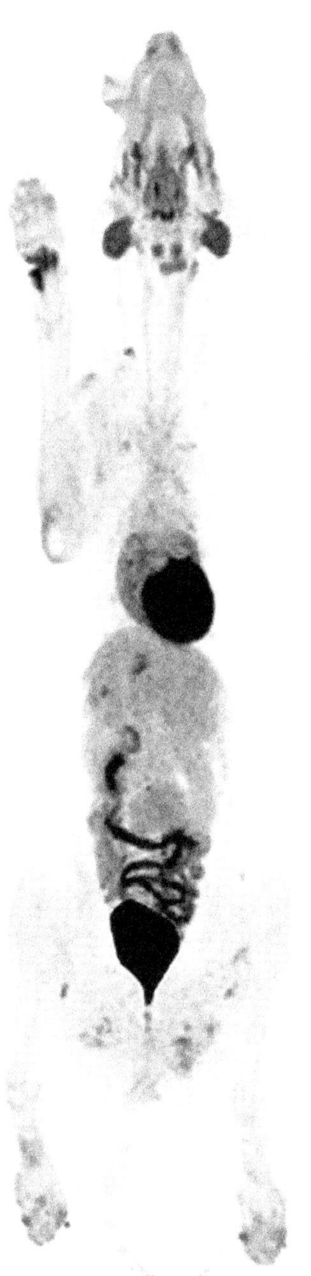

FIG. 6 ^{18}F-FDG PET scan generated on day 363 of a dog diagnosed at day 140 with a cytology confirmed, alkaline phosphatase–positive cutaneous metastatic osteosarcoma (OSA) lesion. No metastatic lesions are visible in this whole-body scan, confirming complete remission. (*From* Flesner BK, Wood GW, Gayheart-Walsten P, Sonderegger FL, Henry CJ, Tate DJ, Bechtel SM, Donnelly LL, Johnson GC, Kim DY, Wahaus TA, Bryan JN, Reyes N. Autologous cancer cell vaccination, adoptive T-cell transfer, and interleukin-2 administration results in long-term survival for companion dogs with osteosarcoma. J Vet Intern Med. 2020 Sep;34(5):2056-2067; with permission.)

serum samples were collected (see Table 1). Serum samples were used to assess any changes in immune-related proinflammatory cytokine levels after T-cell infusion (Fig. 2). Results showed elevated levels from baseline in all examined cytokines (IL-2, IL-6, TNF-α, IFN-γ). The non–cancer-bearing dogs well tolerated the VACT procedures including leukocytapheresis and IL-2 injections. The most commonly reported adverse events were episodes of emesis and gastrointestinal disturbances of a transient nature which did not correlate with any particular VACT procedure.

Safety and efficacy evaluation of vaccine-enhanced adoptive cell therapy procedures in osteosarcoma-bearing dogs

VACT immunotherapy also was evaluated in dogs newly diagnosed with appendicular OSA in a clinical trial [47]. To be eligible for the trial, dogs had to have their affected limb intact, not had any prior treatment for OSA, not received glucocorticoids within 2 weeks of enrollment, have CBC/blood chemistries profiles within normal limits, and have no sign of metastatic disease as evaluated by thoracic radiographs. In this small trial, 18 dogs were evaluated, with 14 OSA-bearing dogs ultimately enrolled in the study. All dogs underwent amputation surgery of the affected limb followed by the VACT treatment described earlier. Dogs were followed up for overall survival for up to 2 years after treatment. The overall median survival at 1-year postdiagnosis and the disease-free intervals were also assessed. The evaluation of these 18 patients and their outcomes are summarized in Fig. 3.

For this study, an overall median overall survival time and disease-free intervals for the "intent-to-treat" populations were 415 days and 213 days, respectively. These results are shown as Kaplan–Meier graphs in Figs. 4 and 5. Dogs on study received no further treatment for their cancer after VACT was completed. Of the 14 dogs undergoing VACT, 5 responded to therapy (36%) and survived disease-free for at least 2 years. One responsive dog had reoccurrence of OSA at 2 years, whereas the other 4 dogs were cancer-free at study conclusion. Among the responders was a dog that developed a cutaneous lesion 140 days after VACT. This lesion was confirmed via cytology as OSA, and the owners decided against further therapy. On recheck

TABLE 3
Toxicoses Summarized by Organ System

	Toxicosis						
Procedure	**Admin Site**	**Gastrointestinal**	**Bone Marrow**	**Cardiac**	**Respiratory**	**Constitutional**	**Fever**
Vaccine	ISR(14) - I	V(1[b])- I					
Leukapheresis			M(1) - II	AV(1)- II			
ACT		V(1[b])- I			C(1[a])- I	L(1[a])- II, W(1[a])- II	F(1[a])- III
IL-2	V(2)- I, N(2)-I D(3)-I/II (2)						

Attributions were assigned by temporal correlation to each phase of the trial. Reactions that occurred before the second dose of IL-2 were attributed to ACT. Reactions that continued after the second dose of IL-2 were attributed to L-2.

Letter indicates toxicosis, (n) is the number of patients, and roman numerals indicate grade of toxicosis. Example: (D3) – I/II/III means 3 patients had grade I, II or III diarrhea.

Abbreviations: AV, AV mock; BR, injection site reaction; C, cough; D, diarrhea; F, fever; L, lethargy; M, myelosupprcssion; N, nausea; V, vomiting; W, weight loss.

[a] Patient treated before premedicants.

[b] Toxicosis unlikely attributable to intervention.

From Flesner BK, Wood GW, Gayheart-Walsten P, Sonderegger FL, Henry CJ, Tate DJ, Bechtel SM, Donnelly LL, Johnson GC, Kim DY, Wahaus TA, Bryan JN, Reyes N. Autologous cancer cell vaccination, adoptive T-cell transfer, and interleukin-2 administration results in long-term survival for companion dogs with osteosarcoma. J Vet Intern Med. 2020 Sep;34(5):2056-2067; with permission.

approximately 2 months afterward, no mass could be identified, and a whole-body PET scan also revealed no cancerous lesions. The appearance and spontaneous resolution of a confirmed metastatic lesion is suggestive of an immunologic response to the new lesion. This dog was among the 5 responsive cancer-free and alive individuals at study completion (Fig. 6).

The median overall survival time of 415 days is improved compared with those reported for standard of care therapy involving amputation followed by chemotherapy (~307 days) [66]. However, this was a small-sized study and did not have a concurrent control group, and thus, additional studies are needed to better characterize the therapy's efficacy. OSA-bearing dogs undergoing VACT tolerated the therapy well.

As can be seen in Table 3, most reported adverse events were characterized as mild to moderate [Veterinary Cooperative Oncology Group (VCOG) ratings I and II], with the exception of one VCOG Grade III (serious) reported incident of fever. Most adverse events also were reported as transitory in nature.

Although 5 of 14 treated study dogs were cancer-free at 2 years posttherapy, response to therapy varied. Potential causes of nonresponding dogs include the patient's own immune response to the vaccines which is reflected in the number of cancer neoantigen–specific T cells present in the mononuclear cell collection, the aggressiveness of the patient's specific cancer, the immunosuppressiveness of the patient's tumor microenvironment, and the patient's remaining cancer tumor burden.

SIGNIFICANCE AND FUTURE DIRECTIONS

Adoptive cell therapies, such as VACT, represent impactful new modalities for the treatment of cancers. These therapies harness the patient's immune system to eliminate their own cancer cells in a highly specific manner. Conditioning of the T cells through autologous tumor vaccines allows for a personalized cancer neoantigen–specific treatment with low toxicity. In human clinical trials, VACT has been shown to improve survival times and, in some cases, generate complete long-term cancer remission in responsive patients [34,35]. The VACT adapted for dogs described here is among the first adoptive T-cell therapies available to veterinarians for the treatment of cancer [67]. Adoptive T-cell therapies such as VACT hold the promise of being able to treat multiple types of cancer as seen human clinical trials and in canine OSA. Further evaluations of VACT in combination with chemotherapy, radiation, or other biologics may provide useful insights into how this treatment modality can be successfully applied in other cancer disease settings.

CLINICS CARE POINTS

- VACT is a personalized immunotherapy which conditions the patient's immune system to recognize cancer neoantigens and eradicate cancer cells in a highly specific manner
- VACT has potential to treat cancers where tumor material can be harvested to manufacture autologous vaccines
- Autologous vaccines provide *in vivo* priming of T cells to cancer neoantigens
- Leukocytapheresis provides a safe and consistent method of collecting large numbers of primed T cells for use in *ex vivo* activation and expansion
- Activated T cells are known to be responsible for cancer cell–killing activities
- VACT was well tolerated in dogs in a clinical trial examining appendicular OSA
- Cytokine release syndrome is a potential sequalae of adoptive T-cell therapies, and patients must be monitored for CRS signs after T-cell infusion
- Intravenously administered dexamethasone (0.25 mg/kg) has been successfully used to control CRS signs
- Cancer burden, overall immune health, and immunosuppressive tumor microenvironment may influence patient response rates
- Fully responsive patients may not need further cancer therapy after VACT

REFERENCES

[1] Rosenberg SA. Lysis of human normal and sarcoma cells in tissue culture by normal human serum: implications for experiments in human tumor immunology. J Natl Cancer Inst 1977;58(5):1233–8.

[2] Cohen CJ, Gartner JJ, Horovitz-Fried M, et al. Isolation of neoantigen-specific T cells from tumor and peripheral lymphocytes. J Clin Invest 2015;125(10):3981–91.

[3] Bianchi V, Alexandre H, Coukos G. Neoantigen-specific adoptive cell therapies for cancer: making T-cell products more personal. Front Immunol 2020;11:1215.

[4] Ott PA, Dotti G, Yee C, et al. An update on adoptive T-cell therapy and neoantigen vaccines. Am Soc Clin Oncol Educ Book 2019;39:e70–8.

[5] Foley EJ. Antigenic properties of methylcholanthrene-induced tumors in mice of the strain of origin. Cancer Res 1953;13(12):835–7.

[6] Dranoff G, Jaffee E, Lazenby A, et al. Vaccination with irradiated tumor cells engineered to secrete murine granulocyte-macrophage colony-stimulating factor stimulates potent, specific, and long-lasting anti-tumor immunity. Proc Natl Acad Sci U S A 1993;90(8):3539–43.

[7] Smith RT. Tumor-specific immune mechanisms. N Engl J Med 1968;278:1207–14.

[8] Baldwin RW. Tumour-associated antigens and tumour-host interactions. Proc R Soc Med 1971;64:1039–42.

[9] Perlmann P, Holm G. Cytotoxic effects of lymphoid cells in vitro. Adv Immunol 1969;11:117–93.

[10] Golstein P, Blomgren H, Svedmyr EA, et al. On T-cell-mediated cytotoxicity. Transpl Proc 1973;5(4):1441–5.

[11] Shu S, Chou T, Rosenberg SA. In vitro sensitization and expansion with viable tumor cells and interleukin 2 in the generation of specific therapeutic effector cells. J Immunol 1986;136(10):3891–8.

[12] Chou T, Shu S. Cellular interactions and the role of interleukin 2 in the expression and induction of immunity against a syngeneic murine sarcoma. J Immunol 1987;139(6):2103–9.

[13] Cheever MA, Greenberg PD, Fefer A. Specificity of adoptive chemoimmunotherapy of established syngeneic tumors. J Immunol 1980;125:711–4.

[14] Eberlein TJ, Rosenstein M, Spiess P, et al. Adoptive chemoimmunotherapy of a syngeneic murine leukemia with long-term lymphoid cell lines expanded in T cell growth factor. Cancer Immunol Immunother 1982;13:5–13.

[15] Blank CU, Haanen JB, Ribas A, et al. Cancer immunology. The cancer immunogram. Science 2016;352:658–60.

[16] Holladay FP, Lopez G, De M, et al. Generation of cytotoxic immune responses against a rat glioma by in vivo priming and secondary in vitro stimulation with tumor cells. Neurosurgery 1992;30:499–505.

[17] Cheever MA, Kempf RA, Fefer A. Tumor neutralization, immunotherapy, and chemoimmmunotherapy of a Friend leukemia with cells secondarily sensitized in vitro. J Immunol 1977;119:714–8.

[18] Holladay FP, Heitz T, Chen Y-L, et al. Successful treatment of a malignant rat glioma with cytotoxic T cells. Neurosurgery 1992;31:528–33.

[19] Aruga E, Aruga A, Arca MJ, et al. Immune responsiveness to a murine mammary carcinoma modified to express B7-1, interleukin-12, or GM-CSF. Cancer Gene Ther 1997;4:157–66.

[20] Tamai H, Watanabe S, Zheng R, et al. Effective treatment of spontaneous metastases derived from a poorly immunogenic murine mammary carcinoma by combined dendritic-tumor hybrid vaccination and adoptive transfer of sensitized T cells. Clin Immunol 2008;127:66–77.

[21] Cha E, Graham L, Manjili MH, et al. IL-7 and IL-15 are superior to IL-2 for the ex vivo expansion of 4T1 mammary carcinoma-specific T cells with greater efficacy against tumors in vivo. Breast Cancer Res Treat 2010;122:359–69.

[22] Saxton ML, Longo DL, Wetzel HE, et al. Adoptive transfer of anti-CD3-activated CD4+ T cells plus cyclophosphamide and liposome-encapsulated interleukin-2 cure murine MC-38 and 3LL tumors and establish tumor-specific immunity. Blood 1997;89:2529–36.

[23] Seki N, Brooks AD, Carter CR, et al. Tumor-specific CTL kill murine renal cancer cells using both perforin and Fas ligand-mediated lysis in vitro, but cause tumor regression in vivo in the absence of perforin. J Immunol 2002;168: 3484–92.

[24] Crossland KD, Lee VK, Chen W, et al. T cells from tumor-immune mice nonspecifically expanded in vitro with anti-CD3 plus IL-2 retain specific function in vitro and can eradicate disseminated leukemia in vivo. J Immunol 1991;146:4414–20.

[25] Kaido T, Maury C, Schirrmacher V, et al. Successful immunotherapy of the highly metastatic murine ESb lymphoma with sensitized CD8+ T cells and IFN-alpha/beta. Int J Cancer 1994;57:538–43.

[26] Geiger JD, Wagner PD, Cameron MJ, et al. Generation of T-cells reactive to the poorly immunogenic B16-BL6 melanoma with efficacy in the treatment of spontaneous metastases. J Immunother Emphasis Tumor Immunol 1993 Apr;13(3):153–65.

[27] Le HK, Graham L, Miller CH, et al. Incubation of antigen-sensitized T lymphocytes activated with bryostatin 1 + ionomycin in IL-7 + IL-15 increases yield of cells capable of inducing regression of melanoma metastases compared to culture in IL-2. Cancer Immunol Immunother 2009;581565–76.

[28] Zhang Q, Yang X, Pins M, et al. Adoptive transfer of tumor-reactive transforming growth factor-beta-insensitive CD8+ T cells: eradication of autologous mouse prostate cancer. Cancer Res 2005;65:1761–9.

[29] Ward-Kavanagh LK, Zhu J, Cooper TK, et al. Whole body irradiation increases the magnitude and persistence of adoptively transferred T cells associated with tumor regression in a mouse model of prostate cancer. Cancer Immunol Res 2014;2:777–88.

[30] Ruttinger D, Li R, Urba WJ, et al. Regression of bone metastases following adoptive transfer of anti-CD3-activated and IL-2-expanded tumor vaccine draining lymph node cells. Clin Exp Metastasis 2004;21:305–12.

[31] Chou T, Bertera S, Chang AE, et al. Adoptive immunotherapy of microscopic and advanced visceral metastases with in vitro sensitized lymphoid cells from mice bearing progressive tumors. J Immunol 1988;141:1775–81.

[32] Peng L, Shu S, Krauss JC. Treatment of subcutaneous tumor with adoptively transferred T-cells. Cell Immunol 1997;178:24–32.

[33] Chang AE, Aruga A, Cameron MJ, et al. Adoptive immunotherapy with vaccine primed lymph node cells secondarily activated with anti-CD3 and interleukin 2. J Clin Oncol 1997;15:796–807.

[34] Sloan AE, Dansey R, Zamorano L, et al. Adoptive immunotherapy in patients with recurrent malignant glioma: preliminary results of using autologous whole-tumor vaccine plus granulocyte-macrophage colony-stimulating factor and adoptive transfer of anti-CD3-activated lymphocytes. Neurosurg Focus 2000;9:1–8.

[35] Chang AE, Jiang GI Sayre DM, Braun TM, et al. Phase II trial of autologous tumor vaccination, anti-CD3-activated vaccine-primed lymphocytes, and interleukin-2 in stage IV renal cell cancer. J Clin Oncol 2003;21:884–90.

[36] Dudley ME, Wunderlich JR, Yang JC, et al. Adoptive cell transfer therapy following non-myeloablative but lymphodepleting chemotherapy for the treatment of patients with refractory metastatic melanoma. J Clin Oncol 2005; 23:2346–57.

[37] Dudley ME, Yang JC, Sherry R, et al. Adoptive cell therapy for patients with metastatic melanoma: evaluation of intensive myeloablative chemoradiation preparative regimens. J Clin Oncol 2008;26:5233–9.

[38] Besser MJ, Shapira-Frommer R, Treves AJ, et al. Clinical responses in a phase II study using adoptive transfer of short-term cultured tumor infiltration lymphocytes in metastatic melanoma patients. Clin Cancer Res 2010; 16:2646–55.

[39] Pilon-Thomas S, Kuhn L, Ellwanger S, et al. Efficacy of adoptive cell transfer of tumor- infiltrating lymphocytes after lymphopenia induction for metastatic melanoma. J Immunother 2012;35:615–20.

[40] Maus MV, Grupp SA, Porter DL, et al. Antibody-modified T cells: CARs take the front seat for hematologic malignancies. Blood 2014;123:2625–35.

[41] Dotti G, Gottschalk S, et al. Design and development of therapies using chimeric antigen receptor-expressing T cells. Immunol Rev 2014;257:107–26.

[42] Greenberg PD, Cheever MA, Fefer A. Eradication of disseminated murine leukemia by chemoimmunotherapy with cyclophosphamide and adoptively transferred immune syngeneic Lyt-1+2- lymphocytes. J Exp Med 1981;154:952–63.

[43] Bookman MA, Swerdlow R, Matis LA. Adoptive chemo-immunotherapy of murine leukemia with helper T lymphocyte clone. J Immunol 1987;139:3166–70.

[44] Awwad M, North RJ. Cyclophosphamide (Cy)-facilitated adoptive immunotherapy of a Cy-resistant tumour. Evidence that Cy permits the expression of adoptive T-cell mediated immunity by removing suppressor T cells rather than by reducing tumour burden. Immunology 1988;65:87–92.

[45] Shu S, Chou T, Sakai K. Lymphocytes generated by in vivo priming and in vitro sensitization demonstrate therapeutic efficacy against a murine tumor that lacks apparent immunogenicity. J Immunol 1989;143(2):740–8.

[46] Geiger JD, Wagner PD, Shu S, et al. A novel role for autologous tumor cell vaccination in the immunotherapy of the poorly immunogenic B16-BL6 melanoma. Surg Oncol 1992;1(3):199–208.

[47] Flesner B, Wood G, Gayheart-Walstein, et al. Autologous cancer cell vaccination, adoptive T-cell transfer,and interleukin-2 administration results in long-term survival for companion dogs with osteosarcoma. J Vet Intern Med 2020;34(5):2056–67.

[48] Sonderegger FL, Fitzpatrick J, Wood G. Phase I clinical trial to evaluate the safety of ELIAS cancer immunotherapy, Research Poster presented at June 08-11, 2016 ACVIM conference;Denver, CO.

[49] Fenger JM, London CA, Kisseberth W. Canine osteosarcoma: a naturally occurring disease to inform pediatric oncology. ILAR J 2014;55(Issue 1):69–85.

[50] Simpson S, Dunning MD, de Brot S. Comparative review of human and canine osteosarcoma: morphology, epidemiology, prognosis, treatment and genetics. Acta Vet Scand 2017;59:71.

[51] Szewczyk M, Lechowski R, Zabielska K. What do we know about canine osteosarcoma treatment? – Review. Vet Res Commun 2015;39:61–7.

[52] Hoover HC Jr, Surdyke M, Dangel RB, et al. Delayed cutaneous hypersensitivity to autologous tumor cells in colorectal cancer patients immunized with an autologous tumor cell: Bacillus Calmette-Guerin vaccine. Cancer Res 1984;44(4):1671–6.

[53] Berd D, Maguire HC, McCue P, et al. Treatment of metastatic melanoma with autologous tumor cell vaccine: clinical and immunologic results in 64 patients. J Clin Oncol 1990;8(11):1858–67.

[54] Simons JW, Jaffee EM, Weber CE, et al. Bioactivity of autologous irradiated renal cell carcinoma vaccines generated by ex vivo granulocyte-macrophage colony-stimulating factor gene transfer. Cancer Res 1997;57(8): 1537–46.

[55] Nelson WG, Simons JW, Mikhak B, et al. Cancer cells engineered to secrete granulocyte-macrophage colony-stimulating factor using ex vivo gene transfer as vaccines for the treatment of genitourinary malignancies. Cancer Chemother Pharmacol 2000;46(Suppl):S67–72.

[56] Salgia R, Lynch T, Skarin A, et al. Vaccination with irradiated autologous tumor cells engineered to secrete granulocyte-macrophage colony-stimulating factor augments antitumor immunity in some patients with metastatic non-small-cell lung carcinoma. J Clin Oncol 2003; 21:624–30.

[57] Chan B, Lee W, Hu CX, et al. Adoptive cellular immunotherapy for non-small cell lung cancer: a pilot study. Cytotherapy 2003;5(1):46–54.

[58] Lipton A, Harvey HA, Balch CM, et al. Corynebacterium parvum versus bacille Calmette-Guérin adjuvant immunotherapy of stage II malignant melanoma. J Clin Oncol 1991;9:1151–6.

[59] Thatcher N, Mene A, Banerjee SS, et al. Randomized study of Corynebacterium parvum adjuvant therapy following surgery for (stage II) malignant melanoma. Br J Surg 1986;73(2):111–5.

[60] Balch CM, Smalley RV, Bartolucci AA, et al. A randomized prospective clinical trial of adjuvant C. parvum immunotherapy in 260 patients with clinically localized melanoma (Stage I): prognostic factors analysis and preliminary results of immunotherapy. Cancer 1982; 49(6):1079–84.

[61] Lipton A, Harvey HA, Lawrence B, et al. Corynebacterium parvum versus BCG adjuvant immunotherapy in human malignant melanoma. Cancer 1983;51:57–60.

[62] Poot J, Janssen LH, van Kasteren-Westerneng TJ, et al. Vaccination of dogs with six different candidate leishmaniasis vaccines composed of a chimerical recombinant protein containing ribosomal and histone protein epitopes in combination with different adjuvants. Vaccine 2009;27(33):4439–46.

[63] Bajnok A, Ivanova M, Rigó J, et al. The distribution of activation markers and selectins on peripheral T lymphocytes in preeclampsia. Mediators Inflamm 2017;2017: 8045161.

[64] National Cancer Institute. Available at: https://www.cancer.gov/publications/dictionaries/cancer-terms/def/cytokine-release-syndrome. Accessed March 3, 2021.

[65] Helfand SC, Modiano JF, Nowell PC. Immunophysiological studies of interleukin-2 and canine lymphocytes. Vet Immunol Immunopathol 1992;33(1–2):1–16.

[66] Phillips B, Powers BE, Dernell WS, et al. Use of single-agent carboplatin as adjuvant or neoadjuvant therapy in conjunction with amputation for appendicular osteosarcoma in dogs. J Am Anim Hosp Assoc 2009;45(1): 33–8.

[67] VACT (ELIAS cancer immunotherapy) is distributed as an experimental product for the treatment of cancer in dogs in accordance with USDA regulations under 9 CFR 103.3. Safety and efficacy have not been established.

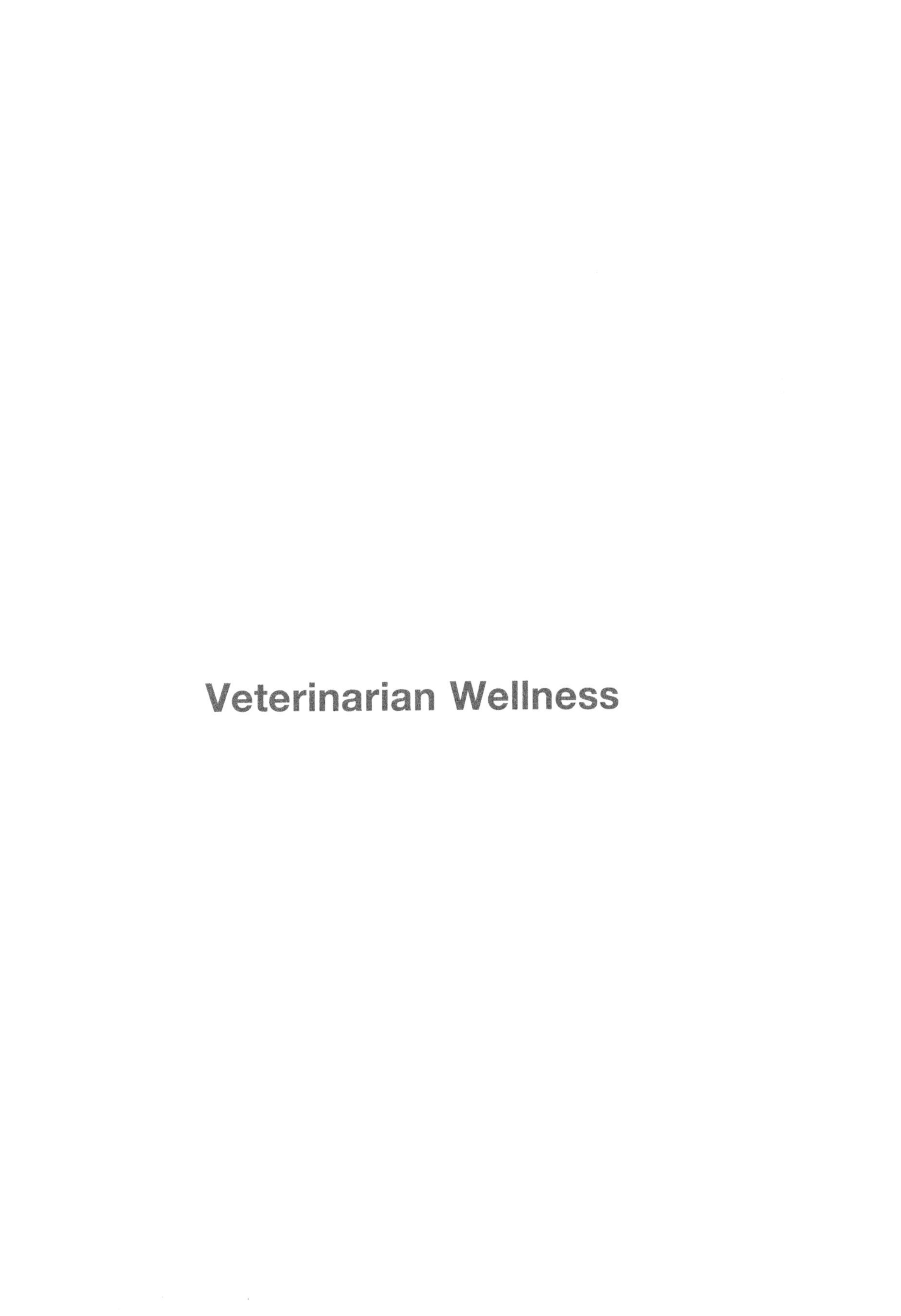

Veterinarian Wellness

Advances in Small Animal Care 2 (2021) 157–162
ADVANCES IN SMALL ANIMAL CARE

How to Toughen Them up Without Roughin' Them Up

Katie Cagel-Holtcamp, PhD[a,b], Pauline Prince, PhD, ABN[b,*]
[a]Mississippi State University College of Veterinary Medicine, Starkville, MS, USA; [b]Office of Academic Affairs, Mississippi State University, PO Box 6100, Mississippi State, MS 39762-6100, USA

KEYWORDS
• Hazing • Hidden curriculum • Problem-focused instruction

KEY POINTS

- There are skills that all veterinarians need to have acquired in order to be successful in professional practice. Not all of those skills come from "formal" classroom learning but as a direct result of a "hidden curriculum." Some of the skills acquired through a hidden learning experience is necessary to allow for one veterinarian to communicate with another or to move from one practice site to another and practice professionally in all settings.
- The practice of veterinary medicine requires long hours, grueling work activities, and the navigation of a wide variety of difficult circumstances around patient care and client interactions. Physical and mental exhaustion can contribute to high stress and interpersonal tensions. In a training environment, these factors can contribute to students feeling like they have been poorly treated and without the proper resources to handle the intensity of the stress of the job demands. From a training site perspective, these experiences are necessary to "toughen them up" for the "real world work" settings.
- There are strategies that can be implemented to "toughen up" our students without "roughin' them up" while preparing them for the difficulties of a real-world work setting.

INTRODUCTION

The process of becoming a skilled, polished veterinarian is somewhat similar to the process of becoming a smooth, polished river stone. River stones start out as a solid material with jagged edges. As the rocks travel down river, the jagged edges are chipped away as they experience some of the harsh realities of the riverbed and the fast-paced course of the flow of the river.

Eventually, though, the rocks emerge solid, well rounded, and polished. Although our students walk through the door with solid skills and the right core qualities to become skilled, polished veterinarians, the fast-paced learning environment and harsh realities of some of the clinical rotations and training demands can leave some students feeling bumped, bruised, and abused.

Most "teaching" veterinarians in our veterinary medical schools are skilled and talented individuals with a passion for their craft. However, for many teaching clinicians, their area of expertise is veterinary medicine—not formal educational principles such as learning, memory, educational assessment, and the influence of emotions on skill acquisition and demonstration. Many teach as they were taught. They pass along the same lessons, rituals, routines, and experiences in the same fashion, sometimes without any consideration as to whether the information or process still holds any relevant value. Formal course content changes as research and technology improve the knowledge base. However, much of the day-to-day practices of veterinary medicine are taught through a hidden curriculum, which changes quite slowly, if at all. All professions have a hidden curriculum that teach the jargon,

*Corresponding author, *E-mail address:* Pjp40@msstate.edu Twitter: @BrainMatters5 (P.P.)

https://doi.org/10.1016/j.yasa.2021.06.004
2666-450X/21/ © 2021 Elsevier Inc. All rights reserved.

routines, and professional culture that allow one member to convey information to other members is an efficient manner. Some lessons of the hidden curriculum can also involve rites of passage, both positive, coating ceremonies for example and negative, such as hazing. Rites of passage and hazing tend to persist for the same reasons—tradition and as evidence that each new member is "worthy" and now deemed capable to withstand the actual and "perceived" real-life demands of the profession. But is hazing a necessary component of the hidden curriculum or is there a better way to "toughen them up" without "roughin' them up"?

HAZING IN THE WORKPLACE

Hazing is defined as a health harming mistreatment of individuals by one or more perceived and/or actual superiors. This behavior can include threats, humiliation, intimidation, sabotage, and/or verbal abuse [1]. In veterinary medicine it is important to remember the rules are different than in other professional work environments. Specifically, veterinary students do not always have the option to report hazing or to find a new placement. Students spend 4 years at an undergraduate university in hopes of being accepted to at least one veterinary school with the odds being stacked against them every step of the way. Once a student is accepted, it is not advised for them to try to find a new placement. A new placement would also require them to start over or sit out a year before another admission cycle was available. Hazing is highly documented in other medical professions such as medical school, nursing, and dentistry. The trouble identifying these tactics is that mostly everyone in these professions is talented to some degree, have a high productivity rate, and are considered exceptional by those who have used them. Because of these factors many cases of hazing go unreported [2].

So, why we are still seeing so many hazing initiatives continuously present in veterinary medicine despite veterinarians who are showings signs of distress? Job satisfaction and career changes in the veterinary world are increasing each year. For those individuals not leaving the field, mental health concerns are becoming more frequent. A review of the literature on the concept of the Hidden Curriculum [3–5] suggests that many veterinary faculty and staff believe students are lacking a specific skill set necessary to be a competent veterinarian outside of the school walls. These skill sets are not specifically defined nor intuitive for many students. A review of the literature on hidden curriculums in veterinary medicine resulted in the identification of 7 skills that were weak or lacking but necessary for veterinary students to master before the end of fourth year. These skills include safety awareness, perspective, open mindedness, problem solving, awareness for life experiences, direct communication, and connective communication.

WAYS TO TEACH THE SKILL SET WITHOUT ROUGHING UP THE STUDENTS

When considering the best way to implement these skillsets within a veterinary school, problem-based learning was at the forefront of effective teaching methods [6]. In problem-based learning the students are the focus of the approach, and group work and team building are used to solve an open-ended problem, which is the motivating factor for the learning. These concepts include critical thinking, self-directed learning, researching, information organization, oral and written communication requirements, and independent work. All of these activities can be used throughout curriculum and clinical portions of veterinary school. Regardless of what skill is being taught, problem-based learning can be used to accomplish the goals.

Not all of our current students enter veterinary medicine school with the same experience with problem-based learning. Two major societal changes occurred that influenced the development of problem-based learning experiences: common core and unstructured play. Much of the current generation of students began their formal grade school education in a system that emphasized, and rewarded, fact-based learning. Memorize these facts and regurgitate them for a test. In 2009, the Common Core State Standards Initiative was released [7]. Common Core uses a problem-solving, abstract reasoning approach: take this fact and that fact and draw a conclusion, make a prediction, or in some manner analyze the information. Many school systems changed overnight without necessarily providing some type of "transition" process to students or their parents. Many of the current generation of students still study from a "fact-based learning" perspective and struggle to switch to the abstract, problem-solving approach that is necessary to survive veterinary medicine [8].

One of the most significant differences between some of the older veterinarians that teach veterinary medicine and their students is the usage prevalence of video games and nonstop access to television or media. For many there is a definite generational gap in the manner of play. Many clinicians who grew up in the 50s, 60s, and 70s played outside. Free, unstructured play, such as stick ball and/or building tree forts, taught abstract problem-solving skills in a manner that is quite different than the skill sets acquired through video gaming. Neuropsychological research has demonstrated that motor play lays the neurocognitive foundation for many executive functioning skills including cognitive problem solving. Teaching the *process* of problem-based learning is an excellent way to ensure that all our students learn to think as veterinarians without assumptions that they automatically have that knowledge base or skill set [8].

SAFETY

Although not every student encounters hazing in veterinary school, each student has been given numerous lectures on safety, which includes safety in the laboratory, safety when handling biohazardous materials, and safety when working with small and large animals. With all of the physical movement in a veterinary school it is easy for safety standards to slip and create a larger concern. Teaching veterinarians are simultaneously responsible for the students and the animals in their care and thus take on an additional level of stress when they are in the clinical learning environment [9]. When students make a mistake that results in a safety concern, it is not uncommon for the teaching clinician to change the tone and increase the intensity and volume of their words to hopefully teach the student what went wrong and how to prevent it from happening again. This necessary form of action, in a stressful moment, can look and feel as if a staff member is yelling at a student, in front of witnesses, and humiliating the individual who made a mistake. These situations will never be totally unavoidable. However, a problem-based learning model provides an opportunity to teach safety routines through anticipatory "walk-throughs" and cognitive rehearsal of some of the more common safety situations and procedures, so that all students can hone intuition for circumstances, even when they have little experience with a particular clinical/treatment event.

PERSPECTIVE

This skill is all about how a student views themselves and uses that understanding to survive in a professional setting. Perspective in this sense encompasses self-awareness and focuses on students' abilities to effectively rank their skills, identify weaknesses, and seek opportunities to improve them [10]. Students are also encouraged to understand things they do well and apply their strengths in all tasks and problem solving. Although this initial idea of self-awareness can be postulated to be a negative experience, research indicates objective self-awareness can improve positive self-evaluation skills, which improve realistic competency identification overall. When students can correctly identify areas of weaker competence, they can seek out specific experiences or knowledge to master the competency.

Another part of perspective is related to emotional well-being and emotional control [11]. Veterinary faculty consider it a beneficial skill when individuals can emotionally regulate in a tough moment, stay focused, and solve the problem at hand. Although it is well documented that an individual's suppression of emotions is damaging to their mental health in the long term, this skill is designed to get through a tough trial in the moment, with emotions being processed more completely after the resolution. In the field of sport and performance psychology, it is well known that one has not truly mastered a skill until they can demonstrate that skill under circumstances of intense emotionality. Quick thinking and effective decision-making are viewed as critical skills for a successful veterinarian. Survival in the profession requires utilization of resources (colleagues, mental health professionals, and so forth) and protective factors (self-care, exercise, and so forth) to process intense emotions that naturally come with a fast-paced, stressful situation, which often requires the making life and death decisions.

The final portion to the perspective skill comes with emotional intelligence [12]. Clinicians are reporting students close to graduations are at a critical low point of being able to understand their client's emotional needs. This inability to connect and create a sense of trust between provider and client can inhibit their ability to do the job to the fullest capacity. Becoming emotionally intelligent allows students to properly calculate risks, navigate challenging social interactions, effectively handle increased pressure in the workplace, and make common-sense decisions in the moment.

Some teaching clinicians, in many professions, believe that hazing behaviors specifically help grow this aspect and teach how to handle increased pressure while navigating challenging social situations. Veterinary medical students tend to be competitive, high achieving, perfectionistic "A" personalities with a tendency toward anxiety disorders. If the teaching situation is known to be intrinsically negative and/or unpredictability threatening, intimidating, and/or humiliating, then students become hypervigilant. Hypervigilance increases distraction and reduces the availability for learning [13]. Hazing sets up circumstances that interfere with the instructional objectives. Problem-focused learning, on the other hand, allows for the teaching of critical thinking skills through case examples and shared problem solving; the group dynamics of a rotation can be used to increase trust and teach how to properly calculate risks, navigate challenging social interactions, effectively handle increased pressure in the workplace, and make common-sense decisions in the moment.

OPEN MINDEDNESS

The skill of open-mindedness came when discussing the transition from specializations to general medicine in the veterinary field [14]. Although many students liked the idea of specializing with their favorite species or job description, each individual who graduates from a veterinary school is expected to be competent with all general animals and in all basic fields. When students start in general medicine and then move to a specialty, the transition is a bit easier; however, when an individual has spent time in their favorite specialization and then has to swap back over to general population medicine, the transition is a bit harder. The idea of open-mindedness does not take away from an individual's personal values or career objectives. This skill simply creates the opportunity for broader thinking and more options with regard to potential first job opportunities. The open-minded approach provides the best chance at identifying false or misleading beliefs. Finally, open mindedness allows conversations and communication to continue even when the stakes are high.

Open mindedness is best taught in an atmosphere free from humiliation, intimidation, and fear of failure. For students to be comfortable asking questions, wagering an educated guess, and/or seeking clarification, the teaching clinicians must also be open minded. Often, teaching clinicians are specialists in the rotation for which they teach. Most are passionate about their field of interest, and this passion is evident in their instruction as well as their conversations. Open-minded clinicians have greater opportunities to inspire students to specialize in their area of expertise when the passion for the specialty is the driving force rather than disparaging remarks toward opposing opinions.

PROBLEM SOLVING

The skill of problem solving is the ability to identify the goal and create a reasonable pattern of behavior to achieve it [15]. A veterinary student is encouraged to be able to make a mental representation of the issue and determine the appropriate steps to move forward. The student is then expected to execute the plan and monitor the resolution status. Veterinary faculty, in previous research, have indicated students lack self-initiative when a problem arises. Students have been described to wait for instruction instead of moving forward with the challenge immediately. Veterinary faculty understand that some of these students will move on to private practice and will not always have a direct supervisor instructing their every move. Therefore, it has been deemed critical for veterinary students to demonstrate appropriate problem-solving skills during their clinical rotations. Veterinary school is an appropriate place for students to take initiative and make mistakes because they do have oversight, and the final responsibility to the animal client does lie on the supervising veterinarian, and this allows the student to have a little leeway in identifying treatment protocols, implementing the plan, and evaluating the outcome.

Some highly anxious students are fearful of making mistakes, especially when there is a life in their hands. Awaiting confirmation from the teaching clinicians is viewed as preferrable to potentially causing harm to an animal. Lack of initiative can be driven by a lack of faith in one's skill set and knowledge base. "Fear of failure," despite having the knowledge and the skills, is a common source of anxiety in veterinary medicine students. This is another example of how a problem-based learning model provides an opportunity to teach through anticipatory "walk-throughs" and cognitive rehearsal of some of the more common medical procedures so that they can be implemented with confidence and independence.

Finally, the skill of problem solving really requires individuals to focus on more than one thing at a time [16]. Veterinarians are consistently given an abundance of information about each client and must be able to pick out the relevant information to make an accurate diagnosis and prognosis. If they are limited to just entertaining one thought at a time, their ability to be holistic in their approach is restricted. The problem-solving teaching model helps build fluency in decision-making by repetition of a process of taking multiple facts, data points, and information to draw a conclusion, make an interfere, and/or determine a treatment path.

AWARENESS OF LIFE EXPERIENCES

This skill is most closely related to the idea of *mentorship* [17]. Veterinary faculty have many years of experience under their belt before becoming a teaching faculty.

This experience might have been in a personal private practice, another vet school, an externship, or through other career opportunities. Regardless of where they have gained understanding and insights, teaching clinicians have experience that their students have not yet acquired. It is important to recognize that mentorship does not mean that they are smarter than their students—it simply means that they have knowledge that their students have not had an opportunity to gain. Veterinary faculty have indicated that the students do not always recognize the value of these work experiences and will brush off suggestions, which hold the potential to make the students' lives a little easier.

For mentorship to be successful, it must be based on mutual respect and a recognition of where each individual is in the development of their career. For example, in this moment the student goal is to learn while the faculty member (mentor) is there to teach, and, if both will recognize their role in the dynamic, the relationship has the potential to be educational for both sides, and this will require both parties to learn what it means to be respectful of the other, as it is imperative for the success of the mentorship. This idea can be a little difficult in the veterinary field due to a power dynamic that is being unequal. Mentors have earned their DVM and become a member of a profession; students still must master goals. Mentoring allows for an exchange of knowledge and experiences that can, at times, place undue stress on the relationship, especially if roles and expectations are not specifically defined at the start of the experience.

DIRECT COMMUNICATION

This skill can also be described as intentional language [18]. The idea of direct communication is to convey precise information in a clear, concise fashion. In our society today, there is a tendency to throw words at a topic until we hit the point of what we are trying to say. In a veterinary medical situation, chaos can lead to inaccuracies being taken as concrete answers. Veterinary faculty simply want students to be able to hear the problem, formulate a solution, and clearly state what plan of action should be followed. Students are encouraged to take a minute, if they do not have the words immediately, to gather their thoughts and then verbalize their response. Anxiety can interfere with a quick and efficient access to our words as well as effective problem solving. Given this information, it is important to understand that independent recall of information is not the ultimate measure of knowledge acquisition. When students struggle to quickly and efficiently retrieve information, and to precisely word their responses, teaching clinicians may wish to consider providing a multiple-choice option. Students who have truly mastered a skill or acquired a knowledge base will recognize the information, even when anxiety interferes with the quick retrieval of the precise wording [8].

This style of communication also speaks to students being able to identify, verbally, if they are uncomfortable or if they need a refresher on a skill. It is a highly valued ability to be able to directly say that you need assistance or that you are unsure about the next step. In veterinary medicine, this skill is imperative; lack of communication can lead to assumptions that can lead to improper diagnosis or animal care [19]. However, highly anxious students with perfectionistic tendencies fear real and perceived failure, the potential for humiliation, and experience imposter syndrome under these circumstances. Veterinary teaching clinicians have the opportunity to encourage help-seeking language as a means of assuring quality instruction.

This skill is also related to the other jobs of veterinary medicine the students do not always consider. Once our students are out of vet school, they will need to communicate with clients who do not always speak the medical language. They will need to be able to deliver difficult news, provide support, handle angry families or patients, and manage conflict in the workplace. The most effective way to do this is through using direct communication. The more our students learn how to effectively communicate test results and evidence-based data compassionately and in everyday language, the greater the opportunities to form positive relationships with their clients and the general public.

CONNECTIVE COMMUNICATION

Connective communication is also a direct form of speaking; however, it is using language in a manner that allows for the development of relationships and grows connections [20]. For example, instead of jumping right to the business of the day, students and clinicians are encouraged to extend an actual greeting and, maybe, a minute of small talk before moving forward. We have become a society that is so busy that we often fail to take time to connect with those who we encounter in our work lives as well as members of our families. We tend to live in our own little bubble with our tasks list and rarely look up to acknowledge others, who in turn are in their bubble with their "to-do" lists. We do not engage with others unless they somehow interfere with our task progress.

Humans are built to connect. Language that connects us is essential for emotional regulation, the building of relationships, and problem solving. When we ask our students about their day, or how things worked out in anatomy class/laboratory, and/or take time to get to know them as individuals, we create a culture of care that has the potential to turn around some of the scary mental health statistics that plague this profession. When we use language that connects, we create safe space to learn and grow. Connective language allows for opportunities to learn how to problem solve, think creatively, seek help, and to create supportive work and learning environments. The ability to connect has been and will always be one of the most important skills a young adult can obtain.

SUMMARY

The process of becoming a veterinarian is much similar to the process of becoming a polished river rock. The fast-paced learning environment and harsh realities of some of the clinical rotations and training demands can leave some students feeling bumped, bruised, and abused. Those who survive emerge from this learning experience as skilled and polished. This article presented 7 skills that were necessary for success in veterinary medicine and how we can teach those skills using a problem-focused teaching model. Hazing is not a necessary component of veterinary medical education to toughen up our students for real-world demands. Problem-focused teaching is a means of providing essential skills that prepare our students for the harsh realities of this career without "roughin' them up" in the process.

CLINICS CARE POINTS

- Teaching the *process* of problem-based learning is an excellent way to ensure that all our students learn to think like veterinarians without assumptions that they automatically have that knowledge base or skill set.
- Hypervigilance increases distraction and reduces the availability for learning.
- Open-mindedness is best taught in an atmosphere free from humiliation, intimidation, and fear of failure.

DISCLOSURE

The authors have nothing to disclose.

REFERENCES

[1] Squires J. Bully tactics 2019. Available at: https://todaysveterinarynurse.com/articles/bully-tactics/ Retrieved 2021. Accessed January 16, 2021.

[2] Available at: Stopbullying.gov. Accessed January 16, 2021.

[3] Mossop, L. The hidden curriculum | veterian key. Available at: https://veteriankey.com/the-hidden-curriculum/. Accessed August 10, 2021.

[4] Whitcomb T. Raising awareness of the hidden curriculum in veterinary medical education: a review and call for research. J Vet Med Educ 2014;41(4):2014.

[5] Andarvahz MR, Afshar L, Yazdani S. Hidden curriculum: an analytical definition. J Med Educ 2017;16(4): 198–207.

[6] DeGraaf E, Kolmos A. Characteristics of problem-based learning. Int J Eng Educ 2003;19(5):657–62.

[7] An in-depth look at common core – what's working and what isn't?. Available at: publicschoolreview.com. Accessed January 16, 2021.

[8] Prince P. From play to problem solving to common core: the development of fluid reasoning. Appl Neuropsychol Child 2017.

[9] Atkinson S, Furnell S, Phippen A. Securing the next generation: enhancing e-safety awareness among young people. Comput Fraud Secur 2009;2009(7):13–9.

[10] Wicklund RA. Objective self-awareness. In: Advances in experimental social psychology, vol. 8. Academic Press; 1975. p. 233–75.

[11] Chapin K. The effect of emotional intelligence on student success. J Adult Educ 2015;44(1):25–31.

[12] Blakemore SJ, Frith C. Self-awareness and action. Curr Opin Neurobiol 2003;13(2):219–24.

[13] Williams A, Prince P. How does anxiety influence fluid reasoning? Appl Neuropsychol Child 2017.

[14] Baehr J. The structure of open-mindedness. Can J Philos 2011;41(2):191–213.

[15] Hesse F, Care E, Buder J, et al. A framework for teachable collaborative problem-solving skills. In: Assessment and teaching of 21st century skills. Dordrecht: Springer; 2015. p. 37–56.

[16] Incebacak BB, Ersoy E. Problem solving skills of secondary school students. China Bus Rev 2016;15(6):275–85.

[17] Merriweather LR, Morgan AJ. Two cultures collide: Bridging the generation gap in a non-traditional mentorship. Qual Rep 2013;18:12.

[18] Schriver K. What we know about expertise in professional communication. In: Berninger VM, editor. Past, present, and future contributions of cognitive writing research to cognitive psychology. 2012. 2012. p. 275–312.

[19] Sargeant J, MacLeod T, Murray A. An interprofessional approach to teaching communication skills. J Contin Educ Health Prof 2011;31(4):265–7.

[20] Dickinson E. Ecocultural conversations: bridging the human-nature divide through connective communication practices. South Commun J 2016;81(1):32–48.

Advances in Small Animal Care 2 (2021) 163–172
ADVANCES IN SMALL ANIMAL CARE

The Myth of Compassion Fatigue and the Reality of Emotional Fatigue

Dani McVety, DVM
Lap of Love Veterinary Hospice

KEYWORDS
• Emotional fatigue • Compassion fatigue • Stress • Mental health • Suicide

KEY POINTS

- The term *emotional fatigue* more accurately describes the stress-related condition that affects many veterinarians, rather than the term *compassion fatigue*.
- Veterinarians do not typically run out of compassion for their patients, but instead struggle with emotional exhaustion related to ethical distress, client frustrations, work-life imbalance, high debt-to-income ratio, and euthanasia-related stress.
- Veterinarians can combat emotional fatigue and relearn to enjoy their profession by continuing to serve pets and people, focusing on their priorities, and reframing conversations about compassion fatigue.

INTRODUCTION

Mental health is an ever-present concern in the veterinary profession, although the true consequences of the burden that veterinary professionals shoulder has been brought to light only in the past 10 to 20 years. Several studies and formal surveys provide concrete evidence that the veterinary profession is suffering. Veterinarians are overwhelmed and emotionally fatigued because of issues such as poor work-life balance, high debt load, low pay, ethical distress, and dealing with client decisions they disagree with. Veterinary technicians and support staff are similarly affected and also experience mental health problems.

One such study, the Merck Animal Health Wellbeing Study 2020, reported that 9.1% of veterinarians suffer from poor well-being, compared with 7.3% of the general population, with female veterinarians more likely to be affected [1]. Poor well-being includes mental health issues, including compassion fatigue, burnout, and depression, which can lead to suicide. A 2014 study conducted by the Centers for Disease Control and Prevention (CDC), which surveyed 11,627 veterinarians, found that 1 in 11 had serious psychological distress and 1 in 6 had experienced suicidal ideation since leaving veterinary school [2]. This finding indicates that a significant number of veterinarians have given serious thought to ending their lives over career-related stress; this a disheartening reality for individuals who competed for a spot in their veterinary class and worked tirelessly for a career they thought they would love.

Mental health is not a new issue for veterinary professionals, and stretches back more than 40 years, according to a retrospective study presented in a 2019 *Journal of the American Veterinary Medical Association (JAVMA)* article. The study, which was conducted by the CDC's National Institute for Occupational Safety and Health, with help from the American Veterinary Medical Association (AVMA), evaluated suicide mortality rates among 11,620 veterinarians who died between 1979 and 2015. Of these veterinary deaths, 398 (3.4%) were from suicide, with proportionate mortality ratios from suicide being 2.1 for male veterinarians and 3.5

E-mail address: DrDani@LapofLove.com

https://doi.org/10.1016/j.yasa.2021.06.003
2666-450X/21/ © 2021 Elsevier Inc. All rights reserved.

for females [3], which means that male veterinarians were 2.1 times more likely to commit suicide than the general public during this time and female veterinarians were 3.5 times more likely. It is reasonable to assume that these statistics also currently apply to veterinarians, because suicide reports are sadly common.

Reports of high burnout and suicide rates are not limited to the United States. Studies conducted in other countries report similar findings. A study of veterinarians in Australia indicated suicide rates approximately four times that of the general population, and 24% of New Zealand veterinarians who responded to a 1999 survey reported feeling depressed at least "reasonably often" [4]. A large-scale 2015 survey of veterinarians and veterinary students conducted by the British Veterinary Association and the Royal College of Veterinary Surgeons (RCVS) reported that 10% of British veterinarians leave the profession each year, and more than half consider a career change [5]. The AVMA and RCVS in 2018 released a joint statement on mental health and well-being in the veterinary profession and emphasized the importance of prioritizing mental health. The statement outlines an approach for supporting mental health and well-being in the veterinary profession by preventing systemic issues that lead to poor mental health, promoting knowledge and skills that can increase well-being, and supporting veterinary professionals who require help in a safe, confidential manner, without judgment [6].

The veterinary profession's state of mental health is clearly in danger, and requires help. Many organizations have provided support and resources for veterinary professionals who struggle with mental health issues, including compassion fatigue, burnout, and depression. Unfortunately, however, statistics indicate that veterinary professionals continue to suffer with these ongoing issues.

Although the ongoing problems of mental distress and suicide have been clearly identified, the veterinary profession has yet to determine how to successfully reduce these problems on a large scale and positively impact the statistics. The number of veterinary professionals who have mental health issues, contemplate suicide, and commit suicide may actually be heading in the wrong direction, and increasing. A strategic plan is necessary to attack this problem and help those who are suffering. The first crucial steps toward truly helping veterinary professionals heal and relearn to love the career they eagerly sought must be to define the type of mental distress veterinary professionals face and identify the sources of their stress.

COMPASSION FATIGUE VERSUS EMOTIONAL FATIGUE

Compassion fatigue is woven throughout studies, statistics, and conversations surrounding mental health and well-being in the veterinary profession. Merriam Webster defines compassion fatigue as "the physical and mental exhaustion and emotional withdrawal experienced by those who care for sick or traumatized people over an extended period of time," and "apathy or indifference toward the suffering of others as the result of overexposure to tragic news stories and images and the subsequent appeals for assistance." The AVMA describes compassion fatigue as "a state of exhaustion and biologic, physiologic, and emotional dysfunction resulting from prolonged exposure to compassion stress." The AVMA goes on to explain that individuals who experience compassion fatigue "feel overwhelmed from bearing the suffering of others, but typically continue to engage in self-sacrifice in the interest of their patients and clients. Factors that place individuals more at risk for experiencing compassion fatigue are high empathy, a history of traumatic experiences, and the existence of unresolved trauma. Factors that affect the severity of compassion fatigue are the duration of the experience, the potential for recurrence, exposure to death and dying, and the presence of a moral conflict [7]."

These definitions indicate that veterinary professionals become exhausted from caring for sick and injured patients and run out of compassion. These definitions imply that veterinarians stop caring about their patients because they have cared so much, for so long, and also that veterinary professionals become disconnected from their patients because they have witnessed so much sickness, trauma, and death. However, do veterinary professionals really run out of compassion for their patients? Do they stop caring about the outcome of difficult cases? Do they really not care whether the parvo puppy on intravenous fluids and medications will survive? Of course they care. Most veterinarians feel great compassion for their patients, despite working long hours, carrying insurmountable debt, and fighting daily ethical battles. So, why does the veterinary profession tend to label all career-related mental distress as "compassion fatigue?"

Compassion fatigue is well documented in human and veterinary medicine and certainly exists. It is possible to become mentally and physically exhausted from caring too much, and it happens to some veterinary professionals. However, labeling the mental anguish many veterinary professionals experience as emotional fatigue, instead of compassion fatigue, seems more appropriate. Caring for patients is one small component of a long list of triggers that regularly lead to emotional exhaustion for many veterinary professionals.

Emotional fatigue describes a state of emotional exhaustion that can result from several factors, including ethical distress, frustration with clients, poor work-life balance, inadequate self-care, high debt-to-income ratio, and euthanasia-related stress. Veterinarians do not typically become overwhelmed with caring for patients. When an emergency presents 15 minutes before the end of a veterinarian's shift, they may be upset with the staff member who did not tell the client to take their pet to the local emergency hospital, or the owner who waited all day to bring in their cat who has not urinated, but they are not upset with the patient, or ambivalent about its survival. The veterinarian still has compassion for the helpless animal who is the victim of circumstances that caused their frustration.

If veterinary professionals truly run out of compassion, then others in caring roles would also run out of compassion. Mothers routinely care for infants who cry through the night, demand their attention, and make mess after mess, yet they do not run out of compassion for their children. Despite their exhaustion from lack of sleep, most new mothers gaze adoringly at their little ones through bleary eyes. If caring for extremely sick and dying patients leads to compassion fatigue, hospice care workers would be expected to have more mental health problems than nurses who work in other capacities. However, a literature review published in the *International Journal of Palliative Nursing* found no strong evidence indicating that palliative care or hospice nurses who routinely care for dying patients experienced higher stress levels than nurses of other disciplines. Instead, the study found that work environment, role conflict, and issues with patients and their families were common stress contributors [8].

If veterinarians do not run out of compassion for patients or their owners, and do not become overwhelmed by caring too much, the *compassion fatigue* label is misleading. Knowing why veterinarians are struggling is an important step toward fixing the problem on a large scale, but chalking up every negative emotion to compassion fatigue is not helpful. Understanding that veterinarians often face emotional fatigue, and identifying contributing factors that trigger emotional fatigue, can help veterinarians move past this career hurdle.

EMOTIONAL FATIGUE IN VETERINARY MEDICINE

People who enter the veterinary field are driven by compassion. These people love animals and work extremely hard for acceptance to veterinary school, often applying to multiple colleges, or applying for years before they are accepted. Their desire to be a veterinarian is their top priority, and they often sacrifice other aspects of their life to meet this goal; they expect veterinary medicine to be an uplifting and rewarding career, but often become disillusioned only years after graduation. Surprisingly, younger veterinarians are more dissatisfied with the profession than older veterinarians, who may be expected to be more fatigued after decades of veterinary work. When asked in the Merck study whether they were suffering, getting by, or flourishing in their career, 13% of veterinarians younger than 35 years reported they were suffering, 41% reported they were getting by, and only 46% said they were flourishing in their career. By comparison, 6% of veterinarians aged 65 years and older reported they were suffering, 21% reported getting by, and 73% said they were flourishing. Overall, 9% of veterinarians in all age groups reported they were suffering, 35% reported only getting by, and 65% said they were flourishing [1]. Young veterinarians seem to feel let down by the career they strived so hard to attain.

Veterinarians follow an educational path similar to human physicians, yet have much lower career satisfaction, which leads to emotional fatigue and burnout. Information gathered during the Merck study about veterinary burnout was compared with information gathered by the Mayo Clinic regarding burnout in human physicians and showed that veterinarians experience higher burnout levels than physicians, despite working fewer hours. Veterinarians who scored highest on the burnout scale included those who consistently worked more than 46 hours per week; worked more evenings, weekends, and holidays; were on call more often that they like; have debt; were wee paid by salary; and were classified as millennials (ie, born between 1981 and 1996) [1].

Also surprising is the portion of veterinarians who are so dissatisfied with their career choice that they would not recommend it to others. Only 48% of veterinarians surveyed in the Merck study would recommend the veterinary profession, citing high student debt, low salary, and high stress as the top 3 reasons [1]. Similarly, only 46% of British veterinarians surveyed would recommend a career in veterinary medicine [5].

Several factors can lead to emotional fatigue among veterinary professionals. An individual's stressors will be unique, but common triggers that affect most of the veterinary profession can be identified. Common contributors include ethical distress, client frustrations, work-life imbalance, high debt-to-income ratio, and euthanasia-related stress.

Ethical Distress

Most of the emotional fatigue veterinarians face on a daily basis likely stems from ethical distress. Veterinarians tend to be high-achieving, hard-working individuals with established moral standards. Yet, patient care is frequently based on decisions made by people who hold different moral standards and who ask veterinarians to compromise their own ethics. Having to adhere repeatedly to someone else's moral standards can cause significant ethical distress, and many veterinarians feel constant guilt about providing what they view as substandard care.

Consider these common situations

- *Being limited by an owner's financial constraints*—A 4-year-old Labrador retriever is presented after being hit by a car. The owner is a single mother of 3 who recently left an abusive marriage. When radiographs reveal a compound fracture that requires surgical repair, she dissolves into tears. She scraped together money to bring the dog in for an examination, and paying for surgical stabilization is not feasible on her limited budget. The dog is otherwise healthy, and surgery will most likely be curative. She contemplates surrendering the dog to a shelter, where it may be euthanized, or selling her car to pay for the dog's surgery. The veterinarian is faced with the dilemma of balancing their obligation to the patient's best interests with their compassion for the owner, who desperately needs her car to transport her 3 children.
- *Pet owner decisions that differ from the veterinarian's*—A 10-year-old cat presents with heart failure signs. The owner does not believe in modern medical practices and has refused vaccines in the past. The veterinarian recommends diagnostics and medical treatment, but the owner wishes to "let nature take its course," and refuses care.
- *Being forced to follow guidelines set by practice management*—A practice's anesthesia protocols do not include preoperative pain management, unless requested by the owner. When the new veterinarian offers preoperative pain management to clients, she must also explain that the medications carry an additional charge. Most owners decline, assuming the anesthesia medications will adequately alleviate their pet's pain. The veterinarian knows that preoperative analgesia is a critical component of an effective pain management protocol, but management refuses, because that would raise procedure costs.

In each of these situations, the veterinarian's desire to provide the best care for their patient is out of their hands because of different limitations. These situations, and hundreds like them, occur every day in veterinary practices around the world.

A 2018 STAT.com article describes the "moral injury" human physicians endure, and compares it with trauma that combat soldiers face. Soldiers leave war with posttraumatic stress disorder. Physicians—and veterinarians—experience burnout. The article explains that "without understanding the critical difference between burnout and moral injury, the wounds will never heal and physicians (veterinarians) and patients alike will continue to suffer the consequences [9]." The term moral injury was first described in a 2009 *Clinical Psychology Review* article as "perpetrating, failing to prevent, or bearing witness to acts that transgress deeply held moral beliefs [10]." For veterinarians, the moral injury is not killing another human during war, but being unable to provide gold-standard health care to the pets they deeply care about. It is euthanizing a perfectly healthy dog with a broken leg instead of letting a single mother sell her car. It is watching an owner walk out the door without life-saving treatment for their pet. It is using a less-than-ideal pain management protocol because a practice owner refuses to institute better practices.

In a 2018 *Journal of Veterinary Internal Medicine* article, more than 70% of 889 North American veterinarians surveyed felt the obstacles that prevented them from providing appropriate patient care caused moderate to severe stress for them or their staff and 79% reported they had been asked to provide care they considered futile [11]. Instead of a large insult, such as a soldier killing another human, persistent, small insults accumulate over time, and contribute greatly to emotional fatigue. Fighting daily ethical battles can quickly wear down the most eager new veterinarian and will certainly take its toll over years.

Client Frustrations

Trying to provide adequate patient care that adheres to the often unreasonable and illogical values of pet owners can also contribute to emotional fatigue. Pet owners often make decisions for their pets that differ from a veterinarian's. Take, for instance, an owner who takes their new puppy to the veterinarian for their first vaccine, but refuses to provide additional vaccines. When the puppy tests positive for parvovirus, many veterinarians would express frustration over the owner's failure to prevent a deadly disease and properly care for their "beloved pet." Likewise, when a pet owner refuses blood work for a sick pet while holding the latest cell phone and carrying a designer purse, veterinarians can find it difficult to empathize when the pet's condition worsens, assuming the owner's priorities are wrong.

The relationships between pet owners and their pets differ significantly. An elderly owner may be willing to spend their life's savings to keep their dog alive for only a few more months, because the pet is their last link to their deceased spouse. On the other hand, a rural client may view their dog as expendable and provide only basic necessities such as food, water, and shelter. Most pet owners' values are somewhere between these extremes—they love their pet and think of them as family, but may be limited by finances, time, or physical or emotional ability to care for their pet as a veterinarian would like.

The common tenet that "people should only have a pet if they can properly care for them," is, unfortunately, somewhat subjective. The definition of "proper care" varies between the groups of pet owners described earlier and may not align with the care a veterinary professional deems appropriate.

In addition, veterinarians often do not receive the respect from clients they feel they deserve. New veterinarians are often surprised that clients follow advice from uneducated sources, question their decisions, and do not always comply with their recommendations. A pet owner who feels they did not receive good service may post a negative online review that can cause significant trauma and injure a veterinarian's self-esteem and confidence.

Work-Life Imbalance

Veterinarians notoriously have a poor work-life balance. Devotion to their patients, an obligation to their practice, and a need to pay off student debt often leads them to work more than 40 hours per week. The Merck study associated working more than 46 hours per week, plus working evenings, weekends, and holidays, with high burnout levels [1]. In addition to in-hospital time, many veterinarians are on call during evenings and weekends, which interferes with their personal time. Veterinarians may also be overwhelmed by calls, texts, and social media messages from clients, friends, and family members asking questions about their pets. In essence, many veterinarians feel they are "on call" all the time, with little time away from their work. It can be worse for practice owners who are solely responsible for their practice and team and may feel that they have to do it all.

The disproportionate women-to-men ratio of veterinarians may contribute to emotional fatigue and burnout. Historically, the veterinary workforce has been dominated by men, but female veterinarians have outnumbered male veterinarians since 2009 [12]. According to AVMA market research statistics that were last published in March 2020, women comprise 62% of the US veterinary population [13]. The Association of American Veterinary Medical Colleges (AAVMC) 2019 to 2020 Annual Data Report shows that approximately 80% of US veterinary students are female [14]. Gone are the days when a male veterinarian worked all day while his wife stayed home with the children, or worked part-time at the practice. Instead, the typical veterinary family now includes a female veterinarian who works more than full time, as well as a full-time working spouse. Women who are away from home so much may feel guilty, particularly if they have children. Many female veterinarians arrive home after dinner and spend only a short time with their children before they go to bed. Weekends may include work or on-call time, and working mothers may miss sporting events, school activities, and birthdays. Missing out on family time may lead to feelings of bitterness toward the veterinary profession.

Working overtime also leaves little time for enjoyable activities that relieve stress, such as self-care, spending time with loved ones, and social events. Many veterinarians rarely take time to decompress and recover from daily ethical and moral distress, which leads to emotional fatigue buildup over time.

High Debt-to-Income Ratio

Eager veterinary students who sacrifice so much to become veterinarians are often shocked to find themselves graduating with hundreds of thousands of dollars of debt. The 2019 class of veterinary students graduated with an average debt of approximately $150,000 and an approximate starting salary of $85,000 [15]. This figure translates to a debt-to-income ratio of 1.76, meaning that the average debt of a new veterinarian is 176% of their starting salary. Although other medical students graduate with high debt, an *American Journal of Pharmaceutical Education* study comparing debt-to-income ratios of dentists, pharmacists, optometrists, physicians, and veterinarians found that veterinarians graduate with the highest debt-to-income ratio. Physicians often graduate with a debt-to-income ratio less than 1, meaning that their starting salary is typically more than their debt load [16].

High student debt was a leading cause of stress among the Merck study participants, second only to the high stress level of veterinarians, with 91% reporting debt as a concern. The study also identified high debt as a predictor for serious psychological distress in veterinarians and cited debt as the top reason 52% of veterinarians would not recommend a veterinary medicine career [1].

A large debt load sets up new veterinarians for high stress levels right as they are starting their anticipated career. These veterinarians suddenly have a large monthly debt payment, which is often more than their mortgage or rent payment, and feel immense pressure to keep up. Some veterinarians work long hours and live frugally to pay off their student loans early, only to end up with prepayment penalties or large tax burdens. For many veterinarians, especially those with families, early repayment is not an option, and they are stuck with a 30-year repayment plan, living for decades with a large debt hanging over their head.

Euthanasia-Related Stress

Euthanasia is a gift that veterinarians can share with pets and their owners, but can create emotionally draining situations. Although veterinarians may be assumed to struggle most with "convenience euthanasia" requests, they more frequently suffer emotional fatigue from trying to diplomatically convince pet owners the time has come to end their pets' suffering. Pet owners put off their pet's euthanasia for a variety of reasons, from wanting more time with them, to not wanting to end their life too soon, to concern that they do not have the right to determine when their pet should die.

As for convenience euthanasia, the author has previously defined 4 different euthanasia types veterinarians face:

- *Convenience euthanasia* is a subjective term used when euthanasia is requested for a pet who would otherwise be deemed adoptable under most circumstances, but the family is unwilling to explore these options. For example, "my cat leaves white fur all over my new dark-colored couch." Many veterinarians refuse to perform true convenience euthanasias and instead offer support and resources to rehome these pets.
- *Nonmedical euthanasia* is a term used to describe a request that is not related to the pet's medical stability. This broad term includes behavior issues, such as aggression or improper elimination in the home, and family-related emotional or lifestyle changes that preclude the pet from experiencing a good quality of life.
- *Nonimminent medical euthanasia* is a term that describes medical situations that may be manageable, or possibly curable, under the right circumstances, but those circumstances do not exist, for whatever reason. Such situations include the parvovirus puppy who may survive with intensive care, the 5-year-old intact female with a pyometra, or the young cat with a broken leg. Without the right conditions and resources for the owner, which may include the expense, this pet would potentially suffer greatly.
- *Medical euthanasia*, which encompasses most euthanasias that occur in veterinary practices, describes a choice made by the family and the veterinarian that the pet's quality of life is unsustainable.

Veterinarians may experience tremendous guilt when they cannot convince an owner to end a pet's suffering, or refuse to fulfill a convenience or nonmedical euthanasia request. In one case, the pet continues to suffer, and in the other, the veterinarian must consider the actions the pet owner may resort to. Will they let the pet go in the parking lot? Or worse, try to euthanize the pet themselves? In both cases, the veterinarian will have failed the pet and their owner, which is the ultimate failure.

SEPARATING EMOTIONAL FATIGUE FROM COMPASSION FATIGUE

The stressors discussed earlier—ethical distress, client frustrations, work-life imbalance, high debt-to-income ratio, and euthanasia-related stress—do not involve compassion for the animals whom veterinarians treat. The list of top stressors does not include treating, caring for, or feeling compassion for pets. The list does include stressors such as coping with decisions that differ from theirs about what they would do for the pet, lack of money, and being overworked. Veterinarians in these situations undoubtedly face emotional fatigue, but they do not run out of compassion for their patients. The author would also argue that they do not run out of compassion for their clients. Although veterinarians may become frustrated with their clients' decisions, their overall goal is to preserve the human-animal bond, which ultimately benefits pets and people.

The AVMA's definition of compassion fatigue includes that veterinarians "typically continue to engage in self-sacrifice in the interest of their patients and clients." This underscores the fact that veterinarians rarely leave the profession. Rather, they continue to care for patients, despite facing frequent ethical dilemmas, client lack of respect, and long hours. Some veterinarians may feel trapped and stay in the field to pay back high student debt, whereas the author believes that most stay out of a moral obligation to their patients. These veterinarians believe that their patients benefit from their presence in the profession and fear that their patients will suffer if they walk away. This decision is based on compassion. Veterinarians do not run out of compassion—compassion drives them to continue, despite their emotional fatigue.

COMBATING EMOTIONAL FATIGUE

A large number of veterinarians are emotionally fatigued, and no longer love the career they worked so hard for. These veterinarians feel betrayed, disrespected, and morally exhausted, but rarely leave the profession. To alleviate the systemic problem of emotional fatigue, veterinarians must identify ways to relearn to love their career; they must use their unending source of compassion (ie, themselves) to drive forward and better themselves, so they can improve their well-being, prevent burnout, and continue caring for the patients they love.

According to the Merck study, predictors of well-being for veterinarians include:

- Enjoying work
- Work-life balance
- Spending time with family and friends
- Invigorating work environment
- Satisfaction with pay [1]

The veterinary profession can be the uplifting and rewarding career that veterinarians desire. However, veterinarians must evaluate their priorities and repair their lives—professionally and personally—to create values and a balance that will allow them to enjoy their career. Veterinarians must not blame veterinary medicine. Achieving the predictors of well-being listed earlier, and enjoying the veterinary profession, is possible, but veterinarians must identify healthy ways to deal with their daily stressors. To combat emotional fatigue, they must deal with ethical distress, client frustrations, work-life imbalance, high debt-to-income ratio, and euthanasia-related stress. Three ways veterinarians can do this include remaining in service to people and pets, focusing on their priorities, and reframing conversations about compassion fatigue.

Remaining in Service to People and Pets

Veterinarians are driven to enter their profession by their dedication to animals and a desire to improve their quality of life and the human-animal bond. To learn how to flourish in the veterinary profession, instead of suffering or merely getting by, veterinarians must find ways to reconnect with the passion that inspired them to pursue their career. One way is to remain in service to people and pets. Research shows that helping others helps combat stress and improve well-being [17]. One study, published in *Clinical Psychological Science*, showed that people who helped others reported higher levels of positive emotions. Conversely, participants reported a more negative emotional reaction to stress during days they helped others less frequently [18]. Veterinary medicine is a service-based profession, and serving pets and their owners is veterinarians' irreplaceable contribution to society. Should they do it without pay, or be available to their clients all hours of the day and night? Definitely not. But, remembering that their greatest talent is serving people and pets to help reinforce the human-animal bond can help them enjoy their career. Practices that have helped the author remain in service to pets include:

- *Keeping a hero mentality*—The veterinary profession's product is not medicine—it is the priceless human-animal bond that every pet deserves, regardless of the owner's financial stability, the level of respect with which they treat their veterinarian, or the decisions they make for their pet. No matter what has occurred before a pet's presentation, a veterinarian is able to better the pet's life while under their care and should work tirelessly to best serve them. Day-to-day stressors can distract veterinarians from remembering their unique position to help animals live longer, healthier lives. Focusing on the pet and having a "hero mentality" can help veterinarians remember their irreplaceable role in a pet's well-being.
- *Being unoffendable*—When a client is difficult, a veterinarian can easily become offended and take their negative attitude personally. Take, for example, a client who accuses a veterinarian of "being in it only for the money" when they cannot afford hospitalization for their sick puppy. "You obviously don't love animals," they may say, frustrated. The veterinarian's first response may be to lecture the owner on vaccinating their puppy to prevent disease or budgeting money for pet emergencies, but those conversations will only drive the client further away. Instead, veterinarians should remember that the client's "disrespect" likely stems from their own

guilt and has nothing to do with the veterinarian. In fact, most negative situations that veterinarians face, from work schedules to a coworker's attitude, likely have little to do with them. Most people are so focused on their own situation and problems that they have little time or desire to purposely offend others. Rude comments or a negative attitude are simply a result of a person's own unhappiness or frustration. Being unoffendable can give veterinarians a different, more compassionate perspective from which to approach clients' situations and help pets.

- *Remembering the ultimate goal*—A veterinarian's ultimate goal is to help pets. This reminder can help veterinarians who struggle with difficult clients or convenience euthanasia requests. Consider a euthanasia request for a cat with early-stage kidney disease. The veterinarian explains that the cat can have a good quality of life for several months—possibly years—with subcutaneous fluids and medications, but the owner refuses, and repeats her euthanasia request. Veterinarians must remember they are not privy to all the factors in a client's decision, nor should they be. Perhaps this client's husband died of kidney failure and she cannot bear to care for her cat with the same disease. The human-animal bond will be damaged, or severed, and the cat and owner will suffer. Clients not only consider their financial budget when making difficult decisions regarding their pet but also must consider their emotional, physical, and time budgets. If a client cannot emotionally handle caring for their pet with kidney disease, or cannot physically carry their heavy dog outside to go to the bathroom during surgical recovery, they cannot afford care, despite sufficient funds. Likewise, a client who is caring for a family member with a chronic illness may not have time to administer daily subcutaneous fluids, or insulin injections, and will suffer from guilt when they miss their pet's treatments. Regardless of the reasons for a euthanasia request, veterinarians should focus on helping the pet and keeping the human-animal bond intact. If euthanasia will not support these goals, veterinarians should be prepared to offer acceptable alternatives, such as taking over the pet's care or finding them another home.

Focusing on Priorities

Veterinarians may be heroes and public servants, but they cannot be expected to devote every moment to their profession. Veterinarians have families, outside priorities, and their own health, which they must consider, in addition to their patients. A 2015 *JAVMA* investigation of suicide risk factors identified practice demands as the most commonly reported stressor among 11,627 veterinarians [2]. Although practice is demanding, veterinarians must draw clear boundaries between their professional and private lives, and unapologetically remain true to their priorities; this will look different for every veterinarian, but may include:

- *Setting clear work hours*—Leaving practice on time each day can have positive mental health benefits, and veterinarians should make this a priority. Finding ways to be more efficient throughout the day, such as employing support staff to help with medical records and making overnight patient treatment plans ahead of time, can help veterinarians get home in time for dinner. Veterinarians should refer clients to an emergency hospital for after-hours care when possible, instead of staying late or being on call. If a veterinarian's current job requires that they miss holidays and family activities, they may consider changing to a job that better aligns with their priorities.
- *Being fully present*—Veterinarians should focus on being fully present wherever they are; they should focus fully on their patients while working and on themselves and their loved ones while outside of work. Many veterinarians are faced with a constant barrage of requests from family and friends for advice, or home visits, which interfere with their personal time. Veterinarians can easily deal with this by kindly responding that they cannot help when out of the office and provide them with their office telephone number to schedule an appointment and the number of a local emergency hospital for immediate help.
- *Making time for self-care*—Self-care is essential to combat emotional fatigue, and every veterinarian should incorporate regular practices that help them heal from daily stressors, such as moral injury. Self-care includes getting adequate sleep, eating a healthy diet, exercising, practicing mindfulness, and spending time with loved ones.
- *Hiring a financial planner*—If student loan debt is a constant stressor, veterinarians should consider consulting a financial planner to help them devise a repayment plan that will allow them to meet their financial goals. A financial planner may also be able to help veterinarians refinance their loans to take advantage of lower interest rates and pay off their loans sooner, so they are better able to enjoy life.

Reframing Conversations about Compassion Fatigue

As previously noted, the term compassion fatigue does not adequately describe the emotional exhaustion many veterinarians deal with regularly. However, this blanket term is often applied to all the negative emotions that veterinarians experience because of practice-related stress. Unfortunately, because running out of compassion is not easily fixed, using this term does not offer a solution. Reframing conversations related to veterinary stress in ways that better describe individual situations, and offering a solution, would be more helpful. For example, a veterinarian who is having a difficult time dealing with challenging clients because they were up at night with a teething child, should say, "I am feeling overwhelmed today because I am tired," which is more accurate than "I have compassion fatigue." Likewise, a veterinarian who does not eat lunch and skips their daily walks during a busy week should think, "I have not taken care of myself this week." Identifying the root of the problem, and not only the resulting stress, allows veterinarians to take steps to alleviate the issue.

SUMMARY

The term *emotional fatigue* describes the stress-related condition that affects many veterinarians more accurately than the term *compassion fatigue*. Veterinarians do not typically run out of compassion for their patients, but instead struggle with emotional exhaustion related to ethical distress, client frustrations, work-life imbalance, high debt-to-income ratio, and euthanasia-related stress. These stressors can cause significant mental health problems for veterinarians and make them feel unfulfilled in their career. Veterinarians can combat emotional fatigue and relearn to enjoy their profession, by remaining in service to pets and people, focusing on their priorities, and reframing conversations about compassion fatigue.

CLINICS CARE POINTS

- Remaining in service to people and pets can help veterinarians combat emotional fatigue. Practices that may help veterinarians include keeping a hero mentality, not taking negative experiences personally, and remembering their ultimate goal of helping pets.
- Veterinarians should also remain unapologetically, but kindly, true to their priorities; tThis may include setting clear work hours, being fully present at work and home, making time for self-care, and hiring a financial advisor.
- Reframing conversations about compassion fatigue can help veterinarians better describe individual situations, and identify possible solutions.

ACKNOWLEDGMENTS

The author would like to acknowledge Angela Beal, DVM, for her help preparing the final manuscript.

REFERENCES

[1] Merck Animal Health. Merck animal health veterinarian wellbeing study 2020 2020. Available at: https://www.merck-animal-health-usa.com/offload-downloads/veterinary-wellbeing-study. Accessed February 5, 2021.

[2] Nett R, Witte T, Holzbauer S, et al. Risk factors for suicide, attitudes toward mental illness, and practice-related stressors among US veterinarians. J Am Vet Med Assoc 2015;247:945–55.

[3] Tomasi S, Fechter-Leggett E, Edwards N, et al. Suicide among veterinarians in the United States from 1979 through 2015. J Am Vet Med Assoc 2019;254:104–12.

[4] Earley M. Veterinarian industry 'crippled' by mental health issues. Stuff; 2018. Available at: https://www.stuff.co.nz/national/health/107696049/veterinarian-industry-crippled-by-mental-health-issues. Accessed February 5, 2021.

[5] Clark C, Knights D. Doubt, depression, anxiety—just some of the problems plaguing the veterinary profession. The Conversation; 2018. Available at: https://theconversation.com/doubt-depression-anxiety-just-some-of-the-problems-plaguing-the-veterinary-profession-96162. Accessed February 5, 2021.

[6] Larkin M. Taking mental health in a positive direction: U.K. vets work with AVMA to promote a culture change in the veterinary profession. JAVMA news; 2018. Available at: https://www.avma.org/javma-news/2018-10-15/taking-mental-health-positive-direction. Accessed February 10, 2021.

[7] Assess your wellbeing. AVMA resources and tools. Available at: https://www.avma.org/resources-tools/wellbeing/assess-your-wellbeing. Accessed February 10, 2021.

[8] Peters L, Cant R, Sellick K, et al. Is work stress in palliative care nurses a cause for concern? A literature review. Int J Palliat Nurs 2012;18:561–7.

[9] Talbot S, Dean W. Physicians aren't 'burning out.' They're suffering from moral injury. Stat news; 2018. Available at: https://www.statnews.com/2018/07/26/physicians-

not-burning-out-they-are-suffering-moral-injury/. Accessed on February 12, 2021.

[10] Litz B, Stein N, Delaney E, et al. Moral injury and moral repair in war veterans: a preliminary model and intervention strategy. Clin Psychol Rev 2009;29:695–706.

[11] Moses L, Malowney M, Boyd J. Ethical conflict and moral distress in veterinary practice: a survey of North American veterinarians. J Vet Intern Med 2018;32:2115–22.

[12] Wuest P. The history of women in veterinary medicine in the U.S. *Today's Veterinary Practice*. Available at: https://todaysveterinarypractice.com/the-history-of-women-in-veterinary-medicine-in-the-us/#:~:text=According%20to%20the%20American%20Veterinary%20Medical%20Association%2C%20the%20current%20ratio,administration%20(i.e.%2C%20leadership. Accessed February 13, 2021.

[13] U.S. veterinarians 2019. In: AVMA reports. 2020. Available at: https://www.avma.org/resources-tools/reports-statistics/market-research-statistics-us-veterinarians-2019 2020. Accessed February 13, 2021.

[14] Association of American Veterinary Medical Colleges annual data report 2019-2020. AAVMC; 2020. Available at: https://www.aavmc.org/wp-content/uploads/2020/10/2020-aavmc-annual-data-report.pdf. Accessed February 13, 2021.

[15] Larkin M. Good news, bad news for educational debt, starting salaries. JAVMA news; 2019. Available at: https://www.avma.org/javma-news/2019-12-15/good-news-bad-news-educational-debt-starting-salaries. Accessed February 13. 2021.

[16] Chisholm-Burns M, Spivey C, Stallworth S, et al. Analysis of educational debt and income among pharmacists and other health professionals. Am J Pharm Educ 2019;83:7460.

[17] Curry O, Rowland L, Van Lissa C, et al. Happy to help? A systematic review and meta-analysis of the effects of performing acts of kindness on the well-being of the actor. J Exp Soc Psychol 2018;76:320–9.

[18] Raposa E, Laws H, Ansell E. Prosocial behavior mitigates the negative effects of stress in everyday life. Clin Psychol Sci 2016;4:691–8.

Sheridan
Hanover, PA USA
October 25, 2021